Desk Reference
to the
Diagnostic Criteria
From

DSM-5-TR™

Desk Reference
to the
Diagnostic Criteria
From

DSM-5-TR™

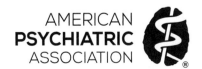

AMERICAN
PSYCHIATRIC
ASSOCIATION

Correspondence regarding copyright permissions should be directed to DSM Permissions, American Psychiatric Association Publishing, 800 Maine Ave. SW, Suite 900, Washington, DC 20024-2812.

Manufactured in the United States of America on acid-free paper.

ISBN 978-0-89042-579-4 (Soft) First Printing, February 2022

ISBN 978-0-89042-580-0 (Spiral) First Printing, February 2022

American Psychiatric Association
800 Maine Ave. SW, Suite 900
Washington, DC 20024-2812
www.psychiatry.org

The correct citation for this book is American Psychiatric Association: Desk Reference to the Diagnostic Criteria From DSM-5-TR. Washington, DC, American Psychiatric Association, 2022.

Library of Congress Cataloging-in-Publication Data
Names: American Psychiatric Association, issuing body.
Title: Desk reference to the diagnostic criteria from DSM-5-TR / American Psychiatric Association.
Other titles: Desk reference to the diagnostic criteria from DSM-5-text revision
Description: Washington, DC : American Psychiatric Association Publishing, [2022] I Includes index.
Identifiers: LCCN 2021051783 (print) I LCCN 2021051784 (ebook) I ISBN 9780890425794 (soft ; alk. paper) I ISBN 9780890425800 (spiral ; alk. paper) I ISBN 9780890425817 (ebook)
Subjects: MESH: Diagnostic and statistical manual of mental disorders. 5th ed. I Mental Disorders—diagnosis I Mental Disorders—classification I Handbook
Classification: LCC RC455.2.C4 (print) I LCC RC455.2.C4 (ebook) I NLM WM 34 IDDC 616.89001/2—dc23/eng/20211124
LC record available at https://lccn.loc.gov/2021051783
LC ebook record available at https://lccn.loc.gov/2021051784

British Library Cataloguing in Publication Data
A CIP record is available from the British Library.

Text Design—Tammy J. Cordova

Contents

Section I
DSM-5 Basics

Section II
Diagnostic Criteria and Codes

Preface

The publication of DSM-5-TR brings updates to the diagnostic classification and coding of DSM-5 mental disorders, as well as clarifications to the diagnostic criteria for more than 70 disorders. For quick reference, clinicians may find useful this small and convenient manual that contains only the DSM-5-TR Classification (i.e., the complete list of disorders, subtypes, specifiers, and diagnostic codes by DSM-5-TR chapter), an updated section describing use of the manual, and updated DSM-5 diagnostic criteria sets and coding notes. The *Desk Reference to the Diagnostic Criteria From DSM-5-TR* is meant to be used in conjunction with the fully updated DSM-5-TR. Proper use of the Desk Reference requires familiarity with the text descriptions for each disorder that accompany the criteria sets. The DSM-5-TR text descriptions have also been comprehensively updated to reflect the most recent literature and the impact of culture, racism, and discrimination on psychiatric diagnosis.

This handy reference provides all updated ICD-10-CM codes, coding notes, and recording procedures included in DSM-5-TR, including diagnostic criteria for the new diagnosis of prolonged grief disorder. Newly available are also symptom codes for indicating current (and past history of) suicidal behavior and nonsuicidal self-injury.

Clinicians will find additional reference information in DSM-5-TR, including Section III: Emerging Measures and Models (containing assessment measures, updated text on psychiatric diagnosis and culture, cultural formulation and interviews, an alternative DSM-5 model for personality disorders, and conditions for further study) and the DSM-5-TR Appendix (containing alphabetical and numerical ICD-10-CM code listings of DSM-5 diagnoses). Assessment measures and additional information are available online at www.psychiatry.org/dsm5.

See www.dsm5.org for periodic DSM-5-TR coding and other updates.

Before each disorder name, ICD-10-CM codes are provided. Blank lines indicate that the ICD-10-CM code depends on the applicable subtype, specifier, or class of substance. For periodic DSM-5-TR coding and other updates, see www.dsm5.org.

Following chapter titles and disorder names, page numbers for the corresponding text or criteria are included in parentheses.

Note for all mental disorders due to another medical condition: Insert the name of the etiological medical condition within the name of the mental disorder due to [the medical condition]. The code and name for the etiological medical condition should be listed first immediately before the mental disorder due to the medical condition.

Neurodevelopmental Disorders (19)

Intellectual Developmental Disorders (19)

Communication Disorders (24)

Autism Spectrum Disorder (27)

F84.0   Autism Spectrum Disorder (27)

Specify current severity: Requiring very substantial support, Requiring substantial support, Requiring support

Specify if: With or without accompanying intellectual impairment, With or without accompanying language impairment

Specify if: Associated with a known genetic or other medical condition or environmental factor (**Coding note:** Use additional code to identify the associated genetic or other medical condition); Associated with a neurodevelopmental, mental, or behavioral problem

Specify if: With catatonia (use additional code F06.1)

Attention-Deficit/Hyperactivity Disorder (31)

___.___   Attention-Deficit/Hyperactivity Disorder (31)

Specify if: In partial remission

Specify current severity: Mild, Moderate, Severe

Specify whether:

F90.2   Combined presentation

F90.0   Predominantly inattentive presentation

F90.1   Predominantly hyperactive/impulsive presentation

F90.8   Other Specified Attention-Deficit/Hyperactivity Disorder (33)

F90.9   Unspecified Attention-Deficit/Hyperactivity Disorder (34)

Specific Learning Disorder (34)

___.___   Specific Learning Disorder (34)

Specify current severity: Mild, Moderate, Severe

Specify if:

F81.0   With impairment in reading (specify if with word reading accuracy, reading rate or fluency, reading comprehension)

F81.81   With impairment in written expression (specify if with spelling accuracy, grammar and punctuation accuracy, clarity or organization of written expression)

F81.2   With impairment in mathematics (specify if with number sense, memorization of arithmetic facts, accurate or fluent calculation, accurate math reasoning)

Motor Disorders (37)

F82   Developmental Coordination Disorder (37)

F98.4   Stereotypic Movement Disorder (37)

Specify if: With self-injurious behavior, Without self-injurious behavior

Specify if: Associated with a known genetic or other medical condition, neurodevelopmental disorder, or environmental factor

Specify current severity: Mild, Moderate, Severe

Tic Disorders (38)

F95.2   Tourette's Disorder (38)

F95.1   Persistent (Chronic) Motor or Vocal Tic Disorder (38)
Specify if: With motor tics only, With vocal tics only

F95.0   Provisional Tic Disorder (39)

F95.8   Other Specified Tic Disorder (39)

F95.9   Unspecified Tic Disorder (39)

Other Neurodevelopmental Disorders (40)

F88   Other Specified Neurodevelopmental Disorder (40)

F89   Unspecified Neurodevelopmental Disorder (40)

Schizophrenia Spectrum
and Other Psychotic Disorders (41)

The following specifiers apply to Schizophrenia Spectrum and Other Psychotic Disorders where indicated:

[a]*Specify* if: The following course specifiers are only to be used after a 1-year duration of the disorder: First episode, currently in acute episode; First episode, currently in partial remission; First episode, currently in full remission; Multiple episodes, currently in acute episode; Multiple episodes, currently in partial remission; Multiple episodes, currently in full remission; Continuous; Unspecified

[b]*Specify* if: With catatonia (use additional code F06.1)

[c]*Specify* current severity of delusions, hallucinations, disorganized speech, abnormal psychomotor behavior, negative symptoms, impaired cognition, depression, and mania symptoms

F21   Schizotypal (Personality) Disorder (41)

F22   Delusional Disorder[a,c] (41)
Specify whether: Erotomanic type, Grandiose type, Jealous type, Persecutory type, Somatic type, Mixed type, Unspecified type
Specify if: With bizarre content

F23   Brief Psychotic Disorder[b,c] (43)
Specify if: With marked stressor(s), Without marked stressor(s), With peripartum onset

F20.81   Schizophreniform Disorder[b,c] (44)
Specify if: With good prognostic features, Without good prognostic features

F20.9   Schizophrenia[a,b,c] (45)

___.___   Schizoaffective Disorder[a,b,c] (47)
Specify whether:

F25.0   Bipolar type

F25.1   Depressive type

____.___   Substance/Medication-Induced Psychotic Disorder[c] (48)
           Note: For applicable ICD-10-CM codes, refer to the substance
               classes under Substance-Related and Addictive Disorders
               for the specific substance/medication-induced psychotic
               disorder. See also the criteria set and corresponding record-
               ing procedures in the manual for more information.
           Coding note: The ICD-10-CM code depends on whether or not
               there is a comorbid substance use disorder present for the
               same class of substance. In any case, an additional separate
               diagnosis of a substance use disorder is not given.
           Specify if: With onset during intoxication, With onset during
               withdrawal, With onset after medication use

____.___   Psychotic Disorder Due to Another Medical Condition[c]
               (51)
           Specify whether:
F06.2   With delusions
F06.0   With hallucinations

F06.1 Catatonia Associated With Another Mental Disorder
               (Catatonia Specifier) (52)

F06.1 Catatonic Disorder Due to Another Medical Condition (52)

F06.1 Unspecified Catatonia (53)
           Note: Code first **R29.818** other symptoms involving nervous
               and musculoskeletal systems.

F28   Other Specified Schizophrenia Spectrum and Other
               Psychotic Disorder (54)

F29   Unspecified Schizophrenia Spectrum and Other Psychotic
               Disorder (55)

Bipolar and Related Disorders (57)

The following specifiers apply to Bipolar and Related Disorders where indicated:
[a]*Specify:* With anxious distress (*specify* current severity: mild, moderate, mod-
    erate-severe, severe); With mixed features; With rapid cycling; With melan-
    cholic features; With atypical features; With mood-congruent psychotic
    features; With mood-incongruent psychotic features; With catatonia (use
    additional code F06.1); With peripartum onset; With seasonal pattern
[b]*Specify:* With anxious distress (*specify* current severity: mild, moderate,
    moderate-severe, severe); With mixed features; With rapid cycling; With
    peripartum onset; With seasonal pattern

____.___   Bipolar I Disorder[a] (57)
____.___   Current or most recent episode manic
F31.11   Mild
F31.12   Moderate
F31.13   Severe
F31.2   With psychotic features

Depressive Disorders (81)

F34.81 Disruptive Mood Dysregulation Disorder (81)

____.__ Major Depressive Disorder (82)

Specify: With anxious distress (*specify* current severity: mild, moderate, moderate-severe, severe); With mixed features; With melancholic features; With atypical features; With mood-congruent psychotic features; With mood-incongruent psychotic features; With catatonia (use additional code F06.1); With peripartum onset; With seasonal pattern

____.__ Single episode

F32.0   Mild
F32.1   Moderate
F32.2   Severe
F32.3   With psychotic features
F32.4   In partial remission
F32.5   In full remission
F32.9   Unspecified

____.__ Recurrent episode

F33.0   Mild
F33.1   Moderate
F33.2   Severe
F33.3   With psychotic features
F33.41   In partial remission
F33.42   In full remission
F33.9   Unspecified

F34.1 Persistent Depressive Disorder (84)

Specify: With anxious distress (*specify* current severity: mild, moderate, moderate-severe, severe); With atypical features
Specify if: In partial remission, In full remission
Specify if: Early onset, Late onset
Specify if: With pure dysthymic syndrome; With persistent major depressive episode; With intermittent major depressive episodes, with current episode; With intermittent major depressive episodes, without current episode
Specify current severity: Mild, Moderate, Severe

F32.81 Premenstrual Dysphoric Disorder (86)

____.__ Substance/Medication-Induced Depressive Disorder (87)

Note: For applicable ICD-10-CM codes, refer to the substance classes under Substance-Related and Addictive Disorders for the specific substance/medication-induced depressive disorder. See also the criteria set and corresponding recording procedures in the manual for more information.

Coding note: The ICD-10-CM code depends on whether or not there is a comorbid substance use disorder present for the same class of substance. In any case, an additional separate diagnosis of a substance use disorder is not given.

Specify if: With onset during intoxication, With onset during withdrawal, With onset after medication use

Anxiety Disorders (99)

Obsessive-Compulsive and Related Disorders (111)

The following specifier applies to Obsessive-Compulsive and Related Disorders where indicated:

[a]*Specify* if: With good or fair insight, With poor insight, With absent insight/delusional beliefs

F42.2   Obsessive-Compulsive Disorder[a] (111)
            Specify if: Tic-related

F45.22 Body Dysmorphic Disorder[a] (112)
            Specify if: With muscle dysmorphia

F42.3   Hoarding Disorder[a] (113)
            Specify if: With excessive acquisition

F63.3   Trichotillomania (Hair-Pulling Disorder) (114)

F42.4   Excoriation (Skin-Picking) Disorder (114)

___.__   Substance/Medication-Induced Obsessive-Compulsive and Related Disorder (114)
            Note: For applicable ICD-10-CM codes, refer to the substance classes under Substance-Related and Addictive Disorders for the specific substance/medication-induced obsessive-compulsive and related disorder. See also the criteria set and corresponding recording procedures in the manual for more information.
            Coding note: The ICD-10-CM code depends on whether or not there is a comorbid substance use disorder present for the same class of substance. In any case, an additional separate diagnosis of a substance use disorder is not given.
            Specify if: With onset during intoxication, With onset during withdrawal, With onset after medication use

F06.8   Obsessive-Compulsive and Related Disorder Due to Another Medical Condition (117)
            Specify if: With obsessive-compulsive disorder–like symptoms, With appearance preoccupations, With hoarding symptoms, With hair-pulling symptoms, With skin-picking symptoms

F42.8   Other Specified Obsessive-Compulsive and Related Disorder (118)

F42.9   Unspecified Obsessive-Compulsive and Related Disorder (119)

Trauma- and Stressor-Related Disorders (121)

F94.1   Reactive Attachment Disorder (121)
            Specify if: Persistent
            Specify current severity: Severe

F94.2   Disinhibited Social Engagement Disorder (122)
            Specify if: Persistent
            Specify current severity: Severe

Dissociative Disorders (133)

Somatic Symptom and Related Disorders (137)

Feeding and Eating Disorders (143)

Elimination Disorders (149)

F98.0   Enuresis (149)
            Specify whether: Nocturnal only, Diurnal only, Nocturnal and
                diurnal
F98.1   Encopresis (149)
            Specify whether: With constipation and overflow incontinence,
                Without constipation and overflow incontinence
___.___   Other Specified Elimination Disorder (150)
N39.498   With urinary symptoms
R15.9   With fecal symptoms
___.___   Unspecified Elimination Disorder (150)
R32   With urinary symptoms
R15.9   With fecal symptoms

Sleep-Wake Disorders (151)

The following specifiers apply to Sleep-Wake Disorders where indicated:
[a]*Specify* if: Episodic, Persistent, Recurrent
[b]*Specify* if: Acute, Subacute, Persistent
[c]*Specify* current severity: Mild, Moderate, Severe

F51.01 Insomnia Disorder[a] (151)
            Specify if: With mental disorder, With medical condition,
                With another sleep disorder
F51.11 Hypersomnolence Disorder[b,c] (152)
            Specify if: With mental disorder, With medical condition,
                With another sleep disorder
___.___   Narcolepsy[c] (153)
            Specify whether:
G47.411   Narcolepsy with cataplexy or hypocretin deficiency
                    (type 1)
G47.419   Narcolepsy without cataplexy and either without
                    hypocretin deficiency or hypocretin unmeasured (type 2)
G47.421   Narcolepsy with cataplexy or hypocretin deficiency due
                    to a medical condition
G47.429   Narcolepsy without cataplexy and without hypocretin
                    deficiency due to a medical condition

Breathing-Related Sleep Disorders (154)

G47.33 Obstructive Sleep Apnea Hypopnea[c] (154)
___.___   Central Sleep Apnea (155)
            Specify current severity
            Specify whether:
G47.31   Idiopathic central sleep apnea
R06.3   Cheyne-Stokes breathing
G47.37   Central sleep apnea comorbid with opioid use
                    Note: First code opioid use disorder, if present.

____.___ Sleep-Related Hypoventilation (156)
          Specify current severity
          Specify whether:
G47.34   Idiopathic hypoventilation
G47.35   Congenital central alveolar hypoventilation
G47.36   Comorbid sleep-related hypoventilation

____.___ Circadian Rhythm Sleep-Wake Disorders[a] (156)
          Specify whether:
G47.21   Delayed sleep phase type (157)
               Specify if: Familial, Overlapping with non-24-hour sleep-wake type
G47.22   Advanced sleep phase type (157)
               Specify if: Familial
G47.23   Irregular sleep-wake type (157)
G47.24   Non-24-hour sleep-wake type (157)
G47.26   Shift work type (157)
G47.20   Unspecified type (157)

Parasomnias (158)

___.___   Non–Rapid Eye Movement Sleep Arousal Disorders (158)
          Specify whether:
F51.3   Sleepwalking type
               Specify if: With sleep-related eating, With sleep-related sexual behavior (sexsomnia)
F51.4   Sleep terror type
F51.5 Nightmare Disorder[b,c] (158)
           Specify if: During sleep onset
           Specify if: With mental disorder, With medical condition, With another sleep disorder

G47.52 Rapid Eye Movement Sleep Behavior Disorder (159)

G25.81 Restless Legs Syndrome (160)

____.___   Substance/Medication-Induced Sleep Disorder (161)
           Note: For applicable ICD-10-CM codes, refer to the substance classes under Substance-Related and Addictive Disorders for the specific substance/medication-induced sleep disorder. See also the criteria set and corresponding recording procedures in the manual for more information.
           Coding note: The ICD-10-CM code depends on whether or not there is a comorbid substance use disorder present for the same class of substance. In any case, an additional separate diagnosis of a substance use disorder is not given.
           Specify whether: Insomnia type, Daytime sleepiness type, Parasomnia type, Mixed type
           Specify if: With onset during intoxication, With onset during withdrawal, With onset after medication use

Sexual Dysfunctions (167)

The following specifiers apply to Sexual Dysfunctions where indicated:
[a]*Specify* whether: Lifelong, Acquired
[b]*Specify* whether: Generalized, Situational
[c]*Specify* current severity: Mild, Moderate, Severe

Gender Dysphoria (177)

The following specifier and note apply to Gender Dysphoria where indicated:
[a]*Specify* if: With a disorder/difference of sex development
[b]**Note:** Code the disorder/difference of sex development if present, in addition to gender dysphoria.

Disruptive, Impulse-Control, and Conduct Disorders (181)

Substance-Related and Addictive Disorders (187)

Substance-Related Disorders (190)

Alcohol-Related Disorders (192)

F10.281	With moderate or severe use disorder
F10.981	Without use disorder
___.___	Alcohol Intoxication Delirium[b,c] (242)
F10.121	With mild use disorder
F10.221	With moderate or severe use disorder
F10.921	Without use disorder
___.___	Alcohol Withdrawal Delirium[b,c] (243)
F10.131	With mild use disorder
F10.231	With moderate or severe use disorder
F10.931	Without use disorder

___.___ Alcohol-Induced Major Neurocognitive Disorder (259)
Specify if: Persistent

___.___	Amnestic-confabulatory type
F10.26	With moderate or severe use disorder
F10.96	Without use disorder
___.___	Nonamnestic-confabulatory type
F10.27	With moderate or severe use disorder
F10.97	Without use disorder

___.___ Alcohol-Induced Mild Neurocognitive Disorder (259)
Specify if: Persistent

F10.188	With mild use disorder
F10.288	With moderate or severe use disorder
F10.988	Without use disorder

F10.99 Unspecified Alcohol-Related Disorder (195)

Caffeine-Related Disorders (195)

F15.920 Caffeine Intoxication (195)

F15.93 Caffeine Withdrawal (196)

___.___ Caffeine-Induced Mental Disorders (196)
Note: Disorders are listed in their order of appearance in the manual.
Specify With onset during intoxication, With onset during withdrawal, With onset after medication use. **Note:** When taken over the counter, substances in this class can also induce the relevant substance-induced mental disorder.

F15.980 Caffeine-Induced Anxiety Disorder (105)

F15.982 Caffeine-Induced Sleep Disorder (161)
Specify whether Insomnia type, Daytime sleepiness type, Mixed type

F15.99 Unspecified Caffeine-Related Disorder (197)

Cannabis-Related Disorders (197)

___.___ Cannabis Use Disorder (197)
Specify if: In a controlled environment
Specify current severity/remission:

F12.10	Mild
F12.11	In early remission
F12.11	In sustained remission

F12.20	Moderate
F12.21	In early remission
F12.21	In sustained remission
F12.20	Severe
F12.21	In early remission
F12.21	In sustained remission

___.___ Cannabis Intoxication (199)

       Without perceptual disturbances

F12.120	With mild use disorder
F12.220	With moderate or severe use disorder
F12.920	Without use disorder

       With perceptual disturbances

F12.122	With mild use disorder
F12.222	With moderate or severe use disorder
F12.922	Without use disorder

___.___ Cannabis Withdrawal (199)

F12.13	With mild use disorder
F12.23	With moderate or severe use disorder
F12.93	Without use disorder

___.___ Cannabis-Induced Mental Disorders (200)

Note: Disorders are listed in their order of appearance in the manual.

[a]*Specify* With onset during intoxication, With onset during withdrawal, With onset after medication use. **Note:** When prescribed as medication, substances in this class can also induce the relevant substance-induced mental disorder.

[b]*Specify* if: Acute, Persistent

[c]*Specify* if: Hyperactive, Hypoactive, Mixed level of activity

___.___   Cannabis-Induced Psychotic Disorder[a] (48)

F12.159	With mild use disorder
F12.259	With moderate or severe use disorder
F12.959	Without use disorder

___.___   Cannabis-Induced Anxiety Disorder[a] (105)

F12.180	With mild use disorder
F12.280	With moderate or severe use disorder
F12.980	Without use disorder

___.___   Cannabis-Induced Sleep Disorder[a] (161)

    Specify whether Insomnia type, Daytime sleepiness type, Mixed type

F12.188	With mild use disorder
F12.288	With moderate or severe use disorder
F12.988	Without use disorder

___.___   Cannabis Intoxication Delirium[b,c] (242)

F12.121	With mild use disorder
F12.221	With moderate or severe use disorder
F12.921	Without use disorder
F12.921	Pharmaceutical Cannabis Receptor Agonist–Induced Delirium[b,c] (244)

> **Note:** When pharmaceutical cannabis receptor agonist medi-
> cation taken as prescribed. The designation "taken as pre-
> scribed" is used to differentiate medication-induced
> delirium from substance intoxication delirium.

F12.99   Unspecified Cannabis-Related Disorder (200)

Hallucinogen-Related Disorders (201)

___.__   Phencyclidine Use Disorder (201)
              Specify if: In a controlled environment
              Specify current severity/remission:
F16.10   Mild
F16.11   In early remission
F16.11   In sustained remission
F16.20   Moderate
F16.21   In early remission
F16.21   In sustained remission
F16.20   Severe
F16.21   In early remission
F16.21   In sustained remission

___.__   Other Hallucinogen Use Disorder (202)
              Specify the particular hallucinogen
              Specify if: In a controlled environment
              Specify current severity/remission:
F16.10   Mild
F16.11   In early remission
F16.11   In sustained remission
F16.20   Moderate
F16.21   In early remission
F16.21   In sustained remission
F16.20   Severe
F16.21   In early remission
F16.21   In sustained remission

___.__   Phencyclidine Intoxication (204)
F16.120   With mild use disorder
F16.220   With moderate or severe use disorder
F16.920   Without use disorder

___.__   Other Hallucinogen Intoxication (205)
F16.120   With mild use disorder
F16.220   With moderate or severe use disorder
F16.920   Without use disorder

F16.983 Hallucinogen Persisting Perception Disorder (206)

___.__   Phencyclidine-Induced Mental Disorders (206)
              Note: Disorders are listed in their order of appearance in the
              manual.
              [a]*Specify* With onset during intoxication, With onset after medica-
              tion use. **Note:** When prescribed as medication, substances in

this class can also induce the relevant substance-induced mental disorder.

	Phencyclidine-Induced Psychotic Disorder[a] (48)
___.___	
F16.159	With mild use disorder
F16.259	With moderate or severe use disorder
F16.959	Without use disorder

	Phencyclidine-Induced Bipolar and Related Disorder[a] (66)
___.___	
F16.14	With mild use disorder
F16.24	With moderate or severe use disorder
F16.94	Without use disorder

	Phencyclidine-Induced Depressive Disorder[a] (87)
___.___	
F16.14	With mild use disorder
F16.24	With moderate or severe use disorder
F16.94	Without use disorder

	Phencyclidine-Induced Anxiety Disorder[a] (105)
___.___	
F16.180	With mild use disorder
F16.280	With moderate or severe use disorder
F16.980	Without use disorder

___.___   Phencyclidine Intoxication Delirium (242)

Specify if: Acute, Persistent

Specify if: Hyperactive, Hypoactive, Mixed level of activity

F16.121	With mild use disorder
F16.221	With moderate or severe use disorder
F16.921	Without use disorder

___.___   Hallucinogen-Induced Mental Disorders (206)

Note: Disorders are listed in their order of appearance in the manual.

[a]*Specify* With onset during intoxication, With onset after medication use. **Note:** When prescribed as medication, substances in this class can also induce the relevant substance-induced mental disorder.

[b]*Specify* if: Acute, Persistent

[c]*Specify* if: Hyperactive, Hypoactive, Mixed level of activity

	Other Hallucinogen–Induced Psychotic Disorder[a] (48)
___.___	
F16.159	With mild use disorder
F16.259	With moderate or severe use disorder
F16.959	Without use disorder

	Other Hallucinogen–Induced Bipolar and Related Disorder[a] (66)
___.___	
F16.14	With mild use disorder
F16.24	With moderate or severe use disorder
F16.94	Without use disorder

	Other Hallucinogen–Induced Depressive Disorder[a] (87)
___.___	
F16.14	With mild use disorder
F16.24	With moderate or severe use disorder
F16.94	Without use disorder

	Other Hallucinogen-Induced Anxiety Disorder[a] (105)
___.___	
F16.180	With mild use disorder

F16.280   With moderate or severe use disorder
F16.980   Without use disorder
___.___   Other Hallucinogen Intoxication Delirium[b,c] (242)
F16.121   With mild use disorder
F16.221   With moderate or severe use disorder
F16.921   Without use disorder
F16.921   Ketamine or Other Hallucinogen–Induced Delirium[b,c]
                    (244)
               Note: When ketamine or other hallucinogen medication taken
                    as prescribed. The designation "taken as prescribed" is
                    used to differentiate medication-induced delirium from
                    substance intoxication delirium.

F16.99   Unspecified Phencyclidine-Related Disorder (207)

F16.99   Unspecified Hallucinogen-Related Disorder (207)

Inhalant-Related Disorders (207)

___.___   Inhalant Use Disorder (207)
               Specify the particular inhalant
               Specify if: In a controlled environment
               Specify current severity/remission:
F18.10   Mild
F18.11   In early remission
F18.11   In sustained remission
F18.20   Moderate
F18.21   In early remission
F18.21   In sustained remission
F18.20   Severe
F18.21   In early remission
F18.21   In sustained remission

___.___   Inhalant Intoxication (209)
F18.120   With mild use disorder
F18.220   With moderate or severe use disorder
F18.920   Without use disorder

___.___   Inhalant-Induced Mental Disorders (210)
               Note: Disorders are listed in their order of appearance in the
                    manual.
               [a]*Specify* With onset during intoxication
___.___   Inhalant-Induced Psychotic Disorder[a] (48)
F18.159   With mild use disorder
F18.259   With moderate or severe use disorder
F18.959   Without use disorder
___.___   Inhalant-Induced Depressive Disorder[a] (87)
F18.14   With mild use disorder
F18.24   With moderate or severe use disorder
F18.94   Without use disorder
___.___   Inhalant-Induced Anxiety Disorder[a] (105)
F18.180   With mild use disorder

F18.280		With moderate or severe use disorder
F18.980		Without use disorder
___.__		Inhalant Intoxication Delirium (242)
		Specify if: Acute, Persistent
		Specify if: Hyperactive, Hypoactive, Mixed level of activity
F18.121		With mild use disorder
F18.221		With moderate or severe use disorder
F18.921		Without use disorder
___.__		Inhalant-Induced Major Neurocognitive Disorder (259)
		Specify if: Persistent
F18.17		With mild use disorder
F18.27		With moderate or severe use disorder
F18.97		Without use disorder
___.__		Inhalant-Induced Mild Neurocognitive Disorder (259)
		Specify if: Persistent
F18.188		With mild use disorder
F18.288		With moderate or severe use disorder
F18.988		Without use disorder
F18.99	Unspecified Inhalant-Related Disorder (210)	

Opioid-Related Disorders (210)

___.__		Opioid Use Disorder (210)
		Specify if: On maintenance therapy, In a controlled environment
		Specify current severity/remission:
F11.10		Mild
F11.11		In early remission
F11.11		In sustained remission
F11.20		Moderate
F11.21		In early remission
F11.21		In sustained remission
F11.20		Severe
F11.21		In early remission
F11.21		In sustained remission
___.__		Opioid Intoxication (212)
		Without perceptual disturbances
F11.120		With mild use disorder
F11.220		With moderate or severe use disorder
F11.920		Without use disorder
		With perceptual disturbances
F11.122		With mild use disorder
F11.222		With moderate or severe use disorder
F11.922		Without use disorder
___.__		Opioid Withdrawal (213)
F11.13		With mild use disorder
F11.23		With moderate or severe use disorder
F11.93		Without use disorder

___.___   Opioid-Induced Mental Disorders (214)
            Note: Disorders are listed in their order of appearance in the
               manual.
            [a]*Specify* With onset during intoxication, With onset during with-
               drawal, With onset after medication use. **Note:** When pre-
               scribed as medication, substances in this class can also induce
               the relevant substance-induced mental disorder.
            [b]*Specify* if: Acute, Persistent
            [c]*Specify* if: Hyperactive, Hypoactive, Mixed level of activity

___.___   Opioid-Induced Depressive Disorder[a] (87)
F11.14   With mild use disorder
F11.24   With moderate or severe use disorder
F11.94   Without use disorder

___.___   Opioid-Induced Anxiety Disorder[a] (105)
F11.180   With mild use disorder
F11.280   With moderate or severe use disorder
F11.980   Without use disorder

___.___   Opioid-Induced Sleep Disorder[a] (161)
            Specify whether Insomnia type, Daytime sleepiness type,
               Mixed type
F11.182   With mild use disorder
F11.282   With moderate or severe use disorder
F11.982   Without use disorder

___.___   Opioid-Induced Sexual Dysfunction[a] (173)
            Specify if: Mild, Moderate, Severe
F11.181   With mild use disorder
F11.281   With moderate or severe use disorder
F11.981   Without use disorder

___.___   Opioid Intoxication Delirium[b,c] (242)
F11.121   With mild use disorder
F11.221   With moderate or severe use disorder
F11.921   Without use disorder

___.___   Opioid Withdrawal Delirium[b,c] (243)
F11.188   With mild use disorder
F11.288   With moderate or severe use disorder
F11.988   Without use disorder

___.___   Opioid-Induced Delirium[b,c] (244)
            Note: The designation "taken as prescribed" is used to differ-
               entiate medication-induced delirium from substance in-
               toxication delirium and substance withdrawal delirium.
F11.921   When opioid medication taken as prescribed (244)
F11.988   During withdrawal from opioid medication taken as
               prescribed (244)

F11.99 Unspecified Opioid-Related Disorder (214)

Sedative-, Hypnotic-, or Anxiolytic-Related Disorders (215)

___.___   Sedative, Hypnotic, or Anxiolytic Use Disorder (215)
            Specify if: In a controlled environment

F13.288	With moderate or severe use disorder
F13.988	Without use disorder
F13.99	Unspecified Sedative-, Hypnotic-, or Anxiolytic-Related Disorder (219)

Stimulant-Related Disorders (220)

___.__	Stimulant Use Disorder (220)
	Specify if: In a controlled environment
	Specify current severity/remission:
___.__	Mild
F15.10	Amphetamine-type substance
F14.10	Cocaine
F15.10	Other or unspecified stimulant
___.__	Mild, In early remission
F15.11	Amphetamine-type substance
F14.11	Cocaine
F15.11	Other or unspecified stimulant
___.__	Mild, In sustained remission
F15.11	Amphetamine-type substance
F14.11	Cocaine
F15.11	Other or unspecified stimulant
___.__	Moderate
F15.20	Amphetamine-type substance
F14.20	Cocaine
F15.20	Other or unspecified stimulant
___.__	Moderate, In early remission
F15.21	Amphetamine-type substance
F14.21	Cocaine
F15.21	Other or unspecified stimulant
___.__	Moderate, In sustained remission
F15.21	Amphetamine-type substance
F14.21	Cocaine
F15.21	Other or unspecified stimulant
___.__	Severe
F15.20	Amphetamine-type substance
F14.20	Cocaine
F15.20	Other or unspecified stimulant
___.__	Severe, In early remission
F15.21	Amphetamine-type substance
F14.21	Cocaine
F15.21	Other or unspecified stimulant
___.__	Severe, In sustained remission
F15.21	Amphetamine-type substance
F14.21	Cocaine
F15.21	Other or unspecified stimulant

Tobacco-Related Disorders (225)

___.__ Tobacco Use Disorder (225)
Specify if: On maintenance therapy, In a controlled environment
Specify current severity/remission:

Z72.0	Mild
F17.200	Moderate
F17.201	In early remission
F17.201	In sustained remission
F17.200	Severe
F17.201	In early remission
F17.201	In sustained remission

F17.203 Tobacco Withdrawal (227)
Note: The ICD-10-CM code indicates the comorbid presence of a moderate or severe tobacco use disorder, which must be present in order to apply the code for tobacco withdrawal.

___.__ Tobacco-Induced Mental Disorders (228)
F17.208 Tobacco-Induced Sleep Disorder, With moderate or severe use disorder (161)
Specify whether Insomnia type, Daytime sleepiness type, Mixed type
Specify With onset during withdrawal, With onset after medication use

F17.209 Unspecified Tobacco-Related Disorder (228)

Other (or Unknown) Substance–Related Disorders (228)

___.__ Other (or Unknown) Substance Use Disorder (228)
Specify if: In a controlled environment
Specify current severity/remission:

F19.10	Mild
F19.11	In early remission
F19.11	In sustained remission
F19.20	Moderate
F19.21	In early remission
F19.21	In sustained remission
F19.20	Severe
F19.21	In early remission
F19.21	In sustained remission

___.__ Other (or Unknown) Substance Intoxication (230)

	Without perceptual disturbances
F19.120	With mild use disorder
F19.220	With moderate or severe use disorder
F19.920	Without use disorder
	With perceptual disturbances
F19.122	With mild use disorder
F19.222	With moderate or severe use disorder
F19.922	Without use disorder

____.____   Other (or Unknown) Substance Withdrawal (231)
               Without perceptual disturbances
F19.130   With mild use disorder
F19.230   With moderate or severe use disorder
F19.930   Without use disorder
               With perceptual disturbances
F19.132   With mild use disorder
F19.232   With moderate or severe use disorder
F19.932   Without use disorder

____.____   Other (or Unknown) Substance–Induced Mental Disorders
               (232)
             Note: Disorders are listed in their order of appearance in the
               manual.
             [a]*Specify* With onset during intoxication, With onset during with-
               drawal, With onset after medication use. **Note:** When pre-
               scribed as medication or taken over the counter, substances
               in this class can also induce the relevant substance-induced
               mental disorder.
             [b]*Specify* if: Acute, Persistent
             [c]*Specify* if: Hyperactive, Hypoactive, Mixed level of activity

____.____   Other (or Unknown) Substance–Induced Psychotic
                   Disorder[a] (48)
F19.159   With mild use disorder
F19.259   With moderate or severe use disorder
F19.959   Without use disorder

____.____   Other (or Unknown) Substance–Induced Bipolar and
                   Related Disorder[a] (66)
F19.14   With mild use disorder
F19.24   With moderate or severe use disorder
F19.94   Without use disorder

____.____   Other (or Unknown) Substance–Induced Depressive
                   Disorder[a] (87)
F19.14   With mild use disorder
F19.24   With moderate or severe use disorder
F19.94   Without use disorder

____.____   Other (or Unknown) Substance–Induced Anxiety
                   Disorder[a] (105)
F19.180   With mild use disorder
F19.280   With moderate or severe use disorder
F19.980   Without use disorder

____.____   Other (or Unknown) Substance–Induced Obsessive-
                   Compulsive and Related Disorder[a] (114)
F19.188   With mild use disorder
F19.288   With moderate or severe use disorder
F19.988   Without use disorder

____.____   Other (or Unknown) Substance–Induced Sleep
                   Disorder[a] (161)
                 Specify whether Insomnia type, Daytime sleepiness type,
                   Parasomnia type, Mixed type

F19.182	With mild use disorder
F19.282	With moderate or severe use disorder
F19.982	Without use disorder
___.___	Other (or Unknown) Substance–Induced Sexual Dysfunction[a] (173)
	Specify if: Mild, Moderate, Severe
F19.181	With mild use disorder
F19.281	With moderate or severe use disorder
F19.981	Without use disorder
___.___	Other (or Unknown) Substance Intoxication Delirium[b,c] (242)
F19.121	With mild use disorder
F19.221	With moderate or severe use disorder
F19.921	Without use disorder
___.___	Other (or Unknown) Substance Withdrawal Delirium[b,c] (243)
F19.131	With mild use disorder
F19.231	With moderate or severe use disorder
F19.931	Without use disorder
___.___	Other (or Unknown) Medication–Induced Delirium[b,c] (244)
	Note: The designation "taken as prescribed" is used to differentiate medication-induced delirium from substance intoxication delirium and substance withdrawal delirium.
F19.921	When other (or unknown) medication taken as prescribed (244)
F19.931	During withdrawal from other (or unknown) medication taken as prescribed (244)
___.___	Other (or Unknown) Substance–Induced Major Neurocognitive Disorder (259)
	Specify if: Persistent
F19.17	With mild use disorder
F19.27	With moderate or severe use disorder
F19.97	Without use disorder
___.___	Other (or Unknown) Substance–Induced Mild Neurocognitive Disorder (259)
	Specify if: Persistent
F19.188	With mild use disorder
F19.288	With moderate or severe use disorder
F19.988	Without use disorder
F19.99	Unspecified Other (or Unknown) Substance–Related Disorder (232)

Non-Substance-Related Disorders (233)

F63.0	Gambling Disorder (233)
	Specify if: Episodic, Persistent
	Specify if: In early remission, In sustained remission
	Specify current severity: Mild, Moderate, Severe

Neurocognitive Disorders (235)

___.___   Delirium (242)
Specify if: Acute, Persistent
Specify if: Hyperactive, Hypoactive, Mixed level of activity
[a]**Note:** For applicable ICD-10-CM codes, refer to the substance
classes under Substance-Related and Addictive Disorders
for the specific substance/medication-induced delirium. See
also the criteria set and corresponding recording procedures
in the manual for more information.
Specify whether:

___.___   Substance intoxication delirium[a]
___.___   Substance withdrawal delirium[a]
___.___   Medication-induced delirium[a]
F05   Delirium due to another medical condition
F05   Delirium due to multiple etiologies
R41.0   Other Specified Delirium (246)
R41.0   Unspecified Delirium (246)

Major and Mild Neurocognitive Disorders (247)

Specify whether due to *[any of the following medical etiologies]*: Alzheimer's
disease, Frontotemporal degeneration, Lewy body disease, Vascular disease, Traumatic brain injury, Substance/medication use, HIV infection,
Prion disease, Parkinson's disease, Huntington's disease, Another medical condition, Multiple etiologies, Unspecified etiology
[a]*Specify* current severity: Mild, Moderate, Severe. *This specifier applies only to
major neurocognitive disorders (including probable and possible).*
[b]*Specify:* Without behavioral disturbance, With behavioral disturbance. *For
all mild neurocognitive disorders, substance/medication-induced major neurocognitive disorder, and unspecified neurocognitive disorder, behavioral disturbance cannot be coded but should still be recorded.*
Note: As indicated for each subtype, an additional medical code is needed
for most major neurocognitive disorders, including those due to probable
and possible medical etiologies. The medical etiology should be coded
first, before the code for the major neurocognitive disorder. An additional
medical code should *not* be used for any mild neurocognitive disorder
and is not used for major or mild vascular neurocognitive disorder, sub-
stance/medication-induced major or mild neurocognitive disorder, and
unspecified neurocognitive disorder.
Coding note: *For major and mild neurocognitive disorders:* Use additional
code(s) to indicate clinically significant psychiatric symptoms due to the
same medical condition causing the major NCD (e.g., F06.2 psychotic disorder due to Alzheimer's disease with delusions; F06.32 depressive disorder due to Parkinson's disease, with major depressive-like episode.)
Note: The additional codes for mental disorders due to another medical
condition are included with disorders with which they share phenomenology (e.g., for depressive disorders due to another medical condition,
see "Depressive Disorders").

Major or Mild Neurocognitive Disorder Due to Alzheimer's Disease (254)

___.__   Major Neurocognitive Disorder Due to Probable
        Alzheimer's Disease[a]
        Note: Code first **G30.9** Alzheimer's disease.

F02.81   With behavioral disturbance
F02.80   Without behavioral disturbance

___.__   Major Neurocognitive Disorder Due to Possible
        Alzheimer's Disease[a]
        Note: Code first **G30.9** Alzheimer's disease.

F02.81   With behavioral disturbance
F02.80   Without behavioral disturbance

G31.84   Mild Neurocognitive Disorder Due to Alzheimer's Disease[b]

Major or Mild Frontotemporal Neurocognitive Disorder (255)

___.__   Major Neurocognitive Disorder Due to Probable
        Frontotemporal Degeneration[a]
        Note: Code first **G31.09** frontotemporal degeneration.

F02.81   With behavioral disturbance
F02.80   Without behavioral disturbance

___.__   Major Neurocognitive Disorder Due to Possible
        Frontotemporal Degeneration[a]
        Note: Code first **G31.09** frontotemporal degeneration.

F02.81   With behavioral disturbance
F02.80   Without behavioral disturbance

G31.84   Mild Neurocognitive Disorder Due to Frontotemporal Degeneration[b]

Major or Mild Neurocognitive Disorder With Lewy Bodies (256)

___.__   Major Neurocognitive Disorder With Probable Lewy
        Bodies[a]
        Note: Code first **G31.83** Lewy body disease.

F02.81   With behavioral disturbance
F02.80   Without behavioral disturbance

___.__   Major Neurocognitive Disorder With Possible Lewy Bodies[a]
        Note: Code first **G31.83** Lewy body disease.

F02.81   With behavioral disturbance
F02.80   Without behavioral disturbance

G31.84   Mild Neurocognitive Disorder With Lewy Bodies[b]

Major or Mild Vascular Neurocognitive Disorder (257)

___.__   Major Neurocognitive Disorder Probably Due to Vascular
        Disease[a]
        Note: No additional medical code for vascular disease.

F01.51   With behavioral disturbance
F01.50   Without behavioral disturbance

___.___   Major Neurocognitive Disorder Possibly Due to Vascular
           Disease[a]
           Note: No additional medical code for vascular disease.
F01.51   With behavioral disturbance
F01.50   Without behavioral disturbance
G31.84   Mild Neurocognitive Disorder Due to Vascular Disease[b]

Major or Mild Neurocognitive Disorder Due to Traumatic Brain Injury (258)

___.___   Major Neurocognitive Disorder Due to Traumatic Brain
           Injury[a]
           Note: For ICD-10-CM, code first **S06.2X9S** diffuse traumatic
           brain injury with loss of consciousness of unspecified dura-
           tion, sequela.
F02.81   With behavioral disturbance
F02.80   Without behavioral disturbance
G31.84   Mild Neurocognitive Disorder Due to Traumatic Brain Injury[b]

Substance/Medication-Induced Major or Mild Neurocognitive Disorder (259)

Note: No additional medical code. For applicable ICD-10-CM codes, refer
to the substance classes under Substance-Related and Addictive Disorders for the specific substance/medication-induced major or mild neurocognitive disorder. See also the criteria set and corresponding recording
procedures in the manual for more information.
Coding note: The ICD-10-CM code depends on whether or not there is a comorbid substance use disorder present for the same class of substance. In
any case, an additional separate diagnosis of a substance use disorder is
not given.
Specify if: Persistent

___.___   Substance/Medication-Induced Major Neurocognitive
           Disorder[a,b]
           Note: If a substance use disorder is present, record mild sub-
           stance use disorder (ICD-10-CM code not available if mild
           substance use disorder does not cause a major neurocogni-
           tive disorder) or moderate or severe substance use disorder;
           if no substance use disorder is present, record only [*specific
           substance*]-induced major neurocognitive disorder.

___.___   Substance/Medication-Induced Mild Neurocognitive
           Disorder[b]
           Note: If a substance use disorder is present, record mild sub-
           stance use disorder or moderate or severe substance use dis-
           order; if no substance use disorder is present, record only
           [*specific substance*]-induced mild neurocognitive disorder.

Major or Mild Neurocognitive Disorder Due to HIV Infection (262)

___.___   Major Neurocognitive Disorder Due to HIV Infection[a]
           Note: Code first **B20** HIV infection.
F02.81   With behavioral disturbance
F02.80   Without behavioral disturbance

G31.84   Mild Neurocognitive Disorder Due to HIV Infection[b]

Major or Mild Neurocognitive Disorder Due to Prion Disease (263)

___.___   Major Neurocognitive Disorder Due to Prion Disease[a]
Note: Code first **A81.9** prion disease.

F02.81   With behavioral disturbance

F02.80   Without behavioral disturbance

G31.84   Mild Neurocognitive Disorder Due to Prion Disease[b]

Major or Mild Neurocognitive Disorder Due to Parkinson's Disease (263)

___.___   Major Neurocognitive Disorder Probably Due to
            Parkinson's Disease[a]
Note: Code first **G20** Parkinson's disease.

F02.81   With behavioral disturbance

F02.80   Without behavioral disturbance

___.___   Major Neurocognitive Disorder Possibly Due to Parkinson's
            Disease[a]
Note: Code first **G20** Parkinson's disease.

F02.81   With behavioral disturbance

F02.80   Without behavioral disturbance

G31.84   Mild Neurocognitive Disorder Due to Parkinson's Disease[b]

Major or Mild Neurocognitive Disorder Due to Huntington's Disease (264)

___.___   Major Neurocognitive Disorder Due to Huntington's
            Disease[a]
Note: Code first **G10** Huntington's disease.

F02.81   With behavioral disturbance

F02.80   Without behavioral disturbance

G31.84   Mild Neurocognitive Disorder Due to Huntington's Disease[b]

Major or Mild Neurocognitive Disorder Due to Another Medical Condition (265)

___.___   Major Neurocognitive Disorder Due to Another Medical
            Condition[a]
Note: Code first the other medical condition.

F02.81   With behavioral disturbance

F02.80   Without behavioral disturbance

G31.84   Mild Neurocognitive Disorder Due to Another Medical
            Condition[b]

Major or Mild Neurocognitive Disorder Due to Multiple Etiologies (266)

___.___   Major Neurocognitive Disorder Due to Multiple Etiologies[a]
Note: Code first all the etiological medical conditions (with the
            exception of vascular disease, which is not coded).

F02.81   With behavioral disturbance
F02.80   Without behavioral disturbance
             Note: If vascular disease is among the multiple etiological med-
             ical conditions, code either **F01.51** for major vascular neuro-
             cognitive disorder, with behavioral disturbance, or **F01.50**
             for major vascular neurocognitive disorder, without behav-
             ioral disturbance.
G31.84   Mild Neurocognitive Disorder Due to Multiple Etiologies[b]

Unspecified Neurocognitive Disorder[b] (267)
Note: No additional medical code.
R41.9   Unspecified Neurocognitive Disorder[b]

Personality Disorders (269)

Cluster A Personality Disorders
F60.0   Paranoid Personality Disorder (269)
F60.1   Schizoid Personality Disorder (270)
F21   Schizotypal Personality Disorder (271)

Cluster B Personality Disorders
F60.2   Antisocial Personality Disorder (271)
F60.3   Borderline Personality Disorder (272)
F60.4   Histrionic Personality Disorder (273)
F60.81   Narcissistic Personality Disorder (273)

Cluster C Personality Disorders
F60.6   Avoidant Personality Disorder (274)
F60.7   Dependent Personality Disorder (274)
F60.5   Obsessive-Compulsive Personality Disorder (275)

Other Personality Disorders
F07.0   Personality Change Due to Another Medical Condition (275)
             Specify whether: Labile type, Disinhibited type, Aggressive type,
                Apathetic type, Paranoid type, Other type, Combined type,
                Unspecified type
F60.89   Other Specified Personality Disorder (276)
F60.9   Unspecified Personality Disorder (277)

Paraphilic Disorders (279)

The following specifier applies to Paraphilic Disorders where indicated:
[a]*Specify* if: In a controlled environment, In full remission
F65.3   Voyeuristic Disorder[a] (279)

Other Mental Disorders and Additional Codes (285)

Medication-Induced Movement Disorders and Other Adverse Effects of Medication (287)

G24.01   Tardive Dyskinesia (297)

G24.09   Tardive Dystonia (299)

G25.71   Tardive Akathisia (299)

G25.1   Medication-Induced Postural Tremor (300)

G25.79   Other Medication-Induced Movement Disorder (301)

___.___   Antidepressant Discontinuation Syndrome (301)
T43.205A   Initial encounter
T43.205D   Subsequent encounter
T43.205S   Sequelae

___.___   Other Adverse Effect of Medication (303)
T50.905A   Initial encounter
T50.905D   Subsequent encounter
T50.905S   Sequelae

Other Conditions That May Be a Focus of Clinical Attention (305)

Suicidal Behavior and Nonsuicidal Self-Injury (306)

Suicidal Behavior (306)

___.___   Current Suicidal Behavior (306)
T14.91A   Initial encounter
T14.91D   Subsequent encounter

Z91.51   History of Suicidal Behavior (307)

Nonsuicidal Self-Injury (307)

R45.88   Current Nonsuicidal Self-Injury (307)

Z91.52   History of Nonsuicidal Self-Injury (307)

Abuse and Neglect (307)

Child Maltreatment and Neglect Problems (308)

Child Physical Abuse (308)

___.___   Child Physical Abuse, Confirmed (308)
T74.12XA   Initial encounter
T74.12XD   Subsequent encounter

___.___   Child Physical Abuse, Suspected (308)
T76.12XA   Initial encounter
T76.12XD   Subsequent encounter

___.___   Other Circumstances Related to Child Physical Abuse (308)
Z69.010   Encounter for mental health services for victim of child physical abuse by parent
Z69.020   Encounter for mental health services for victim of nonparental child physical abuse

Z62.810	Personal history (past history) of physical abuse in childhood
Z69.011	Encounter for mental health services for perpetrator of parental child physical abuse
Z69.021	Encounter for mental health services for perpetrator of nonparental child physical abuse

Child Sexual Abuse (308)

___.__	Child Sexual Abuse, Confirmed (308)
T74.22XA	Initial encounter
T74.22XD	Subsequent encounter
___.__	Child Sexual Abuse, Suspected (309)
T76.22XA	Initial encounter
T76.22XD	Subsequent encounter
___.__	Other Circumstances Related to Child Sexual Abuse (309)
Z69.010	Encounter for mental health services for victim of child sexual abuse by parent
Z69.020	Encounter for mental health services for victim of nonparental child sexual abuse
Z62.810	Personal history (past history) of sexual abuse in childhood
Z69.011	Encounter for mental health services for perpetrator of parental child sexual abuse
Z69.021	Encounter for mental health services for perpetrator of nonparental child sexual abuse

Child Neglect (309)

___.__	Child Neglect, Confirmed (309)
T74.02XA	Initial encounter
T74.02XD	Subsequent encounter
___.__	Child Neglect, Suspected (309)
T76.02XA	Initial encounter
T76.02XD	Subsequent encounter
___.__	Other Circumstances Related to Child Neglect (309)
Z69.010	Encounter for mental health services for victim of child neglect by parent
Z69.020	Encounter for mental health services for victim of nonparental child neglect
Z62.812	Personal history (past history) of neglect in childhood
Z69.011	Encounter for mental health services for perpetrator of parental child neglect
Z69.021	Encounter for mental health services for perpetrator of nonparental child neglect

Child Psychological Abuse (309)

___.__	Child Psychological Abuse, Confirmed (310)
T74.32XA	Initial encounter
T74.32XD	Subsequent encounter

___.__ Child Psychological Abuse, Suspected (310)
T76.32XA Initial encounter
T76.32XD Subsequent encounter

___.__ Other Circumstances Related to Child Psychological Abuse (310)
Z69.010 Encounter for mental health services for victim of child psychological abuse by parent
Z69.020 Encounter for mental health services for victim of nonparental child psychological abuse
Z62.811 Personal history (past history) of psychological abuse in childhood
Z69.011 Encounter for mental health services for perpetrator of parental child psychological abuse
Z69.021 Encounter for mental health services for perpetrator of nonparental child psychological abuse

Adult Maltreatment and Neglect Problems (310)

Spouse or Partner Violence, Physical (310)

___.__ Spouse or Partner Violence, Physical, Confirmed (311)
T74.11XA Initial encounter
T74.11XD Subsequent encounter

___.__ Spouse or Partner Violence, Physical, Suspected (311)
T76.11XA Initial encounter
T76.11XD Subsequent encounter

___.__ Other Circumstances Related to Spouse or Partner Violence, Physical (311)
Z69.11 Encounter for mental health services for victim of spouse or partner violence, physical
Z91.410 Personal history (past history) of spouse or partner violence, physical
Z69.12 Encounter for mental health services for perpetrator of spouse or partner violence, physical

Spouse or Partner Violence, Sexual (311)

___.__ Spouse or Partner Violence, Sexual, Confirmed (311)
T74.21XA Initial encounter
T74.21XD Subsequent encounter

___.__ Spouse or Partner Violence, Sexual, Suspected (311)
T76.21XA Initial encounter
T76.21XD Subsequent encounter

___.__ Other Circumstances Related to Spouse or Partner Violence, Sexual (311)
Z69.81 Encounter for mental health services for victim of spouse or partner violence, sexual

Z91.410   Personal history (past history) of spouse or partner violence, sexual
Z69.12   Encounter for mental health services for perpetrator of spouse or partner violence, sexual

Spouse or Partner Neglect (311)

___.__   Spouse or Partner Neglect, Confirmed (312)
T74.01XA   Initial encounter
T74.01XD   Subsequent encounter

___.__   Spouse or Partner Neglect, Suspected (312)
T76.01XA   Initial encounter
T76.01XD   Subsequent encounter

___.__   Other Circumstances Related to Spouse or Partner Neglect (312)
Z69.11   Encounter for mental health services for victim of spouse or partner neglect
Z91.412   Personal history (past history) of spouse or partner neglect
Z69.12   Encounter for mental health services for perpetrator of spouse or partner neglect

Spouse or Partner Abuse, Psychological (312)

___.__   Spouse or Partner Abuse, Psychological, Confirmed (312)
T74.31XA   Initial encounter
T74.31XD   Subsequent encounter

___.__   Spouse or Partner Abuse, Psychological, Suspected (312)
T76.31XA   Initial encounter
T76.31XD   Subsequent encounter

___.__   Other Circumstances Related to Spouse or Partner Abuse, Psychological (313)
Z69.11   Encounter for mental health services for victim of spouse or partner psychological abuse
Z91.411   Personal history (past history) of spouse or partner psychological abuse
Z69.12   Encounter for mental health services for perpetrator of spouse or partner psychological abuse

Adult Abuse by Nonspouse or Nonpartner (313)

___.__   Adult Physical Abuse by Nonspouse or Nonpartner, Confirmed (313)
T74.11XA   Initial encounter
T74.11XD   Subsequent encounter

___.__   Adult Physical Abuse by Nonspouse or Nonpartner, Suspected (313)
T76.11XA   Initial encounter
T76.11XD   Subsequent encounter

___.___   Adult Sexual Abuse by Nonspouse or Nonpartner,
           Confirmed (313)
T74.21XA   Initial encounter
T74.21XD   Subsequent encounter

___.___   Adult Sexual Abuse by Nonspouse or Nonpartner,
           Suspected (313)
T76.21XA   Initial encounter
T76.21XD   Subsequent encounter

___.___   Adult Psychological Abuse by Nonspouse or Nonpartner,
           Confirmed (313)
T74.31XA   Initial encounter
T74.31XD   Subsequent encounter

___.___   Adult Psychological Abuse by Nonspouse or Nonpartner,
           Suspected (314)
T76.31XA   Initial encounter
T76.31XD   Subsequent encounter

___.___   Other Circumstances Related to Adult Abuse by Nonspouse
           or Nonpartner (314)
Z69.81   Encounter for mental health services for victim of
           nonspousal or nonpartner adult abuse
Z69.82   Encounter for mental health services for perpetrator of
           nonspousal or nonpartner adult abuse

Relational Problems (314)

___.___   Parent-Child Relational Problem (314)
Z62.820   Parent–Biological Child (314)
Z62.821   Parent–Adopted Child (314)
Z62.822   Parent–Foster Child (314)
Z62.898   Other Caregiver–Child (314)
Z62.891 Sibling Relational Problem (315)
Z63.0   Relationship Distress With Spouse or Intimate Partner (315)

Problems Related to the Family Environment (315)
Z62.29   Upbringing Away From Parents (315)
Z62.898 Child Affected by Parental Relationship Distress (315)
Z63.5   Disruption of Family by Separation or Divorce (315)
Z63.8   High Expressed Emotion Level Within Family (315)

Educational Problems (316)
Z55.0   Illiteracy and Low-Level Literacy (316)
Z55.1   Schooling Unavailable and Unattainable (316)
Z55.2   Failed School Examinations (316)
Z55.3   Underachievement in School (316)

Problems Related to Interaction With the Legal System (319)

Problems Related to Other Psychosocial, Personal, and Environmental Circumstances (319)

Problems Related to Access to Medical and Other Health Care (320)

Circumstances of Personal History (320)

Other Health Service Encounters for Counseling and Medical Advice (320)

Additional Conditions or Problems That May Be a Focus of Clinical Attention (320)

SECTION I

DSM-5 Basics

Use of the Manual

This text is designed to provide a practical guide to using DSM-5, particularly in clinical practice.

Approach to Clinical Case Formulation

The primary purpose of DSM-5 is to assist trained clinicians in the diagnosis of mental disorders as part of a case formulation assessment that leads to an informed treatment plan for each individual. The case formulation for any given individual should involve a careful clinical history and concise summary of the social, psychological, and biological factors that may have contributed to developing a given mental disorder. It is not sufficient to simply check off the symptoms in the diagnostic criteria to make a mental disorder diagnosis. A thorough evaluation of these criteria may assure more reliable assessment (which may be aided by the use of dimensional symptom severity assessment tools); the relative severity and salience of an individual's signs and symptoms and their contribution to a diagnosis will ultimately require clinical judgment. Diagnosis requires clinical training to recognize when the combination of predisposing, precipitating, perpetuating, and protective factors has resulted in a psychopathological condition in which the signs and symptoms exceed normal ranges. The ultimate goal of a clinical case formulation is to use the available contextual and diagnostic information in developing a comprehensive treatment plan that is informed by the individual's cultural and social context. However, recommendations for the selection and use of the most appropriate evidence-based treatment options for each disorder are beyond the scope of this manual.

Elements of a Diagnosis

Diagnostic criteria are offered as guidelines for making diagnoses, and their use should be informed by clinical judgment. Text descriptions, including introductory sections of each diagnostic chapter, can help support diagnosis (e.g., describing the criteria more fully under "Diagnostic Features"; providing differential diagnoses).

Following the assessment of diagnostic criteria, clinicians should consider the application of disorder subtypes and/or specifiers as appropriate. Most specifiers are only applicable to the current presentation and may change over the course of the disorder (e.g., with good to fair insight; predominantly inattentive presentation; in a controlled environment) and can be given only if full criteria for the disorder are currently met. Other specifiers are indicative of the lifetime course (e.g., with seasonal pattern, bipolar type in schizoaffective disorder) and can be assigned regardless of current status.

When the symptom presentation does not meet full criteria for any disorder and the symptoms cause clinically significant distress or impairment in social, occupational, or other important areas of functioning, the "other specified" or "unspecified" category corresponding to the predominant symptoms should be considered.

Subtypes and Specifiers

Subtypes and specifiers are provided for increased diagnostic specificity. *Subtypes* define mutually exclusive and jointly exhaustive phenomenological subgroupings within a diagnosis and are indicated by the instruction "*Specify* whether" in the criteria set (e.g., in anorexia nervosa, *Specify* whether restricting type or binge-eating/purging type). In contrast, *specifiers* are not intended to be mutually exclusive or jointly exhaustive, and as a consequence, more than one specifier may be applied to a given diagnosis. Specifiers (as opposed to subtypes) are indicated by the instruction "*Specify*" or "*Specify* if" in the criteria set (e.g., in social anxiety disorder, "*Specify* if: performance only"). Specifiers and subtypes provide an opportunity to define a more homogeneous subgrouping of individuals with the disorder who share certain features (e.g., major depressive disorder, with mixed features) and to convey information that is relevant to the management of the individual's disorder, such as the "with other medical comorbidity" specifier in sleep-wake disorders. Although the fifth character within an ICD-10-CM code is sometimes designated to indicate a particular subtype or specifier (e.g., "0" in the fifth character in the F02.80 diagnostic code for major neurocognitive disorder due to Alzheimer's disease, to indicate the absence of a behavioral disturbance versus a "1" in the fifth character of the F02.81 diagnostic code for major neurocognitive disorder due to Alzheimer's disease to indicate the presence of a behavioral disturbance), the majority of subtypes and specifiers included in DSM-5-TR are not reflected in the ICD-10-CM code and are indicated instead by recording the subtype or specifier after the name of the disorder (e.g., social anxiety disorder, performance type).

Use of Other Specified and Unspecified Mental Disorders

Although decades of scientific effort have gone into developing the diagnostic criteria sets for the disorders included in Section II, it is well recognized that this set of categorical diagnoses does not fully describe the full range of mental disorders that individuals experience and present to clinicians on a daily basis throughout the world. Hence, it is also necessary to include "other specified" or "unspecified" disorder options for presentations that do not fit exactly into the diagnostic boundaries of disorders in each chapter. Moreover, there are settings (e.g., emergency department) where it may only be possible to identify the most prominent symptom expressions associated with a particular chapter (e.g., delusions, hallucinations, mania, depression, anxiety, substance intoxication, neurocognitive symptoms). In such cases, it may be most appropriate to assign the corresponding "unspecified" disorder as a placeholder until a more complete differential diagnosis is possible.

DSM-5 provides two diagnostic options for presentations that do not meet the diagnostic criteria for any of the specific DSM-5 disorders: *other specified disorder* and *unspecified disorder*. The other specified category is provided to allow the clinician to communicate the specific reason that the presentation does not meet the criteria for any specific category within a diagnostic class. This is done by recording the name of the category, followed by the specific reason. For example, with an individual with persistent hallucinations occurring in the absence of any other psychotic symptoms (a presentation that does not meet criteria for any of the specific disorders in the chapter "Schizophrenia Spectrum and Other Psychotic Disorders"), the clinician would record "other specified schizophrenia spectrum and other psychotic disorder, with persistent auditory hallucinations." If the clinician chooses not to specify the reason that the criteria are not met for a specific disorder, then "unspecified schizophrenia spectrum and other psychotic disorder" would be diagnosed. Note that the differentiation between other specified and unspecified disorders is based on the clinician's choice to indicate or not the reasons why the presentation does not meet full criteria, providing maximum flexibility for diagnosis. When the clinician determines that there is enough available clinical information to specify the nature of the presentation, the "other specified" diagnosis can be given. In those cases where the clinician is not able to further specify the clinical presentation (e.g., in emergency room settings), the "unspecified" diagnosis can be given. This is entirely a matter of clinical judgment.

It is a long-standing DSM convention for conditions included in the "Conditions for Further Study" chapter in Section III to be listed as examples of presentations that can be specified using the "other specified" designation. The inclusion of these conditions for further study as examples does not represent endorsement by the American Psychiatric Association that these are valid diagnostic categories.

Use of Clinical Judgment

DSM-5 is a classification of mental disorders that was developed for use in clinical, educational, and research settings. The diagnostic categories, criteria, and textual descriptions are meant to be employed by individuals with appropriate clinical training and experience in diagnosis. It is important that DSM-5 not be applied mechanically by individuals without clinical training. The specific diagnostic criteria included in DSM-5 are meant to serve as guidelines to be informed by clinical judgment and are not meant to be used in a rigid cookbook fashion. For example, the exercise of clinical judgment may justify giving a certain diagnosis to an individual even though the clinical presentation falls just short of meeting the full criteria for the diagnosis as long as the symptoms that are present are persistent and severe. On the other hand, lack of familiarity with DSM-5 or excessively flexible and idiosyncratic application of DSM-5 criteria substantially reduces its utility as a common language for communication.

Clinical Significance Criterion

In the absence of clear biological markers or clinically useful measurements of severity for many mental disorders, it has not been possible to completely separate normal from pathological symptom expressions contained in diagnostic criteria. This gap in information is particularly problematic in clinical situations in which the individual's symptom presentation by itself (particularly in mild forms) is not inherently pathological and may be encountered in those for whom a diagnosis of "mental disorder" would be inappropriate. Therefore, a generic diagnostic criterion requiring distress or disability has been used to establish disorder thresholds, usually worded "the disturbance causes clinically significant distress or impairment in social, occupational, or other important areas of functioning." Assessing whether this criterion is met, especially in terms of role function, is an inherently difficult clinical judgment. The text following the definition of a mental disorder acknowledges that this criterion may be especially helpful in determining an individual's need for treatment. Use of information from the individual as well as from family members and other third parties via interview or self- or informant-reported assessments regarding the individual's performance is often necessary.

Coding and Recording Procedures

The official coding system in use in the United States since October 1, 2015, is the *International Classification of Diseases*, Tenth Revision, Clinical Modification (ICD-10-CM), a version of the World Health Organization's ICD-10 that has been modified for clinical use by the Centers for Disease Control and Prevention's National Center for Health Statistics (NCHS) and provides the only permissible diagnostic codes for mental disorders for clinical use in the United States. Most DSM-5 disorders have an alphanumeric ICD-10-CM code that appears preceding the name of the disorder (or coded subtype or specifier) in the DSM-5-TR Classification and in the accompanying criteria set for each disorder. For some diagnoses (e.g., neurocognitive disorders, substance/medication-induced disorders), the appropriate code depends on further specification and is listed within the criteria set for the disorder with a coding note, and in some cases is further clarified in the text section "Recording Procedures." The names of some disorders are followed by alternative terms enclosed in parentheses.

The use of diagnostic codes is fundamental to medical record keeping. Diagnostic coding facilitates data collection and retrieval and compilation of statistical information. Codes also are often required to report diagnostic data to interested third parties, including governmental agencies, private insurers, and the World Health Organization. For example, in the United States, the use of ICD-10-CM codes for disorders in

DSM-5-TR has been mandated by the Health Care Financing Administration for purposes of reimbursement under the Medicare system.

Principal Diagnosis/Reason for Visit

The general convention in DSM-5 is to allow multiple diagnoses to be assigned for those presentations that meet criteria for more than one DSM-5 disorder. When more than one diagnosis is given in an inpatient setting, the principal diagnosis is the condition established after study to be chiefly responsible for occasioning the admission of the individual. When more than one diagnosis is given for an individual in an outpatient setting, the reason for visit is the condition that is chiefly responsible for the ambulatory medical services received during the visit. In most cases, the principal diagnosis or the reason for visit is also the main focus of attention or treatment. It is often difficult (and somewhat arbitrary) to determine which diagnosis is the principal diagnosis or the reason for visit. For example, it may be unclear which diagnosis should be considered "principal" for an individual hospitalized with both schizophrenia and alcohol use disorder, because each condition may have contributed equally to the need for admission and treatment. The principal diagnosis is indicated by listing it first, and the remaining disorders are listed in order of focus of attention and treatment. When the principal diagnosis or reason for visit is a mental disorder due to another medical condition (e.g., major neurocognitive disorder due to Alzheimer's disease, psychotic disorder due to malignant lung neoplasm), ICD coding rules require that the etiological medical condition be listed first. In that case, the principal diagnosis or reason for visit would be the mental disorder due to the medical condition, the second listed diagnosis. For maximum clarity, the disorder listed as the principal diagnosis or the reason for visit can be followed by the qualifying phrase "(principal diagnosis)" or "(reason for visit)."

Provisional Diagnosis

The modifier "provisional" can be used when there is currently insufficient information to indicate that the diagnostic criteria are met, but there is a strong presumption that the information will become available to allow that determination. The clinician can indicate the diagnostic uncertainty by recording "(provisional)" following the diagnosis. For example, this modifier might be used when an individual who appears to have a presentation consistent with a diagnosis of current major depressive disorder is unable to give an adequate history, but it is expected that such information will become available after interviewing an informant or reviewing medical records. Once that information becomes available and confirms that the diagnostic criteria were met, the modifier "(provisional)" would be removed. Another use of "provisional" is for those situations in which differential diagnosis depends exclusively on whether the duration of illness does not exceed an upper limit as required by the diagnostic criteria. For example, a diagnosis of schizophreniform disorder requires a duration of at least 1 month but less than 6 months. If an individual currently has symptoms consistent with a diagnosis of schizophreniform disorder except that the ultimate duration is unknown because the symptoms are still ongoing, the modifier "(provisional)" would be applied and then removed if the symptoms remit within a period of 6 months. If they do not remit, the diagnosis would be changed to schizophrenia.

Notes About Terminology

Substance/Medication-Induced Mental Disorder

The term "substance/medication-induced mental disorder" refers to symptomatic presentations that are due to the physiological effects of an exogenous substance on the central nervous system, including symptoms that develop during withdrawal from an exogenous substance that is capable of causing physiological dependence. Such exogenous substances include typical intoxicants (e.g., alcohol, inhalants, hallucinogens, cocaine), psychotropic medications (e.g., stimulants; sedatives, hypnotics, anxiolytics), other medications (e.g., steroids), and environmental toxins (e.g., organophosphate insecticides). Editions of DSM from DSM-III to DSM-IV referred to these as "substance-induced mental disorders." To emphasize that medications and not just substances of abuse can cause psychiatric symptoms, the term was changed to "substance/medication-induced" in DSM-5.

Independent Mental Disorders

Historically, mental disorders were divided into those that were termed "organic" (caused by physical factors) versus those that were "nonorganic" (purely of the mind; also referred to as "functional" or "psychogenic"), terms that were included in DSM up through DSM-III-R. Because these dichotomies misleadingly implied that the nonorganic disorders have no biological basis and that mental disorders have no physical basis, DSM-IV updated this terminology as follows: 1) the terms "organic" and "nonorganic" were eliminated from DSM-IV; 2) the disorders formerly called "organic" were divided into those due to the direct physiological effects of a substance (substance-induced) and those due to the direct physiological effects of a medical condition on the central nervous system; and 3) the term "nonorganic mental disorders" (i.e., those disorders not due to either substances or medical conditions) was replaced by "primary mental disorder." In DSM-5, this terminology was further refined, replacing "primary" with "independent" (e.g., Criterion C in substance/medication-induced anxiety disorder starts with "the disturbance is not better accounted for by an anxiety disorder that is not substance-induced. Evidence of an *independent* anxiety disorder could include…" *[italics added for reference]*). This was done to reduce the potential for confusion given that the term "primary" has historically had other meanings (e.g., it is sometimes used to indicate which disorder among several comorbid disorders was the first to occur). The use of "independent mental disorder" should not be construed to mean that the disorder is independent of other potential causal factors such as psychosocial or other environmental stressors.

Other Medical Conditions

Another dichotomy adopted by prior editions of DSM that reflected mind-body dualism was the division of disorders into "mental disorders" and "physical disorders." In conjunction with the elimination of organic/nonorganic terminology, DSM-IV replaced the "mental disorder" versus "physical disorder" dichotomy with a "mental disorder" vs. "general medical condition" dichotomy, based on chapter location within the International Classification of Diseases (ICD). Medical conditions in ICD have been divided into 17 chapters based on a variety of factors, which include etiology (e.g., Neoplasms [Chapter 2]), anatomical location (e.g., Diseases of the ear and mastoid process [Chapter 8]), body system (e.g., Diseases of the circulatory system [Chapter 9]), and context (e.g., Pregnancy, childbirth and the puerperium [Chapter 15]). In the ICD framework, mental disorders are those located in Chapter 5, and general medical conditions are those located within the other 16 chapters. Because of concerns that the term "general medical condition" could be conflated with general practice, DSM-5 uses the term "another medical condition" to emphasize the fact that mental disorders are medical conditions and that mental disorders can be precipitated by other medical conditions. It is important to recognize that "mental disorder" and "another medical condition" are merely terms of convenience and should not be taken to imply that there is any fundamental distinction between mental disorders and other medical conditions, that mental disorders are unrelated to physical or biological factors or processes, or that other medical conditions are unrelated to behavioral or psychosocial factors or processes.

Types of Information in the DSM-5-TR Text

The DSM-5-TR text provides contextual information to aid in diagnostic decision-making. The text appears immediately following the diagnostic criteria for each disorder and systematically describes the disorder under the following headings: Recording Procedures, Subtypes, Specifiers, Diagnostic Features, Associated Features, Prevalence, Development and Course, Risk and Prognostic Factors, Culture-Related Diagnostic Issues, Sex- and Gender-Related Diagnostic Issues, Diagnostic Markers, Association With Suicidal Thoughts or Behavior, Functional Consequences, Differential Diagnosis, and Comorbidity. In general, when limited information is available for a section, that section is not included.

Recording Procedures provides guidelines for reporting the name of the disorder and for selecting and recording the appropriate

ICD-10-CM diagnostic code. It also includes instructions for applying any appropriate subtypes and/or specifiers.

Subtypes and/or **Specifiers** provide brief descriptions of applicable subtypes and/or specifiers.

Diagnostic Features provides descriptive text illustrating the use of the criteria and includes key points on their interpretation. For example, within the diagnostic features for schizophrenia, it is explained that some symptoms that may appear to be negative symptoms could instead be attributable to medication side effects.

Associated Features includes clinical features that are not represented in the criteria but occur significantly more often in individuals with the disorder than those without the disorder. For example, individuals with generalized anxiety disorder may also experience somatic symptoms that are not contained within the disorder criteria.

Prevalence describes rates of the disorder in the community, most often described as 12-month prevalence, although for some disorders point prevalence is noted. Prevalence estimates are also provided by age group and by ethnoracial/cultural group when possible. Sex ratio (prevalence in men vs. women) is also provided in this section. When international data are available, geographic variance in prevalence rates is described. For some disorders, especially those for which there are limited data on rates in the community, prevalence in relevant clinical samples is noted.

Development and Course describes the typical lifetime patterns of presentation and evolution of the disorder. It notes the typical age at onset and whether the presentation may have prodromal/insidious features or may manifest abruptly. Other descriptions may include an episodic versus persistent course as well as a single episode versus a recurrent episodic course. Descriptors in this section may address duration of symptoms or episodes as well as progression of severity and associated functional impact. The general trend of the disorder over time (e.g., stable, worsening, improving) is described here. Variations that may be noted include features related to developmental stage (e.g., infancy, childhood, adolescence, adulthood, late life).

Risk and Prognostic Factors includes a discussion of factors thought to contribute to the development of a disorder. It is divided into subsections addressing *temperamental factors* (e.g., personality features); *environmental factors* (e.g., head trauma, emotional trauma, exposure to toxic substances, substance use); and *genetic and physiological factors* (e.g., *APOE4* for dementia, other known familial genetic risks); this subsection may address familial patterns (traditional) as well as genetic and epigenetic factors. An additional subsection for *course modifiers* includes factors that may incur a deleterious course, and conversely factors that may have ameliorative or protective effects.

Culture-Related Diagnostic Issues includes information on variations in symptom expression, attributions for disorder causes or precipitants, factors associated with differential prevalence across demographic groups, cultural norms that may affect level of perceived pathology, risk of misdiagnosis when evaluating individuals from socially oppressed ethnoracial groups, and other material relevant to culturally informed diagnosis. Prevalence rates in specific cultural/ethnic groups are located in the Prevalence section.

Sex- and Gender-Related Diagnostic Issues includes correlates of the diagnosis that are related to sex or gender, predominance of symptoms or the diagnosis by sex or gender, and any other sex- and gender-related diagnostic implications of the diagnosis, such as differences in the clinical course by sex or gender. Prevalence rates by gender are located in the Prevalence section.

Diagnostic Markers addresses objective measures that have established diagnostic value. These may include physical examination findings (e.g., signs of malnutrition in avoidant/restrictive food intake disorder), laboratory findings (e.g., low CSF hypocretin-1 levels in narcolepsy), or imaging findings (e.g., regionally hypometabolic FDG PET imaging for neurocognitive disorder due to Alzheimer's disease).

Association With Suicidal Thoughts or Behavior provides information about disorder-specific prevalence of suicidal thoughts or behavior, as well as risk factors for suicide that may be associated with the disorder.

Functional Consequences discusses notable functional consequences associated with a disorder that are likely to have an impact on the daily lives of affected individuals; these consequences may affect the ability to engage in tasks related to education, work, and maintaining independent living. These may vary according to age and across the life span.

Differential Diagnosis discusses how to differentiate the disorder from other disorders that have some similar presenting characteristics.

Comorbidity includes descriptions of mental disorders and other medical conditions (i.e., conditions classified outside of the Mental and Behavioral disorders chapter in ICD-10-CM), likely to co-occur with the diagnosis.

Other Conditions and Disorders in Section II

In addition to providing diagnostic criteria and text for DSM-5 mental disorders, Section II also includes two chapters for other conditions that are not mental disorders but may be encountered by mental health clinicians. These conditions may be listed as a reason for a clinical visit in addition to, or in place of, the mental disorders in Section II. The chapter **"Medication-Induced Disorders and Other Adverse Effects of Medication"** includes medication-induced parkinsonism, neuroleptic malignant syndrome, medication-induced acute dystonia, medication-induced acute akathisia, tardive dyskinesia, tardive dystonia/tardive akathisia, medication-induced postural tremor, antidepressant discontinuation syndrome, and other adverse effect of medication. These conditions are included in Section II because of their frequent importance in 1) the management by medication of mental disorders or other medical conditions, and 2) the differential diagnosis with mental disorders (e.g., anxiety disorder vs. medication-induced acute akathisia).

The chapter **"Other Conditions That May Be a Focus of Clinical Attention"** includes conditions and psychosocial or environmental problems that are not considered to be mental disorders but otherwise affect the diagnosis, course, prognosis, or treatment of an individual's mental disorder. These conditions are presented with their corresponding codes from ICD-10-CM (usually Z codes). A condition or problem in this chapter may be coded with or without an accompanying mental disorder diagnosis 1) if it is a reason for the current visit; 2) if it helps to explain the need for a test, procedure, or treatment; 3) if it plays a role in the initiation or exacerbation of a mental disorder; or 4) if it constitutes a problem that should be considered in the overall management plan. These include suicidal behavior and nonsuicidal self-injury; abuse and neglect; relational problems (e.g., Relationship Distress With Spouse or Intimate Partner); educational, occupational, housing, and economic problems; problems related to the social environment, interaction with the legal system, and other psychosocial, personal, and environmental circumstances (e.g., problems related to unwanted pregnancy, being a victim of crime or terrorism); problems related to access to medical and other health care; circumstances of personal history (e.g., Personal History of Psychological Trauma); other health service encounters for counseling and medical advice (e.g., sex counseling); and additional conditions or problems that may be a focus of clinical attention (e.g., wandering associated with a mental disorder, uncomplicated bereavement, phase of life problem).

Online Enhancements

DSM-5-TR is available in online subscriptions at PsychiatryOnline.org, as well as an e-book that reflects the print edition. The online version provides a complete set of supporting in-text citations and references not available in print or e-book; it is also updated periodically to reflect any changes resulting from the DSM-5 iterative revision process, described in the Introduction. DSM-5 will be retained online in an archived format at PsychiatryOnline.org, joining prior versions of DSM.

Clinical rating scales and measures that are in the print edition and e-book (see "Assessment Measures" in Section III) are included online along with additional assessment measures used in the field trials (www.psychiatry.org/dsm5), linked to the relevant disorders. From the Section III chapter "Culture and Psychiatric Diagnosis," the Cultural Formulation Interview, Cultural Formulation Interview—Informant Version (both included in print and e-book), and supplementary modules to the core Cultural Formulation Interview are all available online at www.psychiatry.org/dsm5.

Cautionary Statement for Forensic Use of DSM-5

Although the DSM-5 diagnostic criteria and text are primarily designed to assist clinicians in conducting clinical assessment, case formulation, and treatment planning, DSM-5 is also used as a reference for the courts and attorneys in assessing the legal consequences of mental disorders. As a result, it is important to note that the definition of mental disorder included in DSM-5 was developed to meet the needs of clinicians, public health professionals, and research investigators rather than the technical needs of the courts and legal professionals. It is also important to note that DSM-5 does not provide treatment guidelines for any given disorder.

When used appropriately, diagnoses and diagnostic information can assist legal decision makers in their determinations. For example, when the presence of a mental disorder is the predicate for a subsequent legal determination (e.g., involuntary civil commitment), the use of an established system of diagnosis enhances the value and reliability of the determination. By providing a compendium based on a review of the pertinent clinical and research literature, DSM-5 may facilitate legal decision-makers' understanding of the relevant characteristics of mental disorders. The literature related to diagnoses also serves as a check on ungrounded speculation about mental disorders and about the functioning of a particular individual. Finally, diagnostic information about longitudinal course may improve decision-making when the legal issue concerns an individual's mental functioning at a past or future point in time.

However, the use of DSM-5 in forensic settings should be informed by an awareness of the risks and limitations of its use. When DSM-5 categories, criteria, and textual descriptions are employed for forensic purposes, there is a risk that diagnostic information will be misused or misunderstood. These dangers arise because of the imperfect fit between the questions of ultimate concern to the law and the information contained in a clinical diagnosis. In most situations, the clinical diagnosis of a DSM-5 mental disorder such as intellectual developmental disorder (intellectual disability), schizophrenia, major neurocognitive disorder, gambling disorder, or pedophilic disorder does not imply that an individual with such a condition meets legal criteria for the presence of a mental disorder or "mental illness" as defined in law, or a specified legal standard (e.g., for competence, criminal responsibility, or disability). For the latter, additional information is usually required beyond that contained in the DSM-5 diagnosis, which might include information about the individual's functional impairments and how these impairments affect the particular abilities in question. It is precisely because impairments, abilities, and disabilities vary widely within each diagnostic category that assignment of a particular diagnosis does not imply a specific level of risk, impairment, or disability.

Use of DSM-5 to assess the presence of a mental disorder by non-clinical, nonmedical, or otherwise insufficiently trained individuals is not advised. Nonclinical decision-makers should also be cautioned that a diagnosis does not carry any necessary implications regarding the etiology or causes of the individual's mental disorder or the individual's degree of control over behaviors that may be associated with the disorder. Even when diminished control over the individual's own behavior is a feature of the disorder, having the diagnosis in itself does not demonstrate that a particular individual is (or was) unable to control his or her behavior at a particular time.

SECTION II

Diagnostic Criteria and Codes

Intellectual Developmental Disorders

Intellectual Developmental Disorder (Intellectual Disability)

Intellectual developmental disorder (intellectual disability) is a disorder with onset during the developmental period that includes both intellectual and adaptive functioning deficits in conceptual, social, and practical domains. The following three criteria must be met:

A. Deficits in intellectual functions, such as reasoning, problem solving, planning, abstract thinking, judgment, academic learning, and learning from experience, confirmed by both clinical assessment and individualized, standardized intelligence testing.

B. Deficits in adaptive functioning that result in failure to meet developmental and sociocultural standards for personal independence and social responsibility. Without ongoing support, the adaptive deficits limit functioning in one or more activities of daily life, such as communication, social participation, and independent living, across multiple environments, such as home, school, work, and community.

C. Onset of intellectual and adaptive deficits during the developmental period.

Note: The term *intellectual developmental disorder* is used to clarify its relationship with the WHO ICD-11 classification system, which uses the term *Disorders of Intellectual Development*. The equivalent term *intellectual disability* is placed in parentheses for continued use. The medical and research literature use both terms, while intellectual disability is the term in common use by educational and other professions, advocacy groups, and the lay public. In the United States, Public Law 111-256 (Rosa's Law) changed all references to "mental retardation" in federal laws to "intellectual disability."

Specify current severity (see Table 1):

    F70 Mild
    F71 Moderate
    F72 Severe
    F73 Profound

TABLE 1 Severity levels for intellectual developmental disorder (intellectual disability)

Severity level	Conceptual domain	Social domain	Practical domain
Mild	For preschool children, there may be no obvious conceptual differences. For school-age children and adults, there are difficulties in learning academic skills involving reading, writing, arithmetic, time, or money, with support needed in one or more areas to meet age-related expectations. In adults, abstract thinking, executive function (i.e., planning, strategizing, priority setting, and cognitive flexibility), and short-term memory, as well as functional use of academic skills (e.g., reading, money management), are impaired. There is a somewhat concrete approach to problems and solutions compared with age-mates.	Compared with typically developing age-mates, the individual is immature in social interactions. For example, there may be difficulty in accurately perceiving peers' social cues. Communication, conversation, and language are more concrete or immature than expected for age. There may be difficulties regulating emotion and behavior in age-appropriate fashion; these difficulties are noticed by peers in social situations. There is limited understanding of risk in social situations; social judgment is immature for age, and the person is at risk of being manipulated by others (gullibility).	The individual may function age-appropriately in personal care. Individuals need some support with complex daily living tasks in comparison to peers. In adulthood, supports typically involve grocery shopping, transportation, home and child-care organizing, nutritious food preparation, and banking and money management. Recreational skills resemble those of age-mates, although judgment related to well-being and organization around recreation requires support. In adulthood, competitive employment is often seen in jobs that do not emphasize conceptual skills. Individuals generally need support to make health care decisions and legal decisions, and to learn to perform a skilled vocation competently. Support is typically needed to raise a family.

TABLE 1 Severity levels for intellectual developmental disorder (intellectual disability) *(continued)*

Severity level	Conceptual domain	Social domain	Practical domain
Moderate	All through development, the individual's conceptual skills lag markedly behind those of peers. For preschoolers, language and preacademic skills develop slowly. For school-age children, progress in reading, writing, mathematics, and in understanding time and money occurs slowly across the school years and is markedly limited compared with that of peers. For adults, academic skill development is typically at an elementary level, and support is required for all use of academic skills in work and personal life. Ongoing assistance on a daily basis is needed to complete conceptual tasks of day-to-day life, and others may take over these responsibilities fully for the individual.	The individual shows marked differences from peers in social and communicative behavior across development. Spoken language is typically a primary tool for social communication but is much less complex than that of peers. Capacity for relationships is evident in ties to family and friends, and the individual may have successful friendships across life and sometimes romantic relations in adulthood. However, individuals may not perceive or interpret social cues accurately. Social judgment and decision-making abilities are limited, and caretakers must assist the person with life decisions. Friendships with typically developing peers are often affected by communication or social limitations. Significant social and communicative support is needed in work settings for success.	The individual can care for personal needs involving eating, dressing, elimination, and hygiene as an adult, although an extended period of teaching and time is needed for the individual to become independent in these areas, and reminders may be needed. Similarly, participation in all household tasks can be achieved by adulthood, although an extended period of teaching is needed, and ongoing supports will typically occur for adult-level performance. Independent employment in jobs that require limited conceptual and communication skills can be achieved, but considerable support from co-workers, supervisors, and others is needed to manage social expectations, job complexities, and ancillary responsibilities such as scheduling, transportation, health benefits, and money management. A variety of recreational skills can be developed. These typically require additional supports and learning opportunities over an extended period of time. Maladaptive behavior is present in a significant minority and causes social problems.

TABLE 1   Severity levels for intellectual developmental disorder (intellectual disability) *(continued)*

Severity level	Conceptual domain	Social domain	Practical domain
Severe	Attainment of conceptual skills is limited. The individual generally has little understanding of written language or of concepts involving numbers, quantity, time, and money. Caretakers provide extensive supports for problem solving throughout life.	Spoken language is quite limited in terms of vocabulary and grammar. Speech may be single words or phrases and may be supplemented through augmentative means. Speech and communication are focused on the here and now within everyday events. Language is used for social communication more than for explication. Individuals understand simple speech and gestural communication. Relationships with family members and familiar others are a source of pleasure and help.	The individual requires support for all activities of daily living, including meals, dressing, bathing, and elimination. The individual requires supervision at all times. The individual cannot make responsible decisions regarding well-being of self or others. In adulthood, participation in tasks at home, recreation, and work requires ongoing support and assistance. Skill acquisition in all domains involves long-term teaching and ongoing support. Maladaptive behavior, including self-injury, is present in a significant minority.

TABLE 1   Severity levels for intellectual developmental disorder (intellectual disability) (*continued*)

Severity level	Conceptual domain	Social domain	Practical domain
Profound	Conceptual skills generally involve the physical world rather than symbolic processes. The individual may use objects in goal-directed fashion for self-care, work, and recreation. Certain visuospatial skills, such as matching and sorting based on physical characteristics, may be acquired. However, co-occurring motor and sensory impairments may prevent functional use of objects.	The individual has very limited understanding of symbolic communication in speech or gesture. He or she may understand some simple instructions or gestures. The individual expresses his or her own desires and emotions largely through nonverbal, nonsymbolic communication. The individual enjoys relationships with well-known family members, caretakers, and familiar others, and initiates and responds to social interactions through gestural and emotional cues. Co-occurring sensory and physical impairments may prevent many social activities.	The individual is dependent on others for all aspects of daily physical care, health, and safety, although he or she may be able to participate in some of these activities as well. Individuals without severe physical impairments may assist with some daily work tasks at home, like carrying dishes to the table. Simple actions with objects may be the basis of participation in some vocational activities with high levels of ongoing support. Recreational activities may involve, for example, enjoyment in listening to music, watching movies, going out for walks, or participating in water activities, all with the support of others. Co-occurring physical and sensory impairments are frequent barriers to participation (beyond watching) in home, recreational, and vocational activities. Maladaptive behavior is present in a significant minority.

Global Developmental Delay

F88

This diagnosis is reserved for individuals *under* the age of 5 years when the clinical severity level cannot be reliably assessed during early childhood. This category is diagnosed when an individual fails to meet expected developmental milestones in several areas of intellectual functioning, and applies to individuals who are unable to undergo systematic assessments of intellectual functioning, including children who are too young to participate in standardized testing. This category requires reassessment after a period of time.

Unspecified Intellectual Developmental Disorder (Intellectual Disability)

F79

This category is reserved for individuals *over* the age of 5 years when assessment of the degree of intellectual developmental disorder (intellectual disability) by means of locally available procedures is rendered difficult or impossible because of associated sensory or physical impairments, as in blindness or prelingual deafness; locomotor disability; or presence of severe problem behaviors or co-occurring mental disorder. This category should only be used in exceptional circumstances and requires reassessment after a period of time.

Communication Disorders

Language Disorder

F80.2

A. Persistent difficulties in the acquisition and use of language across modalities (i.e., spoken, written, sign language, or other) due to deficits in comprehension or production that include the following:

1. Reduced vocabulary (word knowledge and use).
2. Limited sentence structure (ability to put words and word endings together to form sentences based on the rules of grammar and morphology).
3. Impairments in discourse (ability to use vocabulary and connect sentences to explain or describe a topic or series of events or have a conversation).

B. Language abilities are substantially and quantifiably below those expected for age, resulting in functional limitations in effective communication, social participation, academic achievement, or occupational performance, individually or in any combination.

C. Onset of symptoms is in the early developmental period.

D. The difficulties are not attributable to hearing or other sensory impairment, motor dysfunction, or another medical or neurological condition and are not better explained by intellectual developmental disorder (intellectual disability) or global developmental delay.

Speech Sound Disorder

F80.0

A. Persistent difficulty with speech sound production that interferes with speech intelligibility or prevents verbal communication of messages.

B. The disturbance causes limitations in effective communication that interfere with social participation, academic achievement, or occupational performance, individually or in any combination.

C. Onset of symptoms is in the early developmental period.

D. The difficulties are not attributable to congenital or acquired conditions, such as cerebral palsy, cleft palate, deafness or hearing loss, traumatic brain injury, or other medical or neurological conditions.

Childhood-Onset Fluency Disorder (Stuttering)

F80.81

A. Disturbances in the normal fluency and time patterning of speech that are inappropriate for the individual's age and language skills, persist over time, and are characterized by frequent and marked occurrences of one (or more) of the following:

1. Sound and syllable repetitions.
2. Sound prolongations of consonants as well as vowels.
3. Broken words (e.g., pauses within a word).
4. Audible or silent blocking (filled or unfilled pauses in speech).
5. Circumlocutions (word substitutions to avoid problematic words).
6. Words produced with an excess of physical tension.
7. Monosyllabic whole-word repetitions (e.g., "I-I-I-I see him").

B. The disturbance causes anxiety about speaking or limitations in effective communication, social participation, or academic or occupational performance, individually or in any combination.

C. The onset of symptoms is in the early developmental period. (**Note:** Later-onset cases are diagnosed as F98.5 adult-onset fluency disorder.)

D. The disturbance is not attributable to a speech-motor or sensory deficit, dysfluency associated with neurological insult (e.g., stroke, tumor, trauma), or another medical condition and is not better explained by another mental disorder.

Social (Pragmatic) Communication Disorder

F80.82

A. Persistent difficulties in the social use of verbal and nonverbal communication as manifested by all of the following:

1. Deficits in using communication for social purposes, such as greeting and sharing information, in a manner that is appropriate for the social context.
2. Impairment of the ability to change communication to match context or the needs of the listener, such as speaking differently in a classroom than on a playground, talking differently to a child than to an adult, and avoiding use of overly formal language.
3. Difficulties following rules for conversation and storytelling, such as taking turns in conversation, rephrasing when misunderstood, and knowing how to use verbal and nonverbal signals to regulate interaction.
4. Difficulties understanding what is not explicitly stated (e.g., making inferences) and nonliteral or ambiguous meanings of language (e.g., idioms, humor, metaphors, multiple meanings that depend on the context for interpretation).

B. The deficits result in functional limitations in effective communication, social participation, social relationships, academic achievement, or occupational performance, individually or in combination.

C. The onset of the symptoms is in the early developmental period (but deficits may not become fully manifest until social communication demands exceed limited capacities).

D. The symptoms are not attributable to another medical or neurological condition or to low abilities in the domains of word structure and grammar, and are not better explained by autism spectrum disorder, intellectual developmental disorder (intellectual disability), global developmental delay, or another mental disorder.

Unspecified Communication Disorder

F80.9

This category applies to presentations in which symptoms characteristic of communication disorder that cause clinically significant distress or impairment in social, occupational, or other important areas of functioning predominate but do not meet the full criteria for communication disorder or for any of the disorders in the neurodevelopmental disorders diagnostic class. The unspecified communication disorder category is used in situations in which the clinician chooses *not* to specify the reason that the criteria are not met for communication disorder or for a specific neurodevelopmental disorder, and includes presentations in which there is insufficient information to make a more specific diagnosis.

Autism Spectrum Disorder

Autism Spectrum Disorder

F84.0

A. Persistent deficits in social communication and social interaction across multiple contexts, as manifested by all of the following, currently or by history (examples are illustrative, not exhaustive):

1. Deficits in social-emotional reciprocity, ranging, for example, from abnormal social approach and failure of normal back-and-forth conversation; to reduced sharing of interests, emotions, or affect; to failure to initiate or respond to social interactions.
2. Deficits in nonverbal communicative behaviors used for social interaction, ranging, for example, from poorly integrated verbal and nonverbal communication; to abnormalities in eye contact and body language or deficits in understanding and use of gestures; to a total lack of facial expressions and nonverbal communication.
3. Deficits in developing, maintaining, and understanding relationships, ranging, for example, from difficulties adjusting behavior to suit various social contexts; to difficulties in sharing imaginative play or in making friends; to absence of interest in peers.

B. Restricted, repetitive patterns of behavior, interests, or activities, as manifested by at least two of the following, currently or by history (examples are illustrative, not exhaustive):

1. Stereotyped or repetitive motor movements, use of objects, or speech (e.g., simple motor stereotypies, lining up toys or flipping objects, echolalia, idiosyncratic phrases).
2. Insistence on sameness, inflexible adherence to routines, or ritualized patterns of verbal or nonverbal behavior (e.g., extreme distress at small changes, difficulties with transitions, rigid

thinking patterns, greeting rituals, need to take same route or eat same food every day).

3. Highly restricted, fixated interests that are abnormal in intensity or focus (e.g., strong attachment to or preoccupation with unusual objects, excessively circumscribed or perseverative interests).

4. Hyper- or hyporeactivity to sensory input or unusual interest in sensory aspects of the environment (e.g., apparent indifference to pain/temperature, adverse response to specific sounds or textures, excessive smelling or touching of objects, visual fascination with lights or movement).

C. Symptoms must be present in the early developmental period (but may not become fully manifest until social demands exceed limited capacities, or may be masked by learned strategies in later life).

D. Symptoms cause clinically significant impairment in social, occupational, or other important areas of current functioning.

E. These disturbances are not better explained by intellectual developmental disorder (intellectual disability) or global developmental delay. Intellectual developmental disorder and autism spectrum disorder frequently co-occur; to make comorbid diagnoses of autism spectrum disorder and intellectual developmental disorder, social communication should be below that expected for general developmental level.

Note: Individuals with a well-established DSM-IV diagnosis of autistic disorder, Asperger's disorder, or pervasive developmental disorder not otherwise specified should be given the diagnosis of autism spectrum disorder. Individuals who have marked deficits in social communication, but whose symptoms do not otherwise meet criteria for autism spectrum disorder, should be evaluated for social (pragmatic) communication disorder.

Specify current severity based on social communication impairments and restricted, repetitive patterns of behavior (see Table 2):

    Requiring very substantial support
    Requiring substantial support
    Requiring support

Specify if:

    With or without accompanying intellectual impairment
    With or without accompanying language impairment

Specify if:

    Associated with a known genetic or other medical condition or environmental factor (**Coding note:** Use additional code to identify the associated genetic or other medical condition.)
    Associated with a neurodevelopmental, mental, or behavioral problem

Specify if:

With catatonia (refer to the criteria for catatonia associated with another mental disorder, p. 52, for definition) (**Coding note:** Use additional code F06.1 catatonia associated with autism spectrum disorder to indicate the presence of the comorbid catatonia.)

Recording Procedures

It may be helpful to note level of support needed for each of the two core psychopathological domains in Table 2 (e.g., "requiring very substantial support for deficits in social communication and requiring substantial support for restricted, repetitive behaviors"). Specification of "with accompanying intellectual impairment" or "without accompanying intellectual impairment" should be recorded next. Language impairment specification should be recorded thereafter. If there is accompanying language impairment, the current level of verbal functioning should be recorded (e.g., "with accompanying language impairment—no intelligible speech" or "with accompanying language impairment—phrase speech").

For autism spectrum disorder for which the specifiers "associated with a known genetic or other medical condition or environmental factor" or "associated with a neurodevelopmental, mental, or behavioral problem" are appropriate, record autism spectrum disorder associated with (name of condition, disorder, or factor) (e.g., autism spectrum disorder associated with tuberous sclerosis complex). These specifiers apply to presentations in which the listed condition or problem is potentially relevant to the clinical care of the individual and do not necessarily indicate that the condition or problem is causally related to the autism spectrum disorder. If the associated neurodevelopmental, mental, or behavioral problem meets criteria for a neurodevelopmental or other mental disorder, both autism spectrum disorder and the other disorder should be diagnosed.

If catatonia is present, record separately "catatonia associated with autism spectrum disorder." For more information, see criteria for catatonia associated with another mental disorder in the chapter "Schizophrenia Spectrum and Other Psychotic Disorders."

TABLE 2   Severity levels for autism spectrum disorder (examples of level of support needs)

Severity level	Social communication	Restricted, repetitive behaviors
Level 3 "Requiring very substantial support"	Severe deficits in verbal and nonverbal social communication skills cause severe impairments in functioning, very limited initiation of social interactions, and minimal response to social overtures from others. For example, a person with few words of intelligible speech who rarely initiates interaction and, when he or she does, makes unusual approaches to meet needs only and responds to only very direct social approaches.	Inflexibility of behavior, extreme difficulty coping with change, or other restricted/repetitive behaviors markedly interfere with functioning in all spheres. Great distress/difficulty changing focus or action.
Level 2 "Requiring substantial support"	Marked deficits in verbal and nonverbal social communication skills; social impairments apparent even with supports in place; limited initiation of social interactions; and reduced or abnormal responses to social overtures from others. For example, a person who speaks simple sentences, whose interaction is limited to narrow special interests, and who has markedly odd nonverbal communication.	Inflexibility of behavior, difficulty coping with change, or other restricted/repetitive behaviors appear frequently enough to be obvious to the casual observer and interfere with functioning in a variety of contexts. Distress and/or difficulty changing focus or action.
Level 1 "Requiring support"	Without supports in place, deficits in social communication cause noticeable impairments. Difficulty initiating social interactions, and clear examples of atypical or unsuccessful responses to social overtures of others. May appear to have decreased interest in social interactions. For example, a person who is able to speak in full sentences and engages in communication but whose to-and-fro conversation with others fails, and whose attempts to make friends are odd and typically unsuccessful.	Inflexibility of behavior causes significant interference with functioning in one or more contexts. Difficulty switching between activities. Problems of organization and planning hamper independence.

Attention-Deficit/Hyperactivity Disorder

Attention-Deficit/Hyperactivity Disorder

A. A persistent pattern of inattention and/or hyperactivity-impulsivity that interferes with functioning or development, as characterized by (1) and/or (2):

1. **Inattention:** Six (or more) of the following symptoms have persisted for at least 6 months to a degree that is inconsistent with developmental level and that negatively impacts directly on social and academic/occupational activities:

    Note: The symptoms are not solely a manifestation of oppositional behavior, defiance, hostility, or failure to understand tasks or instructions. For older adolescents and adults (age 17 and older), at least five symptoms are required.

    a. Often fails to give close attention to details or makes careless mistakes in schoolwork, at work, or during other activities (e.g., overlooks or misses details, work is inaccurate).

    b. Often has difficulty sustaining attention in tasks or play activities (e.g., has difficulty remaining focused during lectures, conversations, or lengthy reading).

    c. Often does not seem to listen when spoken to directly (e.g., mind seems elsewhere, even in the absence of any obvious distraction).

    d. Often does not follow through on instructions and fails to finish schoolwork, chores, or duties in the workplace (e.g., starts tasks but quickly loses focus and is easily sidetracked).

    e. Often has difficulty organizing tasks and activities (e.g., difficulty managing sequential tasks; difficulty keeping materials and belongings in order; messy, disorganized work; has poor time management; fails to meet deadlines).

    f. Often avoids, dislikes, or is reluctant to engage in tasks that require sustained mental effort (e.g., schoolwork or homework; for older adolescents and adults, preparing reports, completing forms, reviewing lengthy papers).

    g. Often loses things necessary for tasks or activities (e.g., school materials, pencils, books, tools, wallets, keys, paperwork, eyeglasses, mobile telephones).

    h. Is often easily distracted by extraneous stimuli (for older adolescents and adults, may include unrelated thoughts).

    i. Is often forgetful in daily activities (e.g., doing chores, running errands; for older adolescents and adults, returning calls, paying bills, keeping appointments).

2. **Hyperactivity and impulsivity:** Six (or more) of the following symptoms have persisted for at least 6 months to a degree that is inconsistent with developmental level and that negatively impacts directly on social and academic/occupational activities:

   Note: The symptoms are not solely a manifestation of oppositional behavior, defiance, hostility, or a failure to understand tasks or instructions. For older adolescents and adults (age 17 and older), at least five symptoms are required.

   a. Often fidgets with or taps hands or feet or squirms in seat.
   b. Often leaves seat in situations when remaining seated is expected (e.g., leaves his or her place in the classroom, in the office or other workplace, or in other situations that require remaining in place).
   c. Often runs about or climbs in situations where it is inappropriate. (**Note:** In adolescents or adults, may be limited to feeling restless.)
   d. Often unable to play or engage in leisure activities quietly.
   e. Is often "on the go," acting as if "driven by a motor" (e.g., is unable to be or uncomfortable being still for extended time, as in restaurants, meetings; may be experienced by others as being restless or difficult to keep up with).
   f. Often talks excessively.
   g. Often blurts out an answer before a question has been completed (e.g., completes people's sentences; cannot wait for turn in conversation).
   h. Often has difficulty waiting his or her turn (e.g., while waiting in line).
   i. Often interrupts or intrudes on others (e.g., butts into conversations, games, or activities; may start using other people's things without asking or receiving permission; for adolescents and adults, may intrude into or take over what others are doing).

B. Several inattentive or hyperactive-impulsive symptoms were present prior to age 12 years.

C. Several inattentive or hyperactive-impulsive symptoms are present in two or more settings (e.g., at home, school, or work; with friends or relatives; in other activities).

D. There is clear evidence that the symptoms interfere with, or reduce the quality of, social, academic, or occupational functioning.

E. The symptoms do not occur exclusively during the course of schizophrenia or another psychotic disorder and are not better explained by another mental disorder (e.g., mood disorder, anxiety disorder, dissociative disorder, personality disorder, substance intoxication or withdrawal).

Specify whether:

F90.2 Combined presentation: If both Criterion A1 (inattention) and Criterion A2 (hyperactivity-impulsivity) are met for the past 6 months.

F90.0 Predominantly inattentive presentation: If Criterion A1 (inattention) is met but Criterion A2 (hyperactivity-impulsivity) is not met for the past 6 months.

F90.1 Predominantly hyperactive/impulsive presentation: If Criterion A2 (hyperactivity-impulsivity) is met and Criterion A1 (inattention) is not met for the past 6 months.

Specify if:

In partial remission: When full criteria were previously met, fewer than the full criteria have been met for the past 6 months, and the symptoms still result in impairment in social, academic, or occupational functioning.

Specify current severity:

Mild: Few, if any, symptoms in excess of those required to make the diagnosis are present, and symptoms result in no more than minor impairments in social or occupational functioning.

Moderate: Symptoms or functional impairment between "mild" and "severe" are present.

Severe: Many symptoms in excess of those required to make the diagnosis, or several symptoms that are particularly severe, are present, or the symptoms result in marked impairment in social or occupational functioning.

Other Specified Attention-Deficit/ Hyperactivity Disorder

F90.8

This category applies to presentations in which symptoms characteristic of attention-deficit/hyperactivity disorder that cause clinically significant distress or impairment in social, occupational, or other important areas of functioning predominate but do not meet the full criteria for attention-deficit/hyperactivity disorder or any of the disorders in the neurodevelopmental disorders diagnostic class. The other specified attention-deficit/hyperactivity disorder category is used in situations in which the clinician chooses to communicate the specific reason that the presentation does not meet the criteria for attention-deficit/ hyperactivity disorder or any specific neurodevelopmental disorder. This is done by recording "other specified attention-deficit/hyperactivity disorder" followed by the specific reason (e.g., "with insufficient inattention symptoms").

Unspecified Attention-Deficit/Hyperactivity Disorder

F90.9

This category applies to presentations in which symptoms charac-teristic of attention-deficit/hyperactivity disorder that cause clinically significant distress or impairment in social, occupational, or other im-portant areas of functioning predominate but do not meet the full cri-teria for attention-deficit/hyperactivity disorder or any of the disorders in the neurodevelopmental disorders diagnostic class. The unspecified attention-deficit/hyperactivity disorder category is used in situations in which the clinician chooses *not* to specify the reason that the criteria are not met for attention-deficit/hyperactivity disorder or for a specific neu-rodevelopmental disorder, and includes presentations in which there is insufficient information to make a more specific diagnosis.

Specific Learning Disorder

Specific Learning Disorder

A. Difficulties learning and using academic skills, as indicated by the presence of at least one of the following symptoms that have per-sisted for at least 6 months, despite the provision of interventions that target those difficulties:

1. Inaccurate or slow and effortful word reading (e.g., reads single words aloud incorrectly or slowly and hesitantly, frequently guesses words, has difficulty sounding out words).
2. Difficulty understanding the meaning of what is read (e.g., may read text accurately but not understand the sequence, re-lationships, inferences, or deeper meanings of what is read).
3. Difficulties with spelling (e.g., may add, omit, or substitute vow-els or consonants).
4. Difficulties with written expression (e.g., makes multiple gram-matical or punctuation errors within sentences; employs poor paragraph organization; written expression of ideas lacks clarity).
5. Difficulties mastering number sense, number facts, or calcula-tion (e.g., has poor understanding of numbers, their magnitude, and relationships; counts on fingers to add single-digit numbers instead of recalling the math fact as peers do; gets lost in the midst of arithmetic computation and may switch procedures).

6. Difficulties with mathematical reasoning (e.g., has severe difficulty applying mathematical concepts, facts, or procedures to solve quantitative problems).

B. The affected academic skills are substantially and quantifiably below those expected for the individual's chronological age, and cause significant interference with academic or occupational performance, or with activities of daily living, as confirmed by individually administered standardized achievement measures and comprehensive clinical assessment. For individuals age 17 years and older, a documented history of impairing learning difficulties may be substituted for the standardized assessment.

C. The learning difficulties begin during school-age years but may not become fully manifest until the demands for those affected academic skills exceed the individual's limited capacities (e.g., as in timed tests, reading or writing lengthy complex reports for a tight deadline, excessively heavy academic loads).

D. The learning difficulties are not better accounted for by intellectual disabilities, uncorrected visual or auditory acuity, other mental or neurological disorders, psychosocial adversity, lack of proficiency in the language of academic instruction, or inadequate educational instruction.

Note: The four diagnostic criteria are to be met based on a clinical synthesis of the individual's history (developmental, medical, family, educational), school reports, and psychoeducational assessment.

Coding note: Specify all academic domains and subskills that are impaired. When more than one domain is impaired, each one should be coded individually according to the following specifiers.

Specify if:

F81.0 With impairment in reading:

Word reading accuracy
Reading rate or fluency
Reading comprehension

Note: *Dyslexia* is an alternative term used to refer to a pattern of learning difficulties characterized by problems with accurate or fluent word recognition, poor decoding, and poor spelling abilities. If dyslexia is used to specify this particular pattern of difficulties, it is important also to specify any additional difficulties that are present, such as difficulties with reading comprehension or math reasoning.

F81.81 With impairment in written expression:

Spelling accuracy
Grammar and punctuation accuracy
Clarity or organization of written expression

F81.2 With impairment in mathematics:

Number sense
Memorization of arithmetic facts
Accurate or fluent calculation
Accurate math reasoning

Note: *Dyscalculia* is an alternative term used to refer to a pattern of difficulties characterized by problems processing numerical information, learning arithmetic facts, and performing accurate or fluent calculations. If dyscalculia is used to specify this particular pattern of mathematic difficulties, it is important also to specify any additional difficulties that are present, such as difficulties with math reasoning or word reasoning accuracy.

Specify current severity:

Mild: Some difficulties learning skills in one or two academic domains, but of mild enough severity that the individual may be able to compensate or function well when provided with appropriate accommodations or support services, especially during the school years.

Moderate: Marked difficulties learning skills in one or more academic domains, so that the individual is unlikely to become proficient without some intervals of intensive and specialized teaching during the school years. Some accommodations or supportive services at least part of the day at school, in the workplace, or at home may be needed to complete activities accurately and efficiently.

Severe: Severe difficulties learning skills, affecting several academic domains, so that the individual is unlikely to learn those skills without ongoing intensive individualized and specialized teaching for most of the school years. Even with an array of appropriate accommodations or services at home, at school, or in the workplace, the individual may not be able to complete all activities efficiently.

Recording Procedures

Each impaired academic domain and subskill of specific learning disorder should be recorded. Because of ICD coding requirements, impairments in reading, impairments in written expression, and impairments in mathematics, with their corresponding impairments in subskills, must be coded and recorded separately. For example, impairments in reading and mathematics and impairments in the subskills of reading rate or fluency, reading comprehension, accurate or fluent calculation, and accurate math reasoning would be coded and recorded as F81.0 specific learning disorder with impairment in reading, with impairment in reading rate or fluency, and impairment in reading comprehension; F81.2 specific learning disorder with impairment in mathematics, with impairment in accurate or fluent calculation and impairment in accurate math reasoning.

Motor Disorders

Developmental Coordination Disorder

F82

A. The acquisition and execution of coordinated motor skills is substantially below that expected given the individual's chronological age and opportunity for skill learning and use. Difficulties are manifested as clumsiness (e.g., dropping or bumping into objects) as well as slowness and inaccuracy of performance of motor skills (e.g., catching an object, using scissors or cutlery, handwriting, riding a bike, or participating in sports).

B. The motor skills deficit in Criterion A significantly and persistently interferes with activities of daily living appropriate to chronological age (e.g., self-care and self-maintenance) and impacts academic/school productivity, prevocational and vocational activities, leisure, and play.

C. Onset of symptoms is in the early developmental period.

D. The motor skills deficits are not better explained by intellectual developmental disorder (intellectual disability) or visual impairment and are not attributable to a neurological condition affecting movement (e.g., cerebral palsy, muscular dystrophy, degenerative disorder).

Stereotypic Movement Disorder

F98.4

A. Repetitive, seemingly driven, and apparently purposeless motor behavior (e.g., hand shaking or waving, body rocking, head banging, self-biting, hitting own body).

B. The repetitive motor behavior interferes with social, academic, or other activities and may result in self-injury.

C. Onset is in the early developmental period.

D. The repetitive motor behavior is not attributable to the physiological effects of a substance or neurological condition and is not better explained by another neurodevelopmental or mental disorder (e.g., trichotillomania [hair-pulling disorder], obsessive-compulsive disorder).

Specify if:

With self-injurious behavior (or behavior that would result in an injury if preventive measures were not used).

Without self-injurious behavior

Specify if:

Associated with a known genetic or other medical condition, neurodevelopmental disorder, or environmental factor (e.g., Lesch-Nyhan syndrome, intellectual developmental disorder [intellectual disability], intrauterine alcohol exposure).

Coding note: Use additional code to identify the associated genetic or other medical condition, neurodevelopmental disorder, or environmental factor.

Specify current severity:

Mild: Symptoms are easily suppressed by sensory stimulus or distraction.
Moderate: Symptoms require explicit protective measures and behavioral modification.
Severe: Continuous monitoring and protective measures are required to prevent serious injury.

Recording Procedures

For stereotypic movement disorder that is associated with a known genetic or other medical condition, neurodevelopmental disorder, or environmental factor, record stereotypic movement disorder associated with (name of condition, disorder, or factor) (e.g., stereotypic movement disorder associated with Lesch-Nyhan syndrome).

Tic Disorders

Note: A tic is a sudden, rapid, recurrent, nonrhythmic motor movement or vocalization.

Tourette's Disorder   F95.2

A. Both multiple motor and one or more vocal tics have been present at some time during the illness, although not necessarily concurrently.
B. The tics may wax and wane in frequency but have persisted for more than 1 year since first tic onset.
C. Onset is before age 18 years.
D. The disturbance is not attributable to the physiological effects of a substance (e.g., cocaine) or another medical condition (e.g., Huntington's disease, postviral encephalitis).

Persistent (Chronic) Motor or
Vocal Tic Disorder   F95.1

A. Single or multiple motor or vocal tics have been present during the illness, but not both motor and vocal.
B. The tics may wax and wane in frequency but have persisted for more than 1 year since first tic onset.
C. Onset is before age 18 years.
D. The disturbance is not attributable to the physiological effects of a substance (e.g., cocaine) or another medical condition (e.g., Huntington's disease, postviral encephalitis).
E. Criteria have never been met for Tourette's disorder.

Specify if:
   With motor tics only
   With vocal tics only

Provisional Tic Disorder   **F95.0**

A. Single or multiple motor and/or vocal tics.
B. The tics have been present for less than 1 year since first tic onset.
C. Onset is before age 18 years.
D. The disturbance is not attributable to the physiological effects of a substance (e.g., cocaine) or another medical condition (e.g., Huntington's disease, postviral encephalitis).
E. Criteria have never been met for Tourette's disorder or persistent (chronic) motor or vocal tic disorder.

Other Specified Tic Disorder

F95.8

This category applies to presentations in which symptoms characteristic of a tic disorder that cause clinically significant distress or impairment in social, occupational, or other important areas of functioning predominate but do not meet the full criteria for a tic disorder or any of the disorders in the neurodevelopmental disorders diagnostic class. The other specified tic disorder category is used in situations in which the clinician chooses to communicate the specific reason that the presentation does not meet the criteria for a tic disorder or any specific neurodevelopmental disorder. This is done by recording "other specified tic disorder" followed by the specific reason (e.g., "with onset after age 18 years").

Unspecified Tic Disorder

F95.9

This category applies to presentations in which symptoms characteristic of a tic disorder that cause clinically significant distress or impairment in social, occupational, or other important areas of functioning predominate but do not meet the full criteria for a tic disorder or for any of the disorders in the neurodevelopmental disorders diagnostic class. The unspecified tic disorder category is used in situations in which the clinician chooses *not* to specify the reason that the criteria are not met for a tic disorder or for a specific neurodevelopmental disorder and includes presentations in which there is insufficient information to make a more specific diagnosis.

Other Neurodevelopmental Disorders

Other Specified Neurodevelopmental Disorder

F88

This category applies to presentations in which symptoms characteristic of a neurodevelopmental disorder that cause impairment in social, occupational, or other important areas of functioning predominate but do not meet the full criteria for any of the disorders in the neurodevelopmental disorders diagnostic class. The other specified neurodevelopmental disorder category is used in situations in which the clinician chooses to communicate the specific reason that the presentation does not meet the criteria for any specific neurodevelopmental disorder. This is done by recording "other specified neurodevelopmental disorder" followed by the specific reason (e.g., "neurodevelopmental disorder associated with prenatal alcohol exposure").

An example of a presentation that can be specified using the "other specified" designation is the following:

Neurodevelopmental disorder associated with prenatal alcohol exposure: Neurodevelopmental disorder associated with prenatal alcohol exposure is characterized by a range of developmental disabilities following exposure to alcohol in utero.

Unspecified Neurodevelopmental Disorder

F89

This category applies to presentations in which symptoms characteristic of a neurodevelopmental disorder that cause impairment in social, occupational, or other important areas of functioning predominate but do not meet the full criteria for any of the disorders in the neurodevelopmental disorders diagnostic class. The unspecified neurodevelopmental disorder category is used in situations in which the clinician chooses *not* to specify the reason that the criteria are not met for a specific neurodevelopmental disorder and includes presentations in which there is insufficient information to make a more specific diagnosis (e.g., in emergency room settings).

Schizophrenia Spectrum and Other Psychotic Disorders

Schizotypal (Personality) Disorder

Criteria for schizotypal personality disorder can be found in the chapter "Personality Disorders." Because this disorder is considered part of the schizophrenia spectrum of disorders, and is labeled in this section of ICD-10 as schizotypal disorder, it is listed in this chapter, and the criteria are presented in the chapter "Personality Disorders."

Delusional Disorder

F22

A. The presence of one (or more) delusions with a duration of 1 month or longer.

B. Criterion A for schizophrenia has never been met.

   Note: Hallucinations, if present, are not prominent and are related to the delusional theme (e.g., the sensation of being infested with insects associated with delusions of infestation).

C. Apart from the impact of the delusion(s) or its ramifications, functioning is not markedly impaired, and behavior is not obviously bizarre or odd.

D. If manic or major depressive episodes have occurred, these have been brief relative to the duration of the delusional periods.

E. The disturbance is not attributable to the physiological effects of a substance or another medical condition and is not better explained by another mental disorder, such as body dysmorphic disorder or obsessive-compulsive disorder.

Specify whether:

   Erotomanic type: This subtype applies when the central theme of the delusion is that another person is in love with the individual.

   Grandiose type: This subtype applies when the central theme of the delusion is the conviction of having some great (but unrecognized) talent or insight or having made some important discovery.

   Jealous type: This subtype applies when the central theme of the individual's delusion is that his or her spouse or lover is unfaithful.

   Persecutory type: This subtype applies when the central theme of the delusion involves the individual's belief that he or she is being conspired against, cheated, spied on, followed, poisoned or drugged, maliciously maligned, harassed, or obstructed in the pursuit of long-term goals.

Somatic type: This subtype applies when the central theme of the delusion involves bodily functions or sensations.

Mixed type: This subtype applies when no one delusional theme predominates.

Unspecified type: This subtype applies when the dominant delusional belief cannot be clearly determined or is not described in the specific types (e.g., referential delusions without a prominent persecutory or grandiose component).

Specify if:

With bizarre content: Delusions are deemed bizarre if they are clearly implausible, not understandable, and not derived from ordinary life experiences (e.g., an individual's belief that a stranger has removed his or her internal organs and replaced them with someone else's organs without leaving any wounds or scars).

Specify if:

The following course specifiers are only to be used after a 1-year duration of the disorder:

First episode, currently in acute episode: First manifestation of the disorder meeting the defining diagnostic symptom and time criteria. An *acute episode* is a time period in which the symptom criteria are fulfilled.

First episode, currently in partial remission: *Partial remission* is a time period during which an improvement after a previous episode is maintained and in which the defining criteria of the disorder are only partially fulfilled.

First episode, currently in full remission: *Full remission* is a period of time after a previous episode during which no disorder-specific symptoms are present.

Multiple episodes, currently in acute episode

Multiple episodes, currently in partial remission

Multiple episodes, currently in full remission

Continuous: Symptoms fulfilling the diagnostic symptom criteria of the disorder are remaining for the majority of the illness course, with subthreshold symptom periods being very brief relative to the overall course.

Unspecified

Specify current severity:

Severity is rated by a quantitative assessment of the primary symptoms of psychosis, including delusions, hallucinations, disorganized speech, abnormal psychomotor behavior, and negative symptoms. Each of these symptoms may be rated for its current severity (most severe in the last 7 days) on a 5-point scale ranging from 0 (not present) to 4 (present and severe). (See Clinician-Rated Dimensions of Psychosis Symptom Severity in the chapter "Assessment Measures" in Section III of DSM-5-TR.)

Note: Diagnosis of delusional disorder can be made without using this severity specifier.

Brief Psychotic Disorder

F23

A. Presence of one (or more) of the following symptoms. At least one of these must be (1), (2), or (3):

  1. Delusions.
  2. Hallucinations.
  3. Disorganized speech (e.g., frequent derailment or incoherence).
  4. Grossly disorganized or catatonic behavior.

  Note: Do not include a symptom if it is a culturally sanctioned response.

B. Duration of an episode of the disturbance is at least 1 day but less than 1 month, with eventual full return to premorbid level of functioning.

C. The disturbance is not better explained by major depressive or bipolar disorder with psychotic features or another psychotic disorder such as schizophrenia or catatonia, and is not attributable to the physiological effects of a substance (e.g., a drug of abuse, a medication) or another medical condition.

Specify if:

  With marked stressor(s) (brief reactive psychosis): If symptoms occur in response to events that, singly or together, would be markedly stressful to almost anyone in similar circumstances in the individual's culture.

  Without marked stressor(s): If symptoms do not occur in response to events that, singly or together, would be markedly stressful to almost anyone in similar circumstances in the individual's culture.

  With peripartum onset: If onset is during pregnancy or within 4 weeks postpartum.

Specify if:

  With catatonia (refer to the criteria for catatonia associated with another mental disorder, p. 52, for definition).

  Coding note: Use additional code F06.1 catatonia associated with brief psychotic disorder to indicate the presence of the comorbid catatonia.

Specify current severity:

  Severity is rated by a quantitative assessment of the primary symptoms of psychosis, including delusions, hallucinations, disorganized speech, abnormal psychomotor behavior, and negative symptoms. Each of these symptoms may be rated for its current severity (most severe in the last 7 days) on a 5-point scale ranging from 0 (not present) to 4 (present and severe). (See Clinician-Rated Dimensions of Psychosis Symptom Severity in the chapter "Assessment Measures" in Section III of DSM-5-TR.)

  Note: Diagnosis of brief psychotic disorder can be made without using this severity specifier.

Schizophreniform Disorder

F20.81

A. Two (or more) of the following, each present for a significant portion of time during a 1-month period (or less if successfully treated). At least one of these must be (1), (2), or (3):

   1. Delusions.
   2. Hallucinations.
   3. Disorganized speech (e.g., frequent derailment or incoherence).
   4. Grossly disorganized or catatonic behavior.
   5. Negative symptoms (i.e., diminished emotional expression or avolition).

B. An episode of the disorder lasts at least 1 month but less than 6 months. When the diagnosis must be made without waiting for recovery, it should be qualified as "provisional."

C. Schizoaffective disorder and depressive or bipolar disorder with psychotic features have been ruled out because either 1) no major depressive or manic episodes have occurred concurrently with the active-phase symptoms, or 2) if mood episodes have occurred during active-phase symptoms, they have been present for a minority of the total duration of the active and residual periods of the illness.

D. The disturbance is not attributable to the physiological effects of a substance (e.g., a drug of abuse, a medication) or another medical condition.

Specify if:

With good prognostic features: This specifier requires the presence of at least two of the following features: onset of prominent psychotic symptoms within 4 weeks of the first noticeable change in usual behavior or functioning; confusion or perplexity; good premorbid social and occupational functioning; and absence of blunted or flat affect.

Without good prognostic features: This specifier is applied if two or more of the above features have not been present.

Specify if:

With catatonia (refer to the criteria for catatonia associated with another mental disorder, p. 52, for definition).

Coding note: Use additional code F06.1 catatonia associated with schizophreniform disorder to indicate the presence of the comorbid catatonia.

Specify current severity:

Severity is rated by a quantitative assessment of the primary symptoms of psychosis, including delusions, hallucinations, disorganized speech, abnormal psychomotor behavior, and negative symptoms. Each of these symptoms may be rated for its current severity (most severe in the last 7 days) on a 5-point scale ranging from 0 (not present) to 4 (present and severe). (See Clinician-Rated Dimensions of Psychosis Symptom Severity in the chapter "Assessment Measures" in Section III of DSM-5-TR.)

Note: Diagnosis of schizophreniform disorder can be made without using this severity specifier.

Schizophrenia

F20.9

A. Two (or more) of the following, each present for a significant portion of time during a 1-month period (or less if successfully treated). At least one of these must be (1), (2), or (3):

1. Delusions.
2. Hallucinations.
3. Disorganized speech (e.g., frequent derailment or incoherence).
4. Grossly disorganized or catatonic behavior.
5. Negative symptoms (i.e., diminished emotional expression or avolition).

B. For a significant portion of the time since the onset of the disturbance, level of functioning in one or more major areas, such as work, interpersonal relations, or self-care, is markedly below the level achieved prior to the onset (or when the onset is in childhood or adolescence, there is failure to achieve expected level of interpersonal, academic, or occupational functioning).

C. Continuous signs of the disturbance persist for at least 6 months. This 6-month period must include at least 1 month of symptoms (or less if successfully treated) that meet Criterion A (i.e., active-phase symptoms) and may include periods of prodromal or residual symptoms. During these prodromal or residual periods, the signs of the disturbance may be manifested by only negative symptoms or by two or more symptoms listed in Criterion A present in an attenuated form (e.g., odd beliefs, unusual perceptual experiences).

D. Schizoaffective disorder and depressive or bipolar disorder with psychotic features have been ruled out because either 1) no major depressive or manic episodes have occurred concurrently with the active-phase symptoms, or 2) if mood episodes have occurred during active-phase symptoms, they have been present for a minority of the total duration of the active and residual periods of the illness.

E. The disturbance is not attributable to the physiological effects of a substance (e.g., a drug of abuse, a medication) or another medical condition.

F. If there is a history of autism spectrum disorder or a communication disorder of childhood onset, the additional diagnosis of schizophrenia is made only if prominent delusions or hallucinations, in addition to the other required symptoms of schizophrenia, are also present for at least 1 month (or less if successfully treated).

Specify if:

The following course specifiers are only to be used after a 1-year duration of the disorder and if they are not in contradiction to the diagnostic course criteria.

First episode, currently in acute episode: First manifestation of the disorder meeting the defining diagnostic symptom and time criteria. An *acute episode* is a time period in which the symptom criteria are fulfilled.

First episode, currently in partial remission: *Partial remission* is a period of time during which an improvement after a previous episode is maintained and in which the defining criteria of the disorder are only partially fulfilled.

First episode, currently in full remission: *Full remission* is a period of time after a previous episode during which no disorder-specific symptoms are present.

Multiple episodes, currently in acute episode: Multiple episodes may be determined after a minimum of two episodes (i.e., after a first episode, a remission and a minimum of one relapse).

Multiple episodes, currently in partial remission

Multiple episodes, currently in full remission

Continuous: Symptoms fulfilling the diagnostic symptom criteria of the disorder are remaining for the majority of the illness course, with subthreshold symptom periods being very brief relative to the overall course.

Unspecified

Specify if:

With catatonia (refer to the criteria for catatonia associated with another mental disorder, p. 52, for definition).

Coding note: Use additional code F06.1 catatonia associated with schizophrenia to indicate the presence of the comorbid catatonia.

Specify current severity:

Severity is rated by a quantitative assessment of the primary symptoms of psychosis, including delusions, hallucinations, disorganized speech, abnormal psychomotor behavior, and negative symptoms. Each of these symptoms may be rated for its current severity (most severe in the last 7 days) on a 5-point scale ranging from 0 (not present) to 4 (present and severe). (See Clinician-Rated Dimensions of Psychosis Symptom Severity in the chapter "Assessment Measures" in Section III of DSM-5-TR.)

Note: Diagnosis of schizophrenia can be made without using this severity specifier.

Schizoaffective Disorder

A. An uninterrupted period of illness during which there is a major mood episode (major depressive or manic) concurrent with Criterion A of schizophrenia.

   Note: The major depressive episode must include Criterion A1: Depressed mood.

B. Delusions or hallucinations for 2 or more weeks in the absence of a major mood episode (depressive or manic) during the lifetime duration of the illness.

C. Symptoms that meet criteria for a major mood episode are present for the majority of the total duration of the active and residual portions of the illness.

D. The disturbance is not attributable to the effects of a substance (e.g., a drug of abuse, a medication) or another medical condition.

Specify whether:

   F25.0 Bipolar type: This subtype applies if a manic episode is part of the presentation. Major depressive episodes may also occur.

   F25.1 Depressive type: This subtype applies if only major depressive episodes are part of the presentation.

Specify if:

   With catatonia (refer to the criteria for catatonia associated with another mental disorder, p. 52, for definition).

   Coding note: Use additional code F06.1 catatonia associated with schizoaffective disorder to indicate the presence of the comorbid catatonia.

Specify if:

The following course specifiers are only to be used after a 1-year duration of the disorder and if they are not in contradiction to the diagnostic course criteria.

   First episode, currently in acute episode: First manifestation of the disorder meeting the defining diagnostic symptom and time criteria. An *acute episode* is a time period in which the symptom criteria are fulfilled.

   First episode, currently in partial remission: *Partial remission* is a time period during which an improvement after a previous episode is maintained and in which the defining criteria of the disorder are only partially fulfilled.

   First episode, currently in full remission: *Full remission* is a period of time after a previous episode during which no disorder-specific symptoms are present.

   Multiple episodes, currently in acute episode: Multiple episodes may be determined after a minimum of two episodes (i.e., after a first episode, a remission and a minimum of one relapse).

   Multiple episodes, currently in partial remission

   Multiple episodes, currently in full remission

Continuous: Symptoms fulfilling the diagnostic symptom criteria of the disorder are remaining for the majority of the illness course, with subthreshold symptom periods being very brief relative to the overall course.

Unspecified

Specify current severity:

Severity is rated by a quantitative assessment of the primary symptoms of psychosis, including delusions, hallucinations, disorganized speech, abnormal psychomotor behavior, and negative symptoms. Each of these symptoms may be rated for its current severity (most severe in the last 7 days) on a 5-point scale ranging from 0 (not present) to 4 (present and severe). (See Clinician-Rated Dimensions of Psychosis Symptom Severity in the chapter "Assessment Measures" in Section III of DSM-5-TR.)

Note: Diagnosis of schizoaffective disorder can be made without using this severity specifier.

Substance/Medication-Induced Psychotic Disorder

A. Presence of one or both of the following symptoms:

1. Delusions.
2. Hallucinations.

B. There is evidence from the history, physical examination, or laboratory findings of both (1) and (2):

1. The symptoms in Criterion A developed during or soon after substance intoxication or withdrawal or after exposure to or withdrawal from a medication.
2. The involved substance/medication is capable of producing the symptoms in Criterion A.

C. The disturbance is not better explained by a psychotic disorder that is not substance/medication-induced. Such evidence of an independent psychotic disorder could include the following:

The symptoms preceded the onset of the substance/medication use; the symptoms persist for a substantial period of time (e.g., about 1 month) after the cessation of acute withdrawal or severe intoxication; or there is other evidence of an independent non-substance/medication-induced psychotic disorder (e.g., a history of recurrent non-substance/medication-related episodes).

D. The disturbance does not occur exclusively during the course of a delirium.

E. The disturbance causes clinically significant distress or impairment in social, occupational, or other important areas of functioning.

Note: This diagnosis should be made instead of a diagnosis of substance intoxication or substance withdrawal only when the symptoms in Criterion A predominate in the clinical picture and when they are sufficiently severe to warrant clinical attention.

Coding note: The ICD-10-CM codes for the [specific substance/medication]-induced psychotic disorders are indicated in the table below. Note that the ICD-10-CM code depends on whether or not there is a comorbid substance use disorder present for the same class of substance. In any case, an additional separate diagnosis of a substance use disorder is not given. If a mild substance use disorder is comorbid with the substance-induced psychotic disorder, the 4th position character is "1," and the clinician should record "mild [substance] use disorder" before the substance-induced psychotic disorder (e.g., "mild cocaine use disorder with cocaine-induced psychotic disorder"). If a moderate or severe substance use disorder is comorbid with the substance-induced psychotic disorder, the 4th position character is "2," and the clinician should record "moderate [substance] use disorder" or "severe [substance] use disorder" depending on the severity of the comorbid substance use disorder. If there is no comorbid substance use disorder (e.g., after a one-time heavy use of the substance), then the 4th position character is "9," and the clinician should record only the substance-induced psychotic disorder.

	ICD-10-CM		
	With mild use disorder	With moderate or severe use disorder	Without use disorder
Alcohol	F10.159	F10.259	F10.959
Cannabis	F12.159	F12.259	F12.959
Phencyclidine	F16.159	F16.259	F16.959
Other hallucinogen	F16.159	F16.259	F16.959
Inhalant	F18.159	F18.259	F18.959
Sedative, hypnotic, or anxiolytic	F13.159	F13.259	F13.959
Amphetamine-type substance (or other stimulant)	F15.159	F15.259	F15.959
Cocaine	F14.159	F14.259	F14.959
Other (or unknown) substance	F19.159	F19.259	F19.959

Specify (see Table 1 in the chapter "Substance-Related and Addictive Disorders," which indicates whether "with onset during intoxication" and/or "with onset during withdrawal" applies to a given substance class; or specify "with onset after medication use"):

With onset during intoxication: If criteria are met for intoxication with the substance and the symptoms develop during intoxication.
With onset during withdrawal: If criteria are met for withdrawal from the substance and the symptoms develop during, or shortly after, withdrawal.
With onset after medication use: If symptoms developed at initiation of medication, with a change in use of medication, or during withdrawal of medication.

Specify current severity:

Severity is rated by a quantitative assessment of the primary symptoms of psychosis, including delusions, hallucinations, abnormal psychomotor behavior, and negative symptoms. Each of these symptoms may be rated for its current severity (most severe in the last 7 days) on a 5-point scale ranging from 0 (not present) to 4 (present and severe). (See Clinician-Rated Dimensions of Psychosis Symptom Severity in the chapter "Assessment Measures" in Section III of DSM-5-TR.)

Note: Diagnosis of substance/medication-induced psychotic disorder can be made without using this severity specifier.

Recording Procedures

The name of the substance/medication-induced psychotic disorder begins with the specific substance (e.g., cocaine, dexamethasone) that is presumed to be causing the delusions or hallucinations. The diagnostic code is selected from the table included in the criteria set, which is based on the drug class and presence or absence of a comorbid substance use disorder. For substances that do not fit into any of the classes (e.g., dexamethasone), the code for "other (or unknown) substance" should be used; and in cases in which a substance is judged to be an etiological factor but the specific class of substance is unknown, the same code should also be used.

When recording the name of the disorder, the comorbid substance use disorder (if any) is listed first, followed by the word "with," followed by the name of the substance-induced psychotic disorder, followed by the specification of onset (i.e., onset during intoxication, onset during withdrawal). For example, in the case of delusions occurring during intoxication in a man with a severe cocaine use disorder, the diagnosis is F14.259 severe cocaine use disorder with cocaine-induced psychotic disorder, with onset during intoxication. A separate diagnosis of the comorbid severe cocaine use disorder is not given. If the substance-induced psychotic disorder occurs without a comorbid substance use disorder (e.g., after a one-time heavy use of the substance), no accompanying substance use disorder is noted (e.g., F16.959 phencyclidine-induced psychotic disorder, with onset during intoxication). When more than one substance is judged to play a significant role in the development of psychotic symptoms, each should be listed separately (e.g., F12.259 severe cannabis use disorder with cannabis-induced psychotic disorder, with onset during intoxication; F16.159 mild phencyclidine use disorder with phencyclidine-induced psychotic disorder, with onset during intoxication).

Psychotic Disorder
Due to Another Medical Condition

A. Prominent hallucinations or delusions.
B. There is evidence from the history, physical examination, or laboratory findings that the disturbance is the direct pathophysiological consequence of another medical condition.
C. The disturbance is not better explained by another mental disorder.
D. The disturbance does not occur exclusively during the course of a delirium.
E. The disturbance causes clinically significant distress or impairment in social, occupational, or other important areas of functioning.

Specify whether:

Code based on predominant symptom:

> **F06.2 With delusions:** If delusions are the predominant symptom.
> **F06.0 With hallucinations:** If hallucinations are the predominant symptom.

Coding note: Include the name of the other medical condition in the name of the mental disorder (e.g., F06.2 psychotic disorder due to malignant lung neoplasm, with delusions). The other medical condition should be coded and listed separately immediately before the psychotic disorder due to the medical condition (e.g., C34.90 malignant lung neoplasm; F06.2 psychotic disorder due to malignant lung neoplasm, with delusions).

Specify current severity:

> Severity is rated by a quantitative assessment of the primary symptoms of psychosis, including delusions, hallucinations, abnormal psychomotor behavior, and negative symptoms. Each of these symptoms may be rated for its current severity (most severe in the last 7 days) on a 5-point scale ranging from 0 (not present) to 4 (present and severe). (See Clinician-Rated Dimensions of Psychosis Symptom Severity in the chapter "Assessment Measures" in Section III of DSM-5-TR.)
> **Note:** Diagnosis of psychotic disorder due to another medical condition can be made without using this severity specifier.

Catatonia

Catatonia Associated With Another Mental Disorder (Catatonia Specifier)

F06.1

A. The clinical picture is dominated by three (or more) of the following symptoms:

1. Stupor (i.e., no psychomotor activity; not actively relating to environment).
2. Catalepsy (i.e., passive induction of a posture held against gravity).
3. Waxy flexibility (i.e., slight, even resistance to positioning by examiner).
4. Mutism (i.e., no, or very little, verbal response [exclude if known aphasia]).
5. Negativism (i.e., opposition or no response to instructions or external stimuli).
6. Posturing (i.e., spontaneous and active maintenance of a posture against gravity).
7. Mannerism (i.e., odd, circumstantial caricature of normal actions).
8. Stereotypy (i.e., repetitive, abnormally frequent, non-goal-directed movements).
9. Agitation, not influenced by external stimuli.
10. Grimacing.
11. Echolalia (i.e., mimicking another's speech).
12. Echopraxia (i.e., mimicking another's movements).

Coding note: Indicate the name of the associated mental disorder when recording the name of the condition (e.g., F06.1 catatonia associated with major depressive disorder). Code first the associated mental disorder (i.e., neurodevelopmental disorder, brief psychotic disorder, schizophreniform disorder, schizophrenia, schizoaffective disorder, bipolar disorder, major depressive disorder, or other mental disorder) (e.g., F25.1 schizoaffective disorder, depressive type; F06.1 catatonia associated with schizoaffective disorder).

Catatonic Disorder Due to Another Medical Condition

F06.1

A. The clinical picture is dominated by three (or more) of the following symptoms:

1. Stupor (i.e., no psychomotor activity; not actively relating to environment).

2. Catalepsy (i.e., passive induction of a posture held against gravity).
3. Waxy flexibility (i.e., slight, even resistance to positioning by examiner).
4. Mutism (i.e., no, or very little, verbal response [Note: not applicable if there is an established aphasia]).
5. Negativism (i.e., opposition or no response to instructions or external stimuli).
6. Posturing (i.e., spontaneous and active maintenance of a posture against gravity).
7. Mannerism (i.e., odd, circumstantial caricature of normal actions).
8. Stereotypy (i.e., repetitive, abnormally frequent, non-goal-directed movements).
9. Agitation, not influenced by external stimuli.
10. Grimacing.
11. Echolalia (i.e., mimicking another's speech).
12. Echopraxia (i.e., mimicking another's movements).

B. There is evidence from the history, physical examination, or laboratory findings that the disturbance is the direct pathophysiological consequence of another medical condition.
C. The disturbance is not better explained by another mental disorder (e.g., a manic episode).
D. The disturbance does not occur exclusively during the course of a delirium.
E. The disturbance causes clinically significant distress or impairment in social, occupational, or other important areas of functioning.

Coding note: Include the name of the medical condition in the name of the mental disorder (e.g., F06.1 catatonic disorder due to hepatic encephalopathy). The other medical condition should be coded and listed separately immediately before the catatonic disorder due to the medical condition (e.g., K72.90 hepatic encephalopathy; F06.1 catatonic disorder due to hepatic encephalopathy).

Unspecified Catatonia

This category applies to presentations in which symptoms characteristic of catatonia cause clinically significant distress or impairment in social, occupational, or other important areas of functioning but either the nature of the underlying mental disorder or other medical condition is unclear, full criteria for catatonia are not met, or there is insufficient information to make a more specific diagnosis (e.g., in emergency room settings).

Coding note: Code first **R29.818** other symptoms involving nervous and musculoskeletal systems, followed by **F06.1** unspecified catatonia.

Other Specified Schizophrenia Spectrum and Other Psychotic Disorder

F28

This category applies to presentations in which symptoms characteristic of a schizophrenia spectrum and other psychotic disorder that cause clinically significant distress or impairment in social, occupational, or other important areas of functioning predominate but do not meet the full criteria for any of the disorders in the schizophrenia spectrum and other psychotic disorders diagnostic class. The other specified schizophrenia spectrum and other psychotic disorder category is used in situations in which the clinician chooses to communicate the specific reason that the presentation does not meet the criteria for any specific schizophrenia spectrum and other psychotic disorder. This is done by recording "other specified schizophrenia spectrum and other psychotic disorder" followed by the specific reason (e.g., "persistent auditory hallucinations").

Examples of presentations that can be specified using the "other specified" designation include the following:

1. **Persistent auditory hallucinations** occurring in the absence of any other features.
2. **Delusions with significant overlapping mood episodes:** This includes persistent delusions with periods of overlapping mood episodes that are present for a substantial portion of the delusional disturbance (such that the criterion stipulating only brief mood disturbance in delusional disorder is not met).
3. **Attenuated psychosis syndrome:** This syndrome is characterized by psychotic-like symptoms that are below a threshold for full psychosis (e.g., the symptoms are less severe and more transient, and insight is relatively maintained).
4. **Delusional symptoms in the context of relationship with an individual with prominent delusions:** In the context of a relationship, the delusional material from the individual with a psychotic disorder provides content for the same delusions held by the other person who may not otherwise have symptoms that meet criteria for a psychotic disorder.

Unspecified Schizophrenia Spectrum and Other Psychotic Disorder

F29

This category applies to presentations in which symptoms characteristic of a schizophrenia spectrum and other psychotic disorder that cause clinically significant distress or impairment in social, occupational, or other important areas of functioning predominate but do not meet the full criteria for any of the disorders in the schizophrenia spectrum and other psychotic disorders diagnostic class. The unspecified schizophrenia spectrum and other psychotic disorder category is used in situations in which the clinician chooses *not* to specify the reason that the criteria are not met for a specific schizophrenia spectrum and other psychotic disorder and includes presentations in which there is insufficient information to make a more specific diagnosis (e.g., in emergency room settings).

Bipolar and Related Disorders

Bipolar I Disorder

For a diagnosis of bipolar I disorder, it is necessary to meet the following criteria for a manic episode. The manic episode may have been preceded by and may be followed by hypomanic or major depressive episodes.

Manic Episode

A. A distinct period of abnormally and persistently elevated, expansive, or irritable mood and abnormally and persistently increased activity or energy, lasting at least 1 week and present most of the day, nearly every day (or any duration if hospitalization is necessary).

B. During the period of mood disturbance and increased energy or activity, three (or more) of the following symptoms (four if the mood is only irritable) are present to a significant degree and represent a noticeable change from usual behavior:

1. Inflated self-esteem or grandiosity.
2. Decreased need for sleep (e.g., feels rested after only 3 hours of sleep).
3. More talkative than usual or pressure to keep talking.
4. Flight of ideas or subjective experience that thoughts are racing.
5. Distractibility (i.e., attention too easily drawn to unimportant or irrelevant external stimuli), as reported or observed.
6. Increase in goal-directed activity (either socially, at work or school, or sexually) or psychomotor agitation (i.e., purposeless non-goal-directed activity).
7. Excessive involvement in activities that have a high potential for painful consequences (e.g., engaging in unrestrained buying sprees, sexual indiscretions, or foolish business investments).

C. The mood disturbance is sufficiently severe to cause marked impairment in social or occupational functioning or to necessitate hospitalization to prevent harm to self or others, or there are psychotic features.

D. The episode is not attributable to the physiological effects of a substance (e.g., a drug of abuse, a medication, other treatment) or another medical condition.

Note: A full manic episode that emerges during antidepressant treatment (e.g., medication, electroconvulsive therapy) but persists at a fully syndromal level beyond the physiological effect of that treatment is sufficient evidence for a manic episode and, therefore, a bipolar I diagnosis.

Note: Criteria A–D constitute a manic episode. At least one lifetime manic episode is required for the diagnosis of bipolar I disorder.

Hypomanic Episode

A. A distinct period of abnormally and persistently elevated, expansive, or irritable mood and abnormally and persistently increased activity or energy, lasting at least 4 consecutive days and present most of the day, nearly every day.

B. During the period of mood disturbance and increased energy and activity, three (or more) of the following symptoms (four if the mood is only irritable) have persisted, represent a noticeable change from usual behavior, and have been present to a significant degree:

   1. Inflated self-esteem or grandiosity.
   2. Decreased need for sleep (e.g., feels rested after only 3 hours of sleep).
   3. More talkative than usual or pressure to keep talking.
   4. Flight of ideas or subjective experience that thoughts are racing.
   5. Distractibility (i.e., attention too easily drawn to unimportant or irrelevant external stimuli), as reported or observed.
   6. Increase in goal-directed activity (either socially, at work or school, or sexually) or psychomotor agitation.
   7. Excessive involvement in activities that have a high potential for painful consequences (e.g., engaging in unrestrained buying sprees, sexual indiscretions, or foolish business investments).

C. The episode is associated with an unequivocal change in functioning that is uncharacteristic of the individual when not symptomatic.

D. The disturbance in mood and the change in functioning are observable by others.

E. The episode is not severe enough to cause marked impairment in social or occupational functioning or to necessitate hospitalization. If there are psychotic features, the episode is, by definition, manic.

F. The episode is not attributable to the physiological effects of a substance (e.g., a drug of abuse, a medication, other treatment) or another medical condition.

   Note: A full hypomanic episode that emerges during antidepressant treatment (e.g., medication, electroconvulsive therapy) but persists at a fully syndromal level beyond the physiological effect of that treatment is sufficient evidence for a hypomanic episode diagnosis. However, caution is indicated so that one or two symptoms (particularly increased irritability, edginess, or agitation following antidepressant use) are not taken as sufficient for diagnosis of a hypomanic episode, nor necessarily indicative of a bipolar diathesis.

Note: Criteria A–F constitute a hypomanic episode. Hypomanic episodes are common in bipolar I disorder but are not required for the diagnosis of bipolar I disorder.

Major Depressive Episode

A. Five (or more) of the following symptoms have been present during the same 2-week period and represent a change from previous functioning; at least one of the symptoms is either (1) depressed mood or (2) loss of interest or pleasure.
    Note: Do not include symptoms that are clearly attributable to another medical condition.

    1. Depressed mood most of the day, nearly every day, as indicated by either subjective report (e.g., feels sad, empty, or hopeless) or observation made by others (e.g., appears tearful). (**Note:** In children and adolescents, can be irritable mood.)
    2. Markedly diminished interest or pleasure in all, or almost all, activities most of the day, nearly every day (as indicated by either subjective account or observation).
    3. Significant weight loss when not dieting or weight gain (e.g., a change of more than 5% of body weight in a month), or decrease or increase in appetite nearly every day. (**Note:** In children, consider failure to make expected weight gain.)
    4. Insomnia or hypersomnia nearly every day.
    5. Psychomotor agitation or retardation nearly every day (observable by others, not merely subjective feelings of restlessness or being slowed down).
    6. Fatigue or loss of energy nearly every day.
    7. Feelings of worthlessness or excessive or inappropriate guilt (which may be delusional) nearly every day (not merely self-reproach or guilt about being sick).
    8. Diminished ability to think or concentrate, or indecisiveness, nearly every day (either by subjective account or as observed by others).
    9. Recurrent thoughts of death (not just fear of dying), recurrent suicidal ideation without a specific plan, or a suicide attempt or a specific plan for committing suicide.

B. The symptoms cause clinically significant distress or impairment in social, occupational, or other important areas of functioning.
C. The episode is not attributable to the physiological effects of a substance or another medical condition.

Note: Criteria A–C constitute a major depressive episode. Major depressive episodes are common in bipolar I disorder but are not required for the diagnosis of bipolar I disorder.

Note: Responses to a significant loss (e.g., bereavement, financial ruin, losses from a natural disaster, a serious medical illness or disability) may include the feelings of intense sadness, rumination about the loss, insomnia, poor appetite, and weight loss noted in Criterion A, which may resemble a depressive episode. Although such symptoms may be understandable or considered appropriate to the loss, the presence of a major depressive episode in addition to the normal response to a significant loss should also be carefully considered. This decision inevitably requires the exercise of clinical judgment based on the individual's history and the cultural norms for the expression of distress in the context of loss.[1]

Bipolar I Disorder

A. Criteria have been met for at least one manic episode (Criteria A–D under "Manic Episode" above).

B. At least one manic episode is not better explained by schizoaffective disorder and is not superimposed on schizophrenia, schizophreniform disorder, delusional disorder, or other specified or unspecified schizophrenia spectrum and other psychotic disorder.

Coding and Recording Procedures

The diagnostic code for bipolar I disorder is based on type of current or most recent episode and its status with respect to current severity, presence of psychotic features, and remission status. Current severity and psychotic features are only indicated if full criteria are currently met for a manic or major depressive episode. Remission specifiers are only indicated if the full criteria are not currently met for a manic, hypomanic, or major depressive episode. Codes are as follows:

---

[1]In distinguishing grief from a major depressive episode (MDE), it is useful to consider that in grief the predominant affect is feelings of emptiness and loss, while in an MDE it is persistent depressed mood and the inability to anticipate happiness or pleasure. The dysphoria in grief is likely to decrease in intensity over days to weeks and occurs in waves, the so-called pangs of grief. These waves tend to be associated with thoughts or reminders of the deceased. The depressed mood of an MDE is more persistent and not tied to specific thoughts or preoccupations. The pain of grief may be accompanied by positive emotions and humor that are uncharacteristic of the pervasive unhappiness and misery characteristic of an MDE. The thought content associated with grief generally features a preoccupation with thoughts and memories of the deceased, rather than the self-critical or pessimistic ruminations seen in an MDE. In grief, self-esteem is generally preserved, whereas in an MDE, feelings of worthlessness and self-loathing are common. If self-derogatory ideation is present in grief, it typically involves perceived failings vis-à-vis the deceased (e.g., not visiting frequently enough, not telling the deceased how much he or she was loved). If a bereaved individual thinks about death and dying, such thoughts are generally focused on the deceased and possibly about "joining" the deceased, whereas in an MDE such thoughts are focused on ending one's own life because of feeling worthless, undeserving of life, or unable to cope with the pain of depression.

Bipolar I disorder	Current or most recent episode manic	Current or most recent episode hypomanic*	Current or most recent episode depressed	Current or most recent episode unspecified**
Mild (p. 79)	F31.11	NA	F31.31	NA
Moderate (p. 79)	F31.12	NA	F31.32	NA
Severe (p. 79)	F31.13	NA	F31.4	NA
With psychotic features*** (p. 76)	F31.2	NA	F31.5	NA
In partial remission (p. 79)	F31.73	F31.71	F31.75	NA
In full remission (p. 79)	F31.74	F31.72	F31.76	NA
Unspecified	F31.9	F31.9	F31.9	NA

*Severity and psychotic specifiers do not apply; code F31.0 for cases not in remission.
**Severity, psychotic, and remission specifiers do not apply. Code F31.9.
***If psychotic features are present, code the "with psychotic features" specifier irrespective of episode severity.

In recording the name of a diagnosis, terms should be listed in the following order: bipolar I disorder, type of current episode (or most recent episode if bipolar I disorder is in partial or full remission), severity/psychotic/remission specifiers, followed by as many of the following specifiers without codes as apply to the current episode (or the most recent episode if bipolar I disorder is in partial or full remission). **Note:** The specifiers "with rapid cycling" and "with seasonal pattern" describe the pattern of mood episodes.

Specify if:
    With anxious distress (pp. 71–72)
    With mixed features (pp. 72–73)
    With rapid cycling (pp. 73–74)
    With melancholic features (pp. 74–75)
    With atypical features (pp. 75–76)
    With mood-congruent psychotic features (p. 76; *applies to manic episode and/or major depressive episode*)
    With mood-incongruent psychotic features (p. 76; *applies to manic episode and/or major depressive episode*)
    With catatonia (pp. 76–77). **Coding note:** Use additional code F06.1.
    With peripartum onset (pp. 77–78)
    With seasonal pattern (pp. 78–79)

Bipolar II Disorder

F31.81

For a diagnosis of bipolar II disorder, it is necessary to meet the following criteria for a current or past hypomanic episode *and* the following criteria for a current or past major depressive episode:

Hypomanic Episode

A. A distinct period of abnormally and persistently elevated, expansive, or irritable mood and abnormally and persistently increased activity or energy, lasting at least 4 consecutive days and present most of the day, nearly every day.

B. During the period of mood disturbance and increased energy and activity, three (or more) of the following symptoms have persisted (four if the mood is only irritable), represent a noticeable change from usual behavior, and have been present to a significant degree:

    1. Inflated self-esteem or grandiosity.
    2. Decreased need for sleep (e.g., feels rested after only 3 hours of sleep).
    3. More talkative than usual or pressure to keep talking.
    4. Flight of ideas or subjective experience that thoughts are racing.
    5. Distractibility (i.e., attention too easily drawn to unimportant or irrelevant external stimuli), as reported or observed.
    6. Increase in goal-directed activity (either socially, at work or school, or sexually) or psychomotor agitation.
    7. Excessive involvement in activities that have a high potential for painful consequences (e.g., engaging in unrestrained buying sprees, sexual indiscretions, or foolish business investments).

C. The episode is associated with an unequivocal change in functioning that is uncharacteristic of the individual when not symptomatic.

D. The disturbance in mood and the change in functioning are observable by others.

E. The episode is not severe enough to cause marked impairment in social or occupational functioning or to necessitate hospitalization. If there are psychotic features, the episode is, by definition, manic.

F. The episode is not attributable to the physiological effects of a substance (e.g., a drug of abuse, a medication, other treatment) or another medical condition.

    Note: A full hypomanic episode that emerges during antidepressant treatment (e.g., medication, electroconvulsive therapy) but persists at a fully syndromal level beyond the physiological effect of that treatment is sufficient evidence for a hypomanic episode diagnosis. However, caution is indicated so that one or two symptoms (particularly increased irritability, edginess, or agitation following antidepressant use) are not taken as sufficient for diagnosis of a hypomanic episode, nor necessarily indicative of a bipolar diathesis.

Major Depressive Episode

A. Five (or more) of the following symptoms have been present during the same 2-week period and represent a change from previous functioning; at least one of the symptoms is either (1) depressed mood or (2) loss of interest or pleasure.

Note: Do not include symptoms that are clearly attributable to a medical condition.

1. Depressed mood most of the day, nearly every day, as indicated by either subjective report (e.g., feels sad, empty, or hopeless) or observation made by others (e.g., appears tearful). (**Note:** In children and adolescents, can be irritable mood.)
2. Markedly diminished interest or pleasure in all, or almost all, activities most of the day, nearly every day (as indicated by either subjective account or observation).
3. Significant weight loss when not dieting or weight gain (e.g., a change of more than 5% of body weight in a month), or decrease or increase in appetite nearly every day. (**Note:** In children, consider failure to make expected weight gain.)
4. Insomnia or hypersomnia nearly every day.
5. Psychomotor agitation or retardation nearly every day (observable by others, not merely subjective feelings of restlessness or being slowed down).
6. Fatigue or loss of energy nearly every day.
7. Feelings of worthlessness or excessive or inappropriate guilt (which may be delusional) nearly every day (not merely self-reproach or guilt about being sick).
8. Diminished ability to think or concentrate, or indecisiveness, nearly every day (either by subjective account or as observed by others).
9. Recurrent thoughts of death (not just fear of dying), recurrent suicidal ideation without a specific plan, or a suicide attempt or a specific plan for committing suicide.

B. The symptoms cause clinically significant distress or impairment in social, occupational, or other important areas of functioning.

C. The episode is not attributable to the physiological effects of a substance or another medical condition.

Note: Criteria A–C constitute a major depressive episode.

Note: Responses to a significant loss (e.g., bereavement, financial ruin, losses from a natural disaster, a serious medical illness or disability) may include the feelings of intense sadness, rumination about the loss, insomnia, poor appetite, and weight loss noted in Criterion A, which may resemble a depressive episode. Although such symptoms may be understandable or considered appropriate to the loss, the presence of a major depressive episode in addition to the normal response to a significant loss should be carefully considered. This decision inevitably requires the exercise of clinical judgment based on the individual's history and the cultural norms for the expression of distress in the context of loss.[2]

Bipolar II Disorder

A. Criteria have been met for at least one hypomanic episode (Criteria A–F under "Hypomanic Episode" above) and at least one major depressive episode (Criteria A–C under "Major Depressive Episode" above).

B. There has never been a manic episode.

C. At least one hypomanic episode and at least one major depressive episode are not better explained by schizoaffective disorder and are not superimposed on schizophrenia, schizophreniform disorder, delusional disorder, or other specified or unspecified schizophrenia spectrum and other psychotic disorder.

D. The symptoms of depression or the unpredictability caused by frequent alternation between periods of depression and hypomania causes clinically significant distress or impairment in social, occupational, or other important areas of functioning.

Coding and Recording Procedures

Bipolar II disorder has one diagnostic code: F31.81. Its status with respect to current severity, presence of psychotic features, course, and other specifiers cannot be coded but should be indicated in writing (e.g., F31.81 bipolar II disorder, current episode depressed, moderate severity, with mixed features; F31.81 bipolar II disorder, most recent episode depressed, in partial remission).

Specify current or most recent episode:

Hypomanic
Depressed

---

[2]In distinguishing grief from a major depressive episode (MDE), it is useful to consider that in grief the predominant affect is feelings of emptiness and loss, while in an MDE it is persistent depressed mood and the inability to anticipate happiness or pleasure. The dysphoria in grief is likely to decrease in intensity over days to weeks and occurs in waves, the so-called pangs of grief. These waves tend to be associated with thoughts or reminders of the deceased. The depressed mood of an MDE is more persistent and not tied to specific thoughts or preoccupations. The pain of grief may be accompanied by positive emotions and humor that are uncharacteristic of the pervasive unhappiness and misery characteristic of an MDE. The thought content associated with grief generally features a preoccupation with thoughts and memories of the deceased, rather than the self-critical or pessimistic ruminations seen in an MDE. In grief, self-esteem is generally preserved, whereas in an MDE feelings of worthlessness and self-loathing are common. If self-derogatory ideation is present in grief, it typically involves perceived failings vis-à-vis the deceased (e.g., not visiting frequently enough, not telling the deceased how much he or she was loved). If a bereaved individual thinks about death and dying, such thoughts are generally focused on the deceased and possibly about "joining" the deceased, whereas in an MDE such thoughts are focused on ending one's own life because of feeling worthless, undeserving of life, or unable to cope with the pain of depression.

If current episode is **hypomanic** (or most recent episode if bipolar II disorder is in partial or full remission):

In recording the diagnosis, terms should be listed in the following order: bipolar II disorder, current or most recent episode hypomanic, in partial remission/in full remission (DSM-5-TR, p. 175) (if full criteria for a hypomanic episode are not currently met), plus any of the following hypomanic episode specifiers that are applicable. **Note:** The specifiers "with rapid cycling" and "with seasonal pattern" describe the pattern of mood episodes.

Specify if:
With anxious distress (p. 71–72)
With mixed features (pp. 72–73)
With rapid cycling (pp. 73–74)
With peripartum onset (pp. 77–78)
With seasonal pattern (pp. 78–79)

If current episode is **depressed** (or most recent episode if bipolar II disorder is in partial or full remission):

In recording the diagnosis, terms should be listed in the following order: bipolar II disorder, current or most recent episode depressed, mild/moderate/severe (if full criteria for a major depressive episode are currently met), in partial remission/in full remission (if full criteria for a major depressive episode are not currently met) (DSM-5-TR, p. 175), plus any of the following major depressive episode specifiers that are applicable. **Note:** The specifiers "with rapid cycling" and "with seasonal pattern" describe the pattern of mood episodes.

Specify if:
With anxious distress (pp. 71–72)
With mixed features (pp. 72–73)
With rapid cycling (pp. 73–74)
With melancholic features (p. 74–75)
With atypical features (pp. 75–76)
With mood-congruent psychotic features (p. 76)
With mood-incongruent psychotic features (p. 76)
With catatonia (pp. 76–77). **Coding note:** Use additional code F06.1.
With peripartum onset (pp. 77–78)
With seasonal pattern (pp. 78–79)

Specify course if full criteria for a mood episode are not currently met:
In partial remission (p. 79)
In full remission (p. 79)

Specify severity if full criteria for a major depressive episode are currently met:
Mild (p. 79)
Moderate (p. 80)
Severe (p. 80)

Cyclothymic Disorder

F34.0

A. For at least 2 years (at least 1 year in children and adolescents) there have been numerous periods with hypomanic symptoms that do not meet criteria for a hypomanic episode and numerous periods with depressive symptoms that do not meet criteria for a major depressive episode.

B. During the above 2-year period (1 year in children and adolescents), Criterion A symptoms have been present for at least half the time and the individual has not been without the symptoms for more than 2 months at a time.

C. Criteria for a major depressive, manic, or hypomanic episode have never been met.

D. The symptoms in Criterion A are not better explained by schizo-affective disorder, schizophrenia, schizophreniform disorder, de-lusional disorder, or other specified or unspecified schizophrenia spectrum and other psychotic disorder.

E. The symptoms are not attributable to the physiological effects of a substance (e.g., a drug of abuse, a medication) or another med-ical condition (e.g., hyperthyroidism).

F. The symptoms cause clinically significant distress or impairment in social, occupational, or other important areas of functioning.

Specify if:
  With anxious distress (see pp. 71–72)

Substance/Medication-Induced Bipolar and Related Disorder

A. A prominent and persistent disturbance in mood that predomi-nates in the clinical picture and is characterized by abnormally el-evated, expansive, or irritable mood and abnormally increased activity or energy.

B. There is evidence from the history, physical examination, or labo-ratory findings of both (1) and (2):

1. The symptoms in Criterion A developed during or soon after substance intoxication or withdrawal or after exposure to or withdrawal from a medication.

2. The involved substance/medication is capable of producing the symptoms in Criterion A.

C. The disturbance is not better explained by a bipolar or related disor-der that is not substance/medication-induced. Such evidence of an independent bipolar or related disorder could include the following:

The symptoms precede the onset of the substance/medication use; the symptoms persist for a substantial period of time (e.g.,

about 1 month) after the cessation of acute withdrawal or severe intoxication; or there is other evidence suggesting the existence of an independent non-substance/medication-induced
bipolar and related disorder (e.g., a history of recurrent non-
substance/medication-related episodes).

D. The disturbance does not occur exclusively during the course of
a delirium.

E. The disturbance causes clinically significant distress or impairment
in social, occupational, or other important areas of functioning.

Note: This diagnosis should be made instead of a diagnosis of substance intoxication or substance withdrawal only when the symptoms
in Criterion A predominate in the clinical picture and when they are
sufficiently severe to warrant clinical attention.

Coding note: The ICD-10-CM codes for the [specific substance/med-
ication]-induced bipolar and related disorders are indicated in the table below. Note that the ICD-10-CM code depends on whether or not
there is a comorbid substance use disorder present for the same class
of substance. In any case, an additional separate diagnosis of a substance use disorder is not given. If a mild substance use disorder is
comorbid with the substance-induced bipolar and related disorder,
the 4th position character is "1," and the clinician should record "mild
[substance] use disorder" before the substance-induced bipolar and
related disorder (e.g., "mild cocaine use disorder with cocaine-
induced bipolar and related disorder"). If a moderate or severe substance
use disorder is comorbid with the substance-induced bipolar and related disorder, the 4th position character is "2," and the clinician should
record "moderate [substance] use disorder" or "severe [substance] use
disorder," depending on the severity of the comorbid substance use
disorder. If there is no comorbid substance use disorder (e.g., after a
one-time heavy use of the substance), then the 4th position character
is "9," and the clinician should record only the substance-induced bipolar and related disorder.

	ICD-10-CM		
	With mild use disorder	With moderate or severe use disorder	Without use disorder
Alcohol	F10.14	F10.24	F10.94
Phencyclidine	F16.14	F16.24	F16.94
Other hallucinogen	F16.14	F16.24	F16.94
Sedative, hypnotic, or anxiolytic	F13.14	F13.24	F13.94

| *(continued)* | ICD-10-CM | | |
	With mild use disorder	With moderate or severe use disorder	Without use disorder
Amphetamine-type substance (or other stimulant)	F15.14	F15.24	F15.94
Cocaine	F14.14	F14.24	F14.94
Other (or unknown) substance	F19.14	F19.24	F19.94

Specify (see Table 1 in the chapter "Substance-Related and Addictive Disorders," which indicates whether "with onset during intoxication" and/or "with onset during withdrawal" applies to a given substance class; or *specify* "with onset after medication use"):

With onset during intoxication: If criteria are met for intoxication with the substance and the symptoms develop during intoxication.

With onset during withdrawal: If criteria are met for withdrawal from the substance and the symptoms develop during, or shortly after, withdrawal.

With onset after medication use: If symptoms developed at initiation of medication, with a change in use of medication, or during withdrawal of medication.

Recording Procedures

The name of the substance/medication-induced bipolar and related disorder begins with the specific substance (e.g., cocaine, dexamethasone) that is presumed to be causing the bipolar mood symptoms. The diagnostic code is selected from the table included in the criteria set, which is based on the drug class and presence or absence of a comorbid substance use disorder. For substances that do not fit into any of the classes (e.g., dexamethasone), the code for "other (or unknown) substance" should be used; and in cases in which a substance is judged to be an etiological factor but the specific class of substance is unknown, the same code should also be used.

When recording the name of the disorder, the comorbid substance use disorder (if any) is listed first, followed by the word "with," followed by the name of the substance-induced bipolar and related disorder, followed by the specification of onset (i.e., onset during intoxication, onset during withdrawal). For example, in the case of irritable symptoms occurring during intoxication in a man with a severe cocaine use disorder, the diagnosis is F14.24 severe cocaine use disorder with cocaine-induced bipolar and related disorder, with onset during intoxication.

A separate diagnosis of the comorbid severe cocaine use disorder is not given. If the substance-induced bipolar and related disorder occurs without a comorbid substance use disorder (e.g., after a one-time heavy use of the substance), no accompanying substance use disorder is noted (e.g., F15.94 amphetamine-induced bipolar and related disorder, with onset during intoxication). When more than one substance is judged to play a significant role in the development of bipolar mood symptoms, each should be listed separately (e.g., F15.24 severe methylphenidate use disorder with methylphenidate-induced bipolar and related disorder, with onset during intoxication; F19.94 dexamethasone-induced bipolar and related disorder, with onset during intoxication).

Bipolar and Related Disorder Due to Another Medical Condition

A. A prominent and persistent disturbance in mood that predominates in the clinical picture and is characterized by abnormally elevated, expansive, or irritable mood and abnormally increased activity or energy.

B. There is evidence from the history, physical examination, or laboratory findings that the disturbance is the direct pathophysiological consequence of another medical condition.

C. The disturbance is not better explained by another mental disorder.

D. The disturbance does not occur exclusively during the course of a delirium.

E. The disturbance causes clinically significant distress or impairment in social, occupational, or other important areas of functioning, or necessitates hospitalization to prevent harm to self or others, or there are psychotic features.

Coding note: The ICD-10-CM code depends on the specifier (see below).

Specify if:

F06.33 With manic features: Full criteria are not met for a manic or hypomanic episode.

F06.33 With manic- or hypomanic-like episode: Full criteria are met except Criterion D for a manic episode or except Criterion F for a hypomanic episode.

F06.34 With mixed features: Symptoms of depression are also present but do not predominate in the clinical picture.

Coding note: Include the name of the other medical condition in the name of the mental disorder (e.g., F06.33 bipolar disorder due to hyperthyroidism, with manic features). The other medical condition should also be coded and listed separately immediately before the bipolar and related disorder due to the medical condition (e.g., E05.90 hyperthyroidism; F06.33 bipolar disorder due to hyperthyroidism, with manic features).

Other Specified Bipolar and Related Disorder

F31.89

This category applies to presentations in which symptoms characteristic of a bipolar and related disorder that cause clinically significant distress or impairment in social, occupational, or other important areas of functioning predominate but do not meet the full criteria for any of the disorders in the bipolar and related disorders diagnostic class. The other specified bipolar and related disorder category is used in situations in which the clinician chooses to communicate the specific reason that the presentation does not meet the criteria for any specific bipolar and related disorder. This is done by recording "other specified bipolar and related disorder" followed by the specific reason (e.g., "short-duration cyclothymia").

Examples of presentations that can be specified using the "other specified" designation include the following:

1. **Short-duration hypomanic episodes (2–3 days) and major depressive episodes:** A lifetime history of one or more major depressive episodes in individuals whose presentation has never met full criteria for a manic or hypomanic episode but who have experienced two or more episodes of short-duration hypomania that meet the full symptomatic criteria for a hypomanic episode but that only last for 2–3 days. The episodes of hypomanic symptoms do not overlap in time with the major depressive episodes, so the disturbance does not meet criteria for major depressive episode, with mixed features.
2. **Hypomanic episodes with insufficient symptoms and major depressive episodes:** A lifetime history of one or more major depressive episodes in individuals whose presentation has never met full criteria for a manic or hypomanic episode but who have experienced one or more episodes of hypomania that do not meet full symptomatic criteria (i.e., at least 4 consecutive days of elevated mood and one or two of the other symptoms of a hypomanic episode, or irritable mood and two or three of the other symptoms of a hypomanic episode). The episodes of hypomanic symptoms do not overlap in time with the major depressive episodes, so the disturbance does not meet criteria for major depressive episode, with mixed features.
3. **Hypomanic episode without prior major depressive episode:** One or more hypomanic episodes in an individual whose presentation has never met full criteria for a major depressive episode or a manic episode.
4. **Short-duration cyclothymia (less than 24 months):** Multiple episodes of hypomanic symptoms that do not meet criteria for a hypomanic episode and multiple episodes of depressive symptoms that do not meet criteria for a major depressive episode that persist over a period of less than 24 months (less than 12 months for children or adolescents) in an individual whose presentation has

never met full criteria for a major depressive, manic, or hypomanic episode and does not meet criteria for any psychotic disorder. During the course of the disorder, the hypomanic or depressive symptoms are present for more days than not, the individual has not been without symptoms for more than 2 months at a time, and the symptoms cause clinically significant distress or impairment.

5. **Manic episode superimposed** on schizophrenia, schizophreniform disorder, delusional disorder, or other specified and unspecified schizophrenia spectrum and other psychotic disorder. **Note:** Manic episodes that are part of schizoaffective disorder do not merit an additional diagnosis of other specified bipolar and related disorder.

Unspecified Bipolar and Related Disorder

F31.9

This category applies to presentations in which symptoms characteristic of a bipolar and related disorder that cause clinically significant distress or impairment in social, occupational, or other important areas of functioning predominate but do not meet the full criteria for any of the disorders in the bipolar and related disorders diagnostic class. The unspecified bipolar and related disorder category is used in situations in which the clinician chooses *not* to specify the reason that the criteria are not met for a specific bipolar and related disorder, and includes presentations in which there is insufficient information to make a more specific diagnosis (e.g., in emergency room settings).

Unspecified Mood Disorder

F39

This category applies to presentations in which symptoms characteristic of a mood disorder that cause clinically significant distress or impairment in social, occupational, or other important areas of functioning predominate but do not at the time of the evaluation meet the full criteria for any of the disorders in either the bipolar or the depressive disorders diagnostic classes and in which it is difficult to choose between unspecified bipolar and related disorder and unspecified depressive disorder (e.g., acute agitation).

Specifiers for Bipolar and Related Disorders

Specify if:

  With anxious distress: The presence of at least two of the following symptoms during the majority of days of the current manic, hypomanic, or major depressive episode in bipolar I disorder (or the most recent episode if bipolar I disorder is in partial or full remission); or of the current hypomanic or major depressive episode in bipolar II disorder (or the most recent episode if bipolar II disorder is in partial or full remission); or during the majority of symptomatic days in cyclothymic disorder:

1. Feeling keyed up or tense.
2. Feeling unusually restless.
3. Difficulty concentrating because of worry.
4. Fear that something awful may happen.
5. Feeling that the individual might lose control of himself or herself.

> *Specify* current severity:
> > **Mild:** Two symptoms.
> > **Moderate:** Three symptoms.
> > **Moderate-severe:** Four or five symptoms.
> > **Severe:** Four or five symptoms with motor agitation.

> **Note:** Anxious distress has been noted as a prominent feature of both bipolar and major depressive disorders in both primary care and specialty mental health settings. High levels of anxiety have been associated with higher suicide risk, longer duration of illness, and greater likelihood of treatment nonresponse. As a result, it is clinically useful to specify accurately the presence and severity levels of anxious distress for treatment planning and monitoring of response to treatment.

With mixed features: The mixed features specifier can apply to the current manic, hypomanic, or major depressive episode in bipolar I disorder (or the most recent episode if bipolar I disorder is in partial or full remission) or to the current hypomanic or major depressive episode in bipolar II disorder (or the most recent episode if bipolar II disorder is in partial or full remission):

Manic or hypomanic episode, with mixed features:

A. Full criteria are met for a manic episode or hypomanic episode, and at least three of the following symptoms are present during the majority of days of the current or most recent episode of mania or hypomania:

1. Prominent dysphoria or depressed mood as indicated by either subjective report (e.g., feels sad or empty) or observation made by others (e.g., appears tearful).
2. Diminished interest or pleasure in all, or almost all, activities (as indicated by either subjective account or observation made by others).
3. Psychomotor retardation nearly every day (observable by others; not merely subjective feelings of being slowed down).
4. Fatigue or loss of energy.
5. Feelings of worthlessness or excessive or inappropriate guilt (not merely self-reproach or guilt about being sick).

6. Recurrent thoughts of death (not just fear of dying), recurrent suicidal ideation without a specific plan, or a suicide attempt or a specific plan for committing suicide.

B. Mixed symptoms are observable by others and represent a change from the person's usual behavior.

C. For individuals whose symptoms meet full episode criteria for both mania and depression simultaneously, the diagnosis should be manic episode, with mixed features, due to the marked impairment and clinical severity of full mania.

D. The mixed symptoms are not attributable to the·physiological effects of a substance (e.g., a drug of abuse, a medication or other treatment).

Depressive episode, with mixed features:

A. Full criteria are met for a major depressive episode, and at least three of the following manic/hypomanic symptoms are present during the majority of days of the current or most recent episode of depression:

1. Elevated, expansive mood.
2. Inflated self-esteem or grandiosity.
3. More talkative than usual or pressure to keep talking.
4. Flight of ideas or subjective experience that thoughts are racing.
5. Increase in energy or goal-directed activity (either socially, at work or school, or sexually).
6. Increased or excessive involvement in activities that have a high potential for painful consequences (e.g., engaging in unrestrained buying sprees, sexual indiscretions, or foolish business investments).
7. Decreased need for sleep (feeling rested despite sleeping less than usual; to be contrasted with insomnia).

B. Mixed symptoms are observable by others and represent a change from the person's usual behavior.

C. For individuals whose symptoms meet full episode criteria for both mania and depression simultaneously, the diagnosis should be manic episode, with mixed features.

D. The mixed symptoms are not attributable to the physiological effects of a substance (e.g., a drug of abuse, a medication or other treatment).

Note: Mixed features associated with a major depressive episode have been found to be a significant risk factor for the development of bipolar I or bipolar II disorder. As a result, it is clinically useful to note the presence of this specifier for treatment planning and monitoring of response to treatment.

With rapid cycling: Presence of at least four mood episodes in the previous 12 months that meet the criteria for manic, hypomanic, or major depressive episode in bipolar I disorder or that meet the criteria for hypomanic or major depressive episode in bipolar II disorder.

Note: Episodes are demarcated by either partial or full remissions of at least 2 months or a switch to an episode of the opposite polarity (e.g., major depressive episode to manic episode).

Note: The essential feature of a rapid-cycling bipolar disorder is the occurrence of at least four mood episodes during the previous 12 months. These episodes can occur in any combination and order. The episodes must meet both the duration and the symptom number criteria for a major depressive, manic, or hypomanic episode and must be demarcated by either a period of full remission or a switch to an episode of the opposite polarity. Manic and hypomanic episodes are counted as being on the same pole. Except for the fact that they occur more frequently, the episodes that occur in a rapid-cycling pattern are no different from those that occur in a non-rapid-cycling pattern. Mood episodes that count toward defining a rapid-cycling pattern exclude those episodes directly caused by a substance (e.g., cocaine, corticosteroids) or another medical condition.

With melancholic features:

A. One of the following is present during the most severe period of the current major depressive episode (or the most recent major depressive episode if bipolar I or bipolar II disorder is currently in partial or full remission):

1. Loss of pleasure in all, or almost all, activities.
2. Lack of reactivity to usually pleasurable stimuli (does not feel much better, even temporarily, when something good happens).

B. Three (or more) of the following:

1. A distinct quality of depressed mood characterized by profound despondency, despair, and/or moroseness or by so-called empty mood.
2. Depression that is regularly worse in the morning.
3. Early-morning awakening (i.e., at least 2 hours before usual awakening).
4. Marked psychomotor agitation or retardation.
5. Significant anorexia or weight loss.
6. Excessive or inappropriate guilt.

Note: The specifier "with melancholic features" is applied if these features are present at the most severe stage of the episode. There is a near-complete absence of the capacity for pleasure, not merely a diminution. A guideline for evaluating the lack of reactivity of mood is that even highly desired events are not associated with marked brightening of mood. Either mood does not brighten at all, or it brightens only partially (e.g., up to 20%–40% of normal for only minutes at a time). The "distinct quality" of mood that is characteristic of the "with melancholic features" specifier is experienced as qualitatively different from that during a nonmelancholic depressive episode. A depressed mood that is described as merely more severe, longer lasting, or present without a reason is not considered distinct in quality. Psychomotor changes are nearly always present and are observable by others.

Melancholic features exhibit only a modest tendency to repeat across episodes in the same individual. They are more frequent in inpatients, as opposed to outpatients; are less likely to occur in milder than in more severe major depressive episodes; and are more likely to occur in individuals with psychotic features.

With atypical features: This specifier is applied when these features predominate during the majority of days of the current major depressive episode (or the most recent major depressive episode if bipolar I or bipolar II disorder is currently in partial or full remission).

A. Mood reactivity (i.e., mood brightens in response to actual or potential positive events).

B. Two (or more) of the following:

   1. Significant weight gain or increase in appetite.
   2. Hypersomnia.
   3. Leaden paralysis (i.e., heavy, leaden feelings in arms or legs).
   4. A long-standing pattern of interpersonal rejection sensitivity (not limited to episodes of mood disturbance) that results in significant social or occupational impairment.

C. Criteria are not met for "with melancholic features" or "with catatonia" during the same episode.

   Note: "Atypical depression" has historical significance (i.e., atypical in contradistinction to the more classical agitated, "endogenous" presentations of depression that were the norm when depression was rarely diagnosed in outpatients and almost never in adolescents or younger adults) and today does not connote an uncommon or unusual clinical presentation as the term might imply.

   Mood reactivity is the capacity to be cheered up when presented with positive events (e.g., a visit from children, compliments from others). Mood may become euthymic (not sad) even for extended periods of time if the external circumstances remain favorable. Increased appetite may be manifested by an obvious increase in food intake or by weight gain. Hypersomnia may include either an extended period of nighttime sleep or daytime napping that totals at least 10 hours of sleep per day (or at least 2 hours more than when not depressed). Leaden paralysis is defined as feeling heavy, leaden, or weighted down, usually in the arms or legs. This sensation is generally present for at least an hour a day but often lasts for many hours at a time. Unlike the other atypical features, pathological sensitivity to perceived interpersonal rejection is a trait that has an early onset and persists throughout most of adult life. Rejection sensitivity occurs both when the person is and is not depressed, though it may be exacerbated during depressive periods.

With psychotic features: Delusions or hallucinations are present at any time in the current manic or major depressive episode in bipolar I disorder (or the most recent manic or major depressive episode if bipolar I disorder is currently in partial or full remission) or in the current major depressive episode in bipolar II disorder (or the most recent major depressive episode if bipolar II disorder is currently in partial or full remission). If psychotic features are present, *specify* if mood-congruent or mood-incongruent:

> *When applied to current or most recent manic episode (in bipolar I disorder):*
>
> > **With mood-congruent psychotic features:** The content of all delusions and hallucinations is consistent with the typical manic themes of grandiosity, invulnerability, etc., but may also include themes of suspiciousness or paranoia, especially with respect to others' doubts about the individual's capacities, accomplishments, and so forth.
> >
> > **With mood-incongruent psychotic features:** The content of the delusions and hallucinations does not involve typical manic themes as described above, or the content is a mixture of mood-incongruent and mood-congruent themes.
>
> *When applied to current or most recent major depressive episode (in bipolar I disorder or bipolar II disorder):*
>
> > **With mood-congruent psychotic features:** The content of all delusions and hallucinations is consistent with the typical depressive themes of personal inadequacy, guilt, disease, death, nihilism, or deserved punishment.
> >
> > **With mood-incongruent psychotic features:** The content of the delusions and hallucinations does not involve typical depressive themes of personal inadequacy, guilt, disease, death, nihilism, or deserved punishment, or the content is a mixture of mood-incongruent and mood-congruent themes.

With catatonia: This specifier is applied to the current manic or major depressive episode in bipolar I disorder (or the most recent manic or major depressive episode if bipolar I disorder is currently in partial or full remission) or to the current major depressive episode in bipolar II disorder (or the most recent major depressive episode if bipolar II disorder is currently in partial or full remission) if catatonic features are present during most of the episode. See criteria for catatonia associated with a mental disorder in the chapter "Schizophrenia Spectrum and Other Psychotic Disorders."

With peripartum onset: This specifier is applied to the current manic, hypomanic, or major depressive episode in bipolar I disorder (or the most recent manic, hypomanic, or major depressive episode if bipolar I disorder is currently in partial or full remission) or to the current hypomanic or major depressive episode in bipolar II disorder (or the most recent hypomanic or major depressive episode if bipolar II disorder is currently in partial or full remission) if onset of mood symptoms occurs during pregnancy or in the 4 weeks following delivery.

> **Note:** Mood episodes can have their onset either during pregnancy or postpartum. About 50% of postpartum major depressive episodes begin prior to delivery. Thus, these episodes are referred to collectively as *peripartum* episodes.
>
> D.Between conception and birth, about 9% of women will experience a major depressive episode. The best estimate for prevalence of a major depressive episode between birth and 12 months postpartum is just below 7%.
>
> Peripartum-onset mood episodes can present either with or without psychotic features. Infanticide (a rare occurrence) is most often associated with postpartum psychotic episodes that are characterized by command hallucinations to kill the infant or delusions that the infant is possessed, but psychotic symptoms can also occur in severe postpartum mood episodes without such specific delusions or hallucinations.
>
> Postpartum mood (major depressive or manic) episodes with psychotic features appear to occur in from 1 in 500 to 1 in 1,000 deliveries and may be more common in primiparous women. The risk of postpartum episodes with psychotic features is particularly increased for women with prior postpartum psychotic mood episodes but is also elevated for those with a prior history of a depressive or bipolar disorder (especially bipolar I disorder) and those with a family history of bipolar disorders.
>
> Once a woman has had a postpartum episode with psychotic features, the risk of recurrence with each subsequent delivery is between 30% and 50%. Postpartum episodes must be differentiated from delirium occurring in the postpartum period, which is distinguished by a fluctuating level of awareness or attention.
>
> Peripartum-onset depressive disorders must be distinguished from the much more common "maternity blues," or what is known in lay terms as "baby blues." Maternity blues is not considered to be a mental disorder and is characterized by sudden changes in mood (e.g., the sudden onset of tearful-

ness in the absence of depression) that do not cause functional impairment and that are likely caused by physiological changes occurring after delivery. It is temporary and self-limited, typically improving quickly (within a week) without the need for treatment. Other symptoms of maternity blues include sleep disturbance and even confusion that can occur shortly after delivery.

Perinatal women may be at higher risk for depressive disorders due to thyroid abnormalities as well as other medical conditions that can cause depressive symptoms. If the depressive symptoms are judged to be due to another medical condition related to the perinatal period, depressive disorder due to another medical condition should be diagnosed instead of a major depressive episode, with peripartum onset.

With seasonal pattern: This specifier applies to the lifetime pattern of mood episodes. The essential feature is a regular seasonal pattern of at least one type of episode (i.e., mania, hypomania, or depression). The other types of episodes may not follow this pattern. For example, an individual may have seasonal manias but have depressions that do not regularly occur at a specific time of year.

A. There has been a regular temporal relationship between the onset of manic, hypomanic, or major depressive episodes and a particular time of the year (e.g., in the fall or winter) in bipolar I or bipolar II disorder.

   Note: Do not include cases in which there is an obvious effect of seasonally related psychosocial stressors (e.g., regularly being unemployed every winter).

B. Full remissions (or a change from major depression to mania or hypomania or vice versa) also occur at a characteristic time of the year (e.g., depression disappears in the spring).

C. In the last 2 years, the individual's manic, hypomanic, or major depressive episodes have demonstrated a temporal seasonal relationship, as defined above, and no nonseasonal episodes of that polarity have occurred during that 2-year period.

D. Seasonal manias, hypomanias, or depressions (as described above) substantially outnumber any nonseasonal manias, hypomanias, or depressions that may have occurred over the individual's lifetime.

   Note: The specifier "with seasonal pattern" can apply to the pattern of major depressive episodes in bipolar I and bipolar II disorders, to the pattern of manic episodes and hypomanic episodes in bipolar I disorder, and to the pattern of hypomanic episodes in bipolar II disorder. The essential feature is the onset and remission of major depressive, manic, or hypomanic episodes at characteristic times of the year. In most cases, the seasonal major depressive episodes begin in fall or winter and remit in spring. Less commonly, there may be recurrent summer depressive episodes. This pattern of onset and remission of episodes must have occurred during at least a 2-year period, without any nonseasonal episodes occurring during this period. In addition, the seasonal depressive, manic, or hypomanic episodes must substantially outnumber any nonseasonal depressive, manic, or hypomanic episodes over the individual's lifetime.

This specifier does not apply to those situations in which the pattern is better explained by seasonally linked psychosocial stressors (e.g., seasonal unemployment or school schedule). It is unclear whether a seasonal pattern of major depressive episodes is more likely in recurrent major depressive disorder or in bipolar disorders. However, within the bipolar disorders group, a seasonal pattern of major depressive episodes appears to be more likely in bipolar II disorder than in bipolar I disorder. In some individuals, the onset of manic or hypomanic episodes may also be linked to a particular season, with peak seasonality of mania or hypomania from spring through summer.

The prevalence of winter-type seasonal pattern appears to vary with latitude, age, and sex. Prevalence increases with higher latitudes. Age is also a strong predictor of seasonality, with younger persons at higher risk for winter depressive episodes.

Specify if:

In partial remission: Symptoms of the immediately previous manic, hypomanic, or major depressive episode are present but full criteria are not met, or there is a period lasting less than 2 months without any significant symptoms of a manic, hypomanic, or major depressive episode following the end of such an episode.

In full remission: During the past 2 months, no significant signs or symptoms of the disturbance were present.

Specify current severity of manic episode:
Severity is based on the number of criterion symptoms, the severity of those symptoms, and the degree of functional disability.

Mild: Minimum symptom criteria are met for a manic episode.
Moderate: Very significant increase in activity or impairment in judgment.
Severe: Almost continual supervision is required in order to prevent physical harm to self or others.

Specify current severity of major depressive episode:
Severity is based on the number of criterion symptoms, the severity of those symptoms, and the degree of functional disability.

Mild: Few, if any, symptoms in excess of those required to make the diagnosis are present, the intensity of the symptoms is distressing but manageable, and the symptoms result in minor impairment in social or occupational functioning.

Moderate: The number of symptoms, intensity of symptoms, and/or functional impairment are between those specified for "mild" and "severe."

Severe: The number of symptoms is substantially in excess of that required to make the diagnosis, the intensity of the symptoms is seriously distressing and unmanageable, and the symptoms markedly interfere with social and occupational functioning.

Depressive Disorders

Disruptive Mood Dysregulation Disorder

F34.81

A. Severe recurrent temper outbursts manifested verbally (e.g., verbal rages) and/or behaviorally (e.g., physical aggression toward people or property) that are grossly out of proportion in intensity or duration to the situation or provocation.

B. The temper outbursts are inconsistent with developmental level.

C. The temper outbursts occur, on average, three or more times per week.

D. The mood between temper outbursts is persistently irritable or angry most of the day, nearly every day, and is observable by others (e.g., parents, teachers, peers).

E. Criteria A–D have been present for 12 or more months. Throughout that time, the individual has not had a period lasting 3 or more consecutive months without all of the symptoms in Criteria A–D.

F. Criteria A and D are present in at least two of three settings (i.e., at home, at school, with peers) and are severe in at least one of these.

G. The diagnosis should not be made for the first time before age 6 years or after age 18 years.

H. By history or observation, the age at onset of Criteria A–E is before 10 years.

I. There has never been a distinct period lasting more than 1 day during which the full symptom criteria, except duration, for a manic or hypomanic episode have been met.

   Note: Developmentally appropriate mood elevation, such as occurs in the context of a highly positive event or its anticipation, should not be considered as a symptom of mania or hypomania.

J. The behaviors do not occur exclusively during an episode of major depressive disorder and are not better explained by another mental disorder (e.g., autism spectrum disorder, posttraumatic stress disorder, separation anxiety disorder, persistent depressive disorder).

   Note: This diagnosis cannot coexist with oppositional defiant disorder, intermittent explosive disorder, or bipolar disorder, though it can coexist with others, including major depressive disorder, attention-deficit/hyperactivity disorder, conduct disorder, and substance use disorders. Individuals whose symptoms meet criteria for both disruptive mood dysregulation disorder and oppositional defiant disorder should only be given the diagnosis of disruptive mood dysregulation disorder. If an individual has ever experienced a manic or hypomanic episode, the diagnosis of disruptive mood dysregulation disorder should not be assigned.

K. The symptoms are not attributable to the physiological effects of a substance or another medical or neurological condition.

Major Depressive Disorder

A. Five (or more) of the following symptoms have been present during the same 2-week period and represent a change from previous functioning; at least one of the symptoms is either (1) depressed mood or (2) loss of interest or pleasure.

Note: Do not include symptoms that are clearly attributable to another medical condition.

1. Depressed mood most of the day, nearly every day, as indicated by either subjective report (e.g., feels sad, empty, hopeless) or observation made by others (e.g., appears tearful). (**Note:** In children and adolescents, can be irritable mood.)
2. Markedly diminished interest or pleasure in all, or almost all, activities most of the day, nearly every day (as indicated by either subjective account or observation).
3. Significant weight loss when not dieting or weight gain (e.g., a change of more than 5% of body weight in a month), or decrease or increase in appetite nearly every day. (**Note:** In children, consider failure to make expected weight gain.)
4. Insomnia or hypersomnia nearly every day.
5. Psychomotor agitation or retardation nearly every day (observable by others, not merely subjective feelings of restlessness or being slowed down).
6. Fatigue or loss of energy nearly every day.
7. Feelings of worthlessness or excessive or inappropriate guilt (which may be delusional) nearly every day (not merely self-reproach or guilt about being sick).
8. Diminished ability to think or concentrate, or indecisiveness, nearly every day (either by subjective account or as observed by others).
9. Recurrent thoughts of death (not just fear of dying), recurrent suicidal ideation without a specific plan, or a suicide attempt or a specific plan for committing suicide.

B. The symptoms cause clinically significant distress or impairment in social, occupational, or other important areas of functioning.

C. The episode is not attributable to the physiological effects of a substance or another medical condition.

Note: Criteria A–C represent a major depressive episode.

Note: Responses to a significant loss (e.g., bereavement, financial ruin, losses from a natural disaster, a serious medical illness or disability) may include the feelings of intense sadness, rumination about the loss, insomnia, poor appetite, and weight loss noted in Criterion A, which may resemble a depressive episode. Although such symptoms may be understandable or considered appropriate to the loss, the presence of a major depressive episode in addition to the normal response to a significant loss should also be carefully considered. This decision inevitably requires the exercise of clinical judgment based on the individual's history and the cultural norms for the expression of distress in the context of loss.[1]

D. At least one major depressive episode is not better explained by schizoaffective disorder and is not superimposed on schizophrenia, schizophreniform disorder, delusional disorder, or other specified and unspecified schizophrenia spectrum and other psychotic disorders.

E. There has never been a manic episode or a hypomanic episode.
   Note: This exclusion does not apply if all of the manic-like or hypomanic-like episodes are substance-induced or are attributable to the physiological effects of another medical condition.

Coding and Recording Procedures

The diagnostic code for major depressive disorder is based on whether this is a single or recurrent episode, current severity, presence of psychotic features, and remission status. Current severity and psychotic features are only indicated if full criteria are currently met for a major depressive episode. Remission specifiers are only indicated if the full criteria are not currently met for a major depressive episode. Codes are as follows:

---

[1]In distinguishing grief from a major depressive episode (MDE), it is useful to consider that in grief the predominant affect is feelings of emptiness and loss, while in an MDE it is persistent depressed mood and the inability to anticipate happiness or pleasure. The dysphoria in grief is likely to decrease in intensity over days to weeks and occurs in waves, the so-called pangs of grief. These waves tend to be associated with thoughts or reminders of the deceased. The depressed mood of an MDE is more persistent and not tied to specific thoughts or preoccupations. The pain of grief may be accompanied by positive emotions and humor that are uncharacteristic of the pervasive unhappiness and misery characteristic of an MDE. The thought content associated with grief generally features a preoccupation with thoughts and memories of the deceased, rather than the self-critical or pessimistic ruminations seen in an MDE. In grief, self-esteem is generally preserved, whereas in an MDE feelings of worthlessness and self-loathing are common. If self-derogatory ideation is present in grief, it typically involves perceived failings vis-à-vis the deceased (e.g., not visiting frequently enough, not telling the deceased how much he or she was loved). If a bereaved individual thinks about death and dying, such thoughts are generally focused on the deceased and possibly about "joining" the deceased, whereas in an MDE such thoughts are focused on ending one's own life because of feeling worthless, undeserving of life, or unable to cope with the pain of depression.

Severity/course specifier	Single episode	Recurrent episode*
Mild (p. 97)	F32.0	F33.0
Moderate (p. 97)	F32.1	F33.1
Severe (p. 98)	F32.2	F33.2
With psychotic features** (p. 95)	F32.3	F33.3
In partial remission (p. 97)	F32.4	F33.41
In full remission (p. 97)	F32.5	F33.42
Unspecified	F32.9	F33.9

*For an episode to be considered recurrent, there must be an interval of at least 2 consecutive months between separate episodes in which criteria are not met for a major depressive episode. The definitions of specifiers are found on the indicated pages.
**If psychotic features are present, code the "with psychotic features" specifier irrespective of episode severity.

In recording the name of a diagnosis, terms should be listed in the following order: major depressive disorder, single or recurrent episode, severity/psychotic/remission specifiers, followed by as many of the following specifiers without codes that apply to the current episode (or the most recent episode if the major depressive disorder is in partial or full remission). **Note:** The specifier "with seasonal pattern" describes the pattern of recurrent major depressive episodes.

Specify:
   With anxious distress (p. 92)
   With mixed features (pp. 92–93)
   With melancholic features (pp. 93–94)
   With atypical features (pp. 94–95)
   With mood-congruent psychotic features (p. 95)
   With mood-incongruent psychotic features (p. 95)
   With catatonia (p. 95). **Coding note:** Use additional code F06.1.
   With peripartum onset (pp. 95–96)
   With seasonal pattern (applies to pattern of recurrent major depressive episodes) (pp. 96–97)

Persistent Depressive Disorder

F34.1

This disorder represents a consolidation of DSM-IV-defined chronic major depressive disorder and dysthymic disorder.
A.   Depressed mood for most of the day, for more days than not, as indicated by either subjective account or observation by others, for at least 2 years.

Note: In children and adolescents, mood can be irritable and duration must be at least 1 year.

B. Presence, while depressed, of two (or more) of the following:

1. Poor appetite or overeating.
2. Insomnia or hypersomnia.
3. Low energy or fatigue.
4. Low self-esteem.
5. Poor concentration or difficulty making decisions.
6. Feelings of hopelessness.

C. During the 2-year period (1 year for children or adolescents) of the disturbance, the individual has never been without the symptoms in Criteria A and B for more than 2 months at a time.

D. Criteria for a major depressive disorder may be continuously present for 2 years.

E. There has never been a manic episode or a hypomanic episode.

F. The disturbance is not better explained by a persistent schizoaffective disorder, schizophrenia, delusional disorder, or other specified or unspecified schizophrenia spectrum and other psychotic disorder.

G. The symptoms are not attributable to the physiological effects of a substance (e.g., a drug of abuse, a medication) or another medical condition (e.g., hypothyroidism).

H. The symptoms cause clinically significant distress or impairment in social, occupational, or other important areas of functioning.

Note: If criteria are sufficient for a diagnosis of a major depressive episode at any time during the 2-year period of depressed mood, then a separate diagnosis of major depression should be made in addition to the diagnosis of persistent depressive disorder along with the relevant specifier (e.g., with intermittent major depressive episodes, with current episode).

Specify if:
> **With anxious distress** (p. 92)
> **With atypical features** (pp. 94–95)

Specify if:
> **In partial remission** (p. 97)
> **In full remission** (p. 97)

Specify if:
> **Early onset:** If onset is before age 21 years.
> **Late onset:** If onset is at age 21 years or older.

Specify if (for most recent 2 years of persistent depressive disorder):
> **With pure dysthymic syndrome:** Full criteria for a major depressive episode have not been met in at least the preceding 2 years.
> **With persistent major depressive episode:** Full criteria for a major depressive episode have been met throughout the preceding 2-year period.
> **With intermittent major depressive episodes, with current episode:** Full criteria for a major depressive episode are currently

met, but there have been periods of at least 8 weeks in at least the preceding 2 years with symptoms below the threshold for a full major depressive episode.

With intermittent major depressive episodes, without current episode: Full criteria for a major depressive episode are not currently met, but there has been one or more major depressive episodes in at least the preceding 2 years.

Specify current severity:

Mild (p. 97)
Moderate (p. 97)
Severe (p. 98)

Premenstrual Dysphoric Disorder

F32.81

A. In the majority of menstrual cycles, at least five symptoms must be present in the final week before the onset of menses, start to *improve* within a few days after the onset of menses, and become *minimal* or absent in the week postmenses.

B. One (or more) of the following symptoms must be present:

1. Marked affective lability (e.g., mood swings; feeling suddenly sad or tearful, or increased sensitivity to rejection).
2. Marked irritability or anger or increased interpersonal conflicts.
3. Marked depressed mood, feelings of hopelessness, or self-deprecating thoughts.
4. Marked anxiety, tension, and/or feelings of being keyed up or on edge.

C. One (or more) of the following symptoms must additionally be present, to reach a total of *five* symptoms when combined with symptoms from Criterion B.

1. Decreased interest in usual activities (e.g., work, school, friends, hobbies).
2. Subjective difficulty in concentration.
3. Lethargy, easy fatigability, or marked lack of energy.
4. Marked change in appetite; overeating; or specific food cravings.
5. Hypersomnia or insomnia.
6. A sense of being overwhelmed or out of control.
7. Physical symptoms such as breast tenderness or swelling, joint or muscle pain, a sensation of "bloating," or weight gain.

Note: The symptoms in Criteria A–C must have been met for most menstrual cycles that occurred in the preceding year.

D. The symptoms cause clinically significant distress or interference with work, school, usual social activities, or relationships with others (e.g., avoidance of social activities; decreased productivity and efficiency at work, school, or home).

E. The disturbance is not merely an exacerbation of the symptoms of another disorder, such as major depressive disorder, panic disorder, persistent depressive disorder, or a personality disorder (although it may co-occur with any of these disorders).

F. Criterion A should be confirmed by prospective daily ratings during at least two symptomatic cycles. (**Note:** The diagnosis may be made provisionally prior to this confirmation.)

G. The symptoms are not attributable to the physiological effects of a substance (e.g., a drug of abuse, a medication, other treatment) or another medical condition (e.g., hyperthyroidism).

Recording Procedures

If symptoms have not been confirmed by prospective daily ratings of at least two symptomatic cycles, "provisional" should be noted after the name of the diagnosis (i.e., "premenstrual dysphoric disorder, provisional").

Substance/Medication-Induced Depressive Disorder

A. A prominent and persistent disturbance in mood that predominates in the clinical picture and is characterized by depressed mood or markedly diminished interest or pleasure in all, or almost all, activities.

B. There is evidence from the history, physical examination, or laboratory findings of both (1) and (2):

1. The symptoms in Criterion A developed during or soon after substance intoxication or withdrawal or after exposure to or withdrawal from a medication.

2. The involved substance/medication is capable of producing the symptoms in Criterion A.

C. The disturbance is not better explained by a depressive disorder that is not substance/medication-induced. Such evidence of an independent depressive disorder could include the following:

The symptoms preceded the onset of the substance/medication use; the symptoms persist for a substantial period of time (e.g., about 1 month) after the cessation of acute withdrawal or severe intoxication; or there is other evidence suggesting the existence of an independent non-substance/medication-induced depressive disorder (e.g., a history of recurrent non-substance/medication-related episodes).

D. The disturbance does not occur exclusively during the course of a delirium.

E. The disturbance causes clinically significant distress or impairment in social, occupational, or other important areas of functioning.

Note: This diagnosis should be made instead of a diagnosis of substance intoxication or substance withdrawal only when the symptoms in Criterion A predominate in the clinical picture and when they are sufficiently severe to warrant clinical attention.

Coding note: The ICD-10-CM codes for the [specific substance/medication]-induced depressive disorders are indicated in the table below. Note that the ICD-10-CM code depends on whether or not there is a comorbid substance use disorder present for the same class of substance. In any case, an additional separate diagnosis of a substance use disorder is not given. If a mild substance use disorder is comorbid with the substance-induced depressive disorder, the 4th position character is "1," and the clinician should record "mild [substance] use disorder" before the substance-induced depressive disorder (e.g., "mild cocaine use disorder with cocaine-induced depressive disorder"). If a moderate or severe substance use disorder is comorbid with the substance-induced depressive disorder, the 4th position character is "2," and the clinician should record "moderate [substance] use disorder" or "severe [substance] use disorder," depending on the severity of the comorbid substance use disorder. If there is no comorbid substance use disorder (e.g., after a one-time heavy use of the substance), then the 4th position character is "9," and the clinician should record only the substance-induced depressive disorder.

	ICD-10-CM		
	With mild use disorder	With moderate or severe use disorder	Without use disorder
Alcohol	F10.14	F10.24	F10.94
Phencyclidine	F16.14	F16.24	F16.94
Other hallucinogen	F16.14	F16.24	F16.94
Inhalant	F18.14	F18.24	F18.94
Opioid	F11.14	F11.24	F11.94
Sedative, hypnotic, or anxiolytic	F13.14	F13.24	F13.94
Amphetamine-type substance (or other stimulant)	F15.14	F15.24	F15.94
Cocaine	F14.14	F14.24	F14.94
Other (or unknown) substance	F19.14	F19.24	F19.94

Specify (see Table 1 in the chapter "Substance-Related and Addictive Disorders," which indicates whether "with onset during intoxication" and/or "with onset during withdrawal" applies to a given substance class; or *specify* "with onset after medication use"):

With onset during intoxication: If criteria are met for intoxication with the substance and the symptoms develop during intoxication.
With onset during withdrawal: If criteria are met for withdrawal from the substance and the symptoms develop during, or shortly after, withdrawal.
With onset after medication use: If symptoms developed at initiation of medication, with a change in use of medication, or during withdrawal of medication.

Recording Procedures

The name of the substance/medication-induced depressive disorder begins with the specific substance (e.g., cocaine, dexamethasone) that is presumed to be causing the depressive symptoms. The diagnostic code is selected from the table included in the criteria set, which is based on the drug class and presence or absence of a comorbid substance use disorder. For substances that do not fit into any of the classes (e.g., dexamethasone), the code for "other (or unknown) substance" should be used; and in cases in which a substance is judged to be an etiological factor but the specific class of substance is unknown, the same code should also be used.

When recording the name of the disorder, the comorbid substance use disorder (if any) is listed first, followed by the word "with," followed by the name of the substance-induced depressive disorder, followed by the specification of onset (i.e., onset during intoxication, onset during withdrawal). For example, in the case of depressive symptoms occurring during withdrawal in a man with a severe cocaine use disorder, the diagnosis is F14.24 severe cocaine use disorder with cocaine-induced depressive disorder, with onset during withdrawal. A separate diagnosis of the comorbid severe cocaine use disorder is not given. If the substance-induced depressive disorder occurs without a comorbid substance use disorder (e.g., after a one-time heavy use of the substance), no accompanying substance use disorder is noted (e.g., F16.94 phencyclidine-induced depressive disorder, with onset during intoxication). When more than one substance is judged to play a significant role in the development of depressive mood symptoms, each should be listed separately (e.g., F15.24 severe methylphenidate use disorder with methylphenidate-induced depressive disorder, with onset during withdrawal; F19.94 dexamethasone-induced depressive disorder, with onset during intoxication).

Depressive Disorder
Due to Another Medical Condition

A. A prominent and persistent disturbance in mood that predominates in the clinical picture and is characterized by depressed mood or markedly diminished interest or pleasure in all, or almost all, activities.

B. There is evidence from the history, physical examination, or laboratory findings that the disturbance is the direct pathophysiological consequence of another medical condition.

C. The disturbance is not better explained by another mental disorder (e.g., adjustment disorder, with depressed mood, in which the stressor is a serious medical condition).

D. The disturbance does not occur exclusively during the course of a delirium.

E. The disturbance causes clinically significant distress or impairment in social, occupational, or other important areas of functioning.

Coding note: The ICD-10-CM code depends on the specifier (see below).

Specify if:

> **F06.31 With depressive features:** Full criteria are not met for a major depressive episode.
>
> **F06.32 With major depressive–like episode:** Full criteria are met (except Criterion C) for a major depressive episode.
>
> **F06.34 With mixed features**: Symptoms of mania or hypomania are also present but do not predominate in the clinical picture.

Coding note: Include the name of the other medical condition in the name of the mental disorder (e.g., F06.31 depressive disorder due to hypothyroidism, with depressive features). The other medical condition should also be coded and listed separately immediately before the depressive disorder due to the medical condition (e.g., E03.9 hypothyroidism; F06.31 depressive disorder due to hypothyroidism, with depressive features).

Other Specified Depressive Disorder
F32.89

This category applies to presentations in which symptoms characteristic of a depressive disorder that cause clinically significant distress or impairment in social, occupational, or other important areas of functioning predominate but do not meet the full criteria for any of the disorders in the depressive disorders diagnostic class and do not meet criteria for adjustment disorder with depressed mood or adjustment disorder with mixed anxiety and depressed mood. The other specified depressive disorder category is used in situations in which the clinician chooses to communicate the specific reason that the presentation does not meet the criteria for any specific depressive disorder. This is done by recording "other specified depressive disorder" followed by the specific reason (e.g., "short-duration depressive episode").

Examples of presentations that can be specified using the "other specified" designation include the following:

1. **Recurrent brief depression:** Concurrent presence of depressed mood and at least four other symptoms of depression for 2–13 days

at least once per month (not associated with the menstrual cycle) for at least 12 consecutive months in an individual whose presentation has never met criteria for any other depressive or bipolar disorder and does not currently meet active or residual criteria for any psychotic disorder.

2. **Short-duration depressive episode (4–13 days):** Depressed affect and at least four of the other eight symptoms of a major depressive episode associated with clinically significant distress or impairment that persists for more than 4 days, but less than 14 days, in an individual whose presentation has never met criteria for any other depressive or bipolar disorder, does not currently meet active or residual criteria for any psychotic disorder, and does not meet criteria for recurrent brief depression.

3. **Depressive episode with insufficient symptoms:** Depressed affect and at least one of the other eight symptoms of a major depressive episode associated with clinically significant distress or impairment that persist for at least 2 weeks in an individual whose presentation has never met criteria for any other depressive or bipolar disorder, does not currently meet active or residual criteria for any psychotic disorder, and does not meet criteria for mixed anxiety and depressive disorder symptoms.

4. **Major depressive episode superimposed** on schizophrenia, schizophreniform disorder, delusional disorder, or other specified and unspecified schizophrenia spectrum and other psychotic disorder. **Note:** Major depressive episodes that are part of schizoaffective disorder do not merit an additional diagnosis of other specified depressive disorder.

Unspecified Depressive Disorder

F32.A

This category applies to presentations in which symptoms characteristic of a depressive disorder that cause clinically significant distress or impairment in social, occupational, or other important areas of functioning predominate but do not meet the full criteria for any of the disorders in the depressive disorders diagnostic class and do not meet criteria for adjustment disorder with depressed mood or adjustment disorder with mixed anxiety and depressed mood. The unspecified depressive disorder category is used in situations in which the clinician chooses *not* to specify the reason that the criteria are not met for a specific depressive disorder, and includes presentations for which there is insufficient information to make a more specific diagnosis (e.g., in emergency room settings).

Unspecified Mood Disorder

F39

This category applies to presentations in which symptoms characteristic of a mood disorder that cause clinically significant distress or impairment in social, occupational, or other important areas of functioning predominate but do not at the time of the evaluation meet the full criteria for any of the disorders in either the bipolar or the depressive disorders diagnostic classes and in which it is difficult to choose between unspecified bipolar and related disorder and unspecified depressive disorder (e.g., acute agitation).

Specifiers for Depressive Disorders

Specify if:

With anxious distress: Anxious distress is defined as the presence of at least two of the following symptoms during the majority of days of the current major depressive episode (or the most recent major depressive episode if major depressive disorder is currently in partial or full remission) or current persistent depressive disorder:

1. Feeling keyed up or tense.
2. Feeling unusually restless.
3. Difficulty concentrating because of worry.
4. Fear that something awful may happen.
5. Feeling that the individual might lose control of himself or herself.

Specify current severity:

Mild: Two symptoms.
Moderate: Three symptoms.
Moderate-severe: Four or five symptoms.
Severe: Four or five symptoms and with motor agitation.

Note: Anxious distress has been noted as a prominent feature of both bipolar and major depressive disorder in both primary care and specialty mental health settings. High levels of anxiety have been associated with higher suicide risk, longer duration of illness, and greater likelihood of treatment nonresponse. As a result, it is clinically useful to specify accurately the presence and severity levels of anxious distress for treatment planning and monitoring of response to treatment.

With mixed features:

A. At least three of the following manic/hypomanic symptoms are present during the majority of days of the current major depressive episode (or the most recent major depressive episode if major depressive disorder is currently in partial or full remission):

   1. Elevated, expansive mood.
   2. Inflated self-esteem or grandiosity.
   3. More talkative than usual or pressure to keep talking.
   4. Flight of ideas or subjective experience that thoughts are racing.
   5. Increase in energy or goal-directed activity (either socially, at work or school, or sexually).
   6. Increased or excessive involvement in activities that have a high potential for painful consequences (e.g., engaging in unrestrained buying sprees, sexual indiscretions, or foolish business investments).
   7. Decreased need for sleep (feeling rested despite sleeping less than usual; to be contrasted with insomnia).

B. Mixed symptoms are observable by others and represent a change from the person's usual behavior.
C. For individuals whose symptoms meet full criteria for either mania or hypomania, the diagnosis should be bipolar I or bipolar II disorder.
D. The mixed symptoms are not attributable to the physiological effects of a substance (e.g., a drug of abuse, a medication or other treatment).

   Note: Mixed features associated with a major depressive episode have been found to be a significant risk factor for the development of bipolar I or bipolar II disorder. As a result, it is clinically useful to note the presence of this specifier for treatment planning and monitoring of response to treatment.

With melancholic features:

A. One of the following is present during the most severe period of the current major depressive episode (or the most recent major depressive episode if major depressive disorder is currently in partial or full remission):

   1. Loss of pleasure in all, or almost all, activities.
   2. Lack of reactivity to usually pleasurable stimuli (does not feel much better, even temporarily, when something good happens).

B. Three (or more) of the following:

   1. A distinct quality of depressed mood characterized by profound despondency, despair, and/or moroseness or by so-called empty mood.
   2. Depression that is regularly worse in the morning.
   3. Early-morning awakening (i.e., at least 2 hours before usual awakening).
   4. Marked psychomotor agitation or retardation.
   5. Significant anorexia or weight loss.
   6. Excessive or inappropriate guilt.

Note: The specifier "with melancholic features" is applied if these features are present at the most severe stage of the episode. There is a near-complete absence of the capacity for pleasure, not merely a diminution. A guideline for evaluating the lack of reactivity of mood is that even highly desired events are not associated with marked brightening of mood. Either mood does not brighten at all, or it brightens only partially (e.g., up to 20%–40% of normal for only minutes at a time). The "distinct quality" of mood that is characteristic of the "with melancholic features" specifier is experienced as qualitatively different from that during a nonmelancholic depressive episode. A depressed mood that is described as merely more severe, longer lasting, or present without a reason is not considered distinct in quality. Psychomotor changes are nearly always present and are observable by others.

Melancholic features exhibit only a modest tendency to repeat across episodes in the same individual. They are more frequent in inpatients, as opposed to outpatients; are less likely to occur in milder than in more severe major depressive episodes; and are more likely to occur in individuals with psychotic features.

With atypical features: This specifier is applied when these features predominate during the majority of days of the current major depressive episode (or the most recent major depressive episode if major depressive disorder is currently in partial or full remission) or current persistent depressive disorder.

A. Mood reactivity (i.e., mood brightens in response to actual or potential positive events).
B. Two (or more) of the following:
    1. Significant weight gain or increase in appetite.
    2. Hypersomnia.
    3. Leaden paralysis (i.e., heavy, leaden feelings in arms or legs).
    4. A long-standing pattern of interpersonal rejection sensitivity (not limited to episodes of mood disturbance) that results in significant social or occupational impairment.
C. Criteria are not met for "with melancholic features" or "with catatonia" during the same episode.

Note: "Atypical depression" has historical significance (i.e., atypical in contradistinction to the more classical agitated, "endogenous" presentations of depression that were the norm when depression was rarely diagnosed in outpatients and almost never in adolescents or younger adults) and today does not connote an uncommon or unusual clinical presentation as the term might imply.

Mood reactivity is the capacity to be cheered up when presented with positive events (e.g., a visit from children, compliments from others). Mood may become euthymic (not sad) even for extended periods of time if the external circumstances remain favorable. Increased appetite may be manifested by an obvious increase in food intake or by weight gain. Hypersomnia may include either an extended period of nighttime sleep or daytime napping that totals at least 10 hours of sleep per day (or at least 2 hours more than when not depressed). Leaden paralysis is defined as feeling heavy, leaden, or weighted down, usually in the arms or legs. This sensation is generally present for at least an hour a day but often lasts for many hours at a time. Unlike the other atypical features, pathological sensitivity to perceived interpersonal rejection is a trait that has an early onset and persists throughout most of adult life. Rejection sensitivity occurs when the person is and is not depressed, though it may be exacerbated during depressive periods.

With psychotic features: Delusions and/or hallucinations are present at any time in the current major depressive episode (or the most recent major depressive episode if major depressive disorder is currently in partial or full remission). If psychotic features are present, *specify* if mood-congruent or mood-incongruent.

> **With mood-congruent psychotic features:** The content of all delusions and hallucinations is consistent with the typical depressive themes of personal inadequacy, guilt, disease, death, nihilism, or deserved punishment.
> **With mood-incongruent psychotic features:** The content of the delusions or hallucinations does not involve typical depressive themes of personal inadequacy, guilt, disease, death, nihilism, or deserved punishment, or the content is a mixture of mood-incongruent and mood-congruent themes.

With catatonia: This specifier is applied to the current major depressive episode (or the most recent major depressive episode if major depressive disorder is currently in partial or full remission) if catatonic features are present during most of the episode. See criteria for catatonia associated with a mental disorder in the chapter "Schizophrenia Spectrum and Other Psychotic Disorders."

With peripartum onset: This specifier is applied to the current major depressive episode (or the most recent major depressive episode if major depressive disorder is currently in partial or full remission) if onset of mood symptoms occurs during pregnancy or in the 4 weeks following delivery.

> **Note:** Mood episodes can have their onset either during pregnancy or postpartum. About 50% of postpartum major depressive episodes begin prior to delivery. Thus, these episodes are referred to collectively as *peripartum* episodes.
> Between conception and birth, about 9% of women will experience a major depressive episode. The best estimate for prevalence of a major depressive episode between birth and 12 months postpartum is just below 7%.
> Peripartum-onset mood episodes can present either with or without psychotic features. Infanticide (a rare occurrence) is most often associated with postpartum psychotic episodes that are characterized by command hallucinations to kill the infant or delusions that the infant is possessed, but psychotic symptoms

can also occur in severe postpartum mood episodes without such specific delusions or hallucinations.

Postpartum mood (major depressive or manic) episodes with psychotic features appear to occur in from 1 in 500 to 1 in 1,000 deliveries and may be more common in primiparous women. The risk of postpartum episodes with psychotic features is particularly increased for women with prior postpartum psychotic mood episodes but is also elevated for those with a prior history of a depressive or bipolar disorder (especially bipolar I disorder) and those with a family history of bipolar disorders.

Once a woman has had a postpartum episode with psychotic features, the risk of recurrence with each subsequent delivery is between 30% and 50%. Postpartum episodes must be differentiated from delirium occurring in the postpartum period, which is distinguished by a fluctuating level of awareness or attention.

Peripartum-onset depressive disorders must be distinguished from the much more common "maternity blues," or what is known in lay terms as "baby blues." Maternity blues is not considered to be a mental disorder and is characterized by sudden changes in mood (e.g., the sudden onset of tearfulness in the absence of depression) that do not cause functional impairment and that are likely caused by physiological changes occurring after delivery. It is temporary and self-limited, typically improving quickly (within a week) without the need for treatment. Other symptoms of maternity blues include sleep disturbance and even confusion that can occur shortly after delivery.

Perinatal women may be at higher risk for depressive disorders due to thyroid abnormalities as well as other medical conditions that can cause depressive symptoms. If the depressive symptoms are judged to be due to another medical condition related to the perinatal period, depressive disorder due to another medical condition should be diagnosed instead of a major depressive episode, with peripartum onset.

With seasonal pattern: This specifier applies to recurrent major depressive disorder.

A. There has been a regular temporal relationship between the onset of major depressive episodes in major depressive disorder and a particular time of the year (e.g., in the fall or winter).
    Note: Do not include cases in which there is an obvious effect of seasonally related psychosocial stressors (e.g., regularly being unemployed every winter).
B. Full remissions also occur at a characteristic time of the year (e.g., depression disappears in the spring).
C. In the last 2 years, two major depressive episodes have occurred that demonstrate the temporal seasonal relationships defined above and no nonseasonal major depressive episodes have occurred during that same period.

D. Seasonal major depressive episodes (as described above) substantially outnumber the nonseasonal major depressive episodes that may have occurred over the individual's lifetime.

Note: The specifier "with seasonal pattern" can apply to the pattern of major depressive episodes in major depressive disorder, recurrent. The essential feature is the onset and remission of major depressive episodes at characteristic times of the year. In most cases, the episodes begin in fall or winter and remit in spring. Less commonly, there may be recurrent summer depressive episodes. This pattern of onset and remission of episodes must have occurred during at least a 2-year period, without any nonseasonal episodes occurring during this period. In addition, the seasonal depressive episodes must substantially outnumber any nonseasonal depressive episodes over the individual's lifetime.

This specifier does not apply to those situations in which the pattern is better explained by seasonally linked psychosocial stressors (e.g., seasonal unemployment or school schedule). Major depressive episodes that occur in a seasonal pattern are often characterized by loss of energy, hypersomnia, overeating, weight gain, and a craving for carbohydrates.

The prevalence of winter-type seasonal pattern appears to vary with latitude, age, and sex. Prevalence increases with higher latitudes. Age is also a strong predictor of seasonality, with younger persons at higher risk for winter depressive episodes.

Specify if:

In partial remission: Symptoms of the immediately previous major depressive episode are present but full criteria are not met, or there is a period lasting less than 2 months without any significant symptoms of a major depressive episode following the end of such an episode.

In full remission: During the past 2 months, no significant signs or symptoms of the disturbance were present.

Specify current severity:

Severity is based on the number of criterion symptoms, the severity of those symptoms, and the degree of functional disability.

Mild: Few, if any, symptoms in excess of those required to make the diagnosis are present, the intensity of the symptoms is distressing but manageable, and the symptoms result in minor impairment in social or occupational functioning.

Moderate: The number of symptoms, intensity of symptoms, and/or functional impairment are between those specified for "mild" and "severe."

Severe: The number of symptoms is substantially in excess of that required to make the diagnosis, the intensity of the symptoms is seriously distressing and unmanageable, and the symptoms markedly interfere with social and occupational functioning.

Anxiety Disorders

Separation Anxiety Disorder

F93.0

A. Developmentally inappropriate and excessive fear or anxiety concerning separation from those to whom the individual is attached, as evidenced by at least three of the following:

1. Recurrent excessive distress when anticipating or experiencing separation from home or from major attachment figures.
2. Persistent and excessive worry about losing major attachment figures or about possible harm to them, such as illness, injury, disasters, or death.
3. Persistent and excessive worry about experiencing an untoward event (e.g., getting lost, being kidnapped, having an accident, becoming ill) that causes separation from a major attachment figure.
4. Persistent reluctance or refusal to go out, away from home, to school, to work, or elsewhere because of fear of separation.
5. Persistent and excessive fear of or reluctance about being alone or without major attachment figures at home or in other settings.
6. Persistent reluctance or refusal to sleep away from home or to go to sleep without being near a major attachment figure.
7. Repeated nightmares involving the theme of separation.
8. Repeated complaints of physical symptoms (e.g., headaches, stomachaches, nausea, vomiting) when separation from major attachment figures occurs or is anticipated.

B. The fear, anxiety, or avoidance is persistent, lasting at least 4 weeks in children and adolescents and typically 6 months or more in adults.

C. The disturbance causes clinically significant distress or impairment in social, academic, occupational, or other important areas of functioning.

D. The disturbance is not better explained by another mental disorder, such as refusing to leave home because of excessive resistance to change in autism spectrum disorder; delusions or hallucinations concerning separation in psychotic disorders; refusal to go outside without a trusted companion in agoraphobia; worries about ill health or other harm befalling significant others in generalized anxiety disorder; or concerns about having an illness in illness anxiety disorder.

Selective Mutism

F94.0

A. Consistent failure to speak in specific social situations in which there is an expectation for speaking (e.g., at school) despite speaking in other situations.

B. The disturbance interferes with educational or occupational achievement or with social communication.

C. The duration of the disturbance is at least 1 month (not limited to the first month of school).

D. The failure to speak is not attributable to a lack of knowledge of, or comfort with, the spoken language required in the social situation.

E. The disturbance is not better explained by a communication disorder (e.g., childhood-onset fluency disorder) and does not occur exclusively during the course of autism spectrum disorder, schizophrenia, or another psychotic disorder.

Specific Phobia

A. Marked fear or anxiety about a specific object or situation (e.g., flying, heights, animals, receiving an injection, seeing blood).

Note: In children, the fear or anxiety may be expressed by crying, tantrums, freezing, or clinging.

B. The phobic object or situation almost always provokes immediate fear or anxiety.

C. The phobic object or situation is actively avoided or endured with intense fear or anxiety.

D. The fear or anxiety is out of proportion to the actual danger posed by the specific object or situation and to the sociocultural context.

E. The fear, anxiety, or avoidance is persistent, typically lasting for 6 months or more.

F. The fear, anxiety, or avoidance causes clinically significant distress or impairment in social, occupational, or other important areas of functioning.

G. The disturbance is not better explained by the symptoms of another mental disorder, including fear, anxiety, and avoidance of situations associated with panic-like symptoms or other incapacitating symptoms (as in agoraphobia); objects or situations related to obsessions (as in obsessive-compulsive disorder); reminders of traumatic events (as in posttraumatic stress disorder); separation from home or attachment figures (as in separation anxiety disorder); or social situations (as in social anxiety disorder).

Specify if:

Code based on the phobic stimulus:

F40.218 Animal (e.g., spiders, insects, dogs)

F40.228 Natural environment (e.g., heights, storms, water)

F40.23x Blood-injection-injury (e.g., needles, invasive medical procedures)

> **Coding note:** Select specific ICD-10-CM code as follows: **F40.230** fear of blood; **F40.231** fear of injections and transfusions; **F40.232** fear of other medical care; or **F40.233** fear of injury.

F40.248 Situational (e.g., airplanes, elevators, enclosed places)

F40.298 Other (e.g., situations that may lead to choking or vomiting; in children, e.g., loud sounds or costumed characters)

Coding note. When more than one phobic stimulus is present, code all ICD-10-CM codes that apply (e.g., for fear of snakes and flying, F40.218 specific phobia, animal, and F40.248 specific phobia, situational).

Social Anxiety Disorder

F40.10

A. Marked fear or anxiety about one or more social situations in which the individual is exposed to possible scrutiny by others. Examples include social interactions (e.g., having a conversation, meeting unfamiliar people), being observed (e.g., eating or drinking), and performing in front of others (e.g., giving a speech).

   Note: In children, the anxiety must occur in peer settings and not just during interactions with adults.

B. The individual fears that he or she will act in a way or show anxiety symptoms that will be negatively evaluated (i.e., will be humiliating or embarrassing; will lead to rejection or offend others).

C. The social situations almost always provoke fear or anxiety.

   Note: In children, the fear or anxiety may be expressed by crying, tantrums, freezing, clinging, shrinking, or failing to speak in social situations.

D. The social situations are avoided or endured with intense fear or anxiety.

E. The fear or anxiety is out of proportion to the actual threat posed by the social situation and to the sociocultural context.

F. The fear, anxiety, or avoidance is persistent, typically lasting for 6 months or more.

G. The fear, anxiety, or avoidance causes clinically significant distress or impairment in social, occupational, or other important areas of functioning.

H. The fear, anxiety, or avoidance is not attributable to the physiolog-
    ical effects of a substance (e.g., a drug of abuse, a medication) or
    another medical condition.
I. The fear, anxiety, or avoidance is not better explained by the symp-
    toms of another mental disorder, such as panic disorder, body dys-
    morphic disorder, or autism spectrum disorder.
J. If another medical condition (e.g., Parkinson's disease, obesity,
    disfigurement from burns or injury) is present, the fear, anxiety, or
    avoidance is clearly unrelated or is excessive.

Specify if:
   Performance only: If the fear is restricted to speaking or performing in public.

Panic Disorder

F41.0

A. Recurrent unexpected panic attacks. A panic attack is an abrupt
    surge of intense fear or intense discomfort that reaches a peak
    within minutes, and during which time four (or more) of the follow-
    ing symptoms occur:

    Note: The abrupt surge can occur from a calm state or an anxious
    state.

    1. Palpitations, pounding heart, or accelerated heart rate.
    2. Sweating.
    3. Trembling or shaking.
    4. Sensations of shortness of breath or smothering.
    5. Feelings of choking.
    6. Chest pain or discomfort.
    7. Nausea or abdominal distress.
    8. Feeling dizzy, unsteady, light-headed, or faint.
    9. Chills or heat sensations.
   10. Paresthesias (numbness or tingling sensations).
   11. Derealization (feelings of unreality) or depersonalization
        (being detached from oneself).
   12. Fear of losing control or "going crazy."
   13. Fear of dying.

    Note: Culture-specific symptoms (e.g., tinnitus, neck soreness,
    headache, uncontrollable screaming or crying) may be seen. Such
    symptoms should not count as one of the four required symptoms.

B. At least one of the attacks has been followed by 1 month (or more)
    of one or both of the following:

    1. Persistent concern or worry about additional panic attacks or
        their consequences (e.g., losing control, having a heart at-
        tack, "going crazy").

2. A significant maladaptive change in behavior related to the attacks (e.g., behaviors designed to avoid having panic attacks, such as avoidance of exercise or unfamiliar situations).

C. The disturbance is not attributable to the physiological effects of a substance (e.g., a drug of abuse, a medication) or another medical condition (e.g., hyperthyroidism, cardiopulmonary disorders).

D. The disturbance is not better explained by another mental disorder (e.g., the panic attacks do not occur only in response to feared social situations, as in social anxiety disorder; in response to circumscribed phobic objects or situations, as in specific phobia; in response to obsessions, as in obsessive-compulsive disorder; in response to reminders of traumatic events, as in posttraumatic stress disorder; or in response to separation from attachment figures, as in separation anxiety disorder).

Panic Attack Specifier

Note: Symptoms are presented for the purpose of identifying a panic attack; however, panic attack is not a mental disorder and cannot be coded. Panic attacks can occur in the context of any anxiety disorder as well as other mental disorders (e.g., depressive disorders, posttraumatic stress disorder, substance use disorders) and some medical conditions (e.g., cardiac, respiratory, vestibular, gastrointestinal). When the presence of a panic attack is identified, it should be noted as a specifier (e.g., "posttraumatic stress disorder with panic attacks"). For panic disorder, the presence of panic attack is contained within the criteria for the disorder and panic attack is not used as a specifier.

An abrupt surge of intense fear or intense discomfort that reaches a peak within minutes, and during which time four (or more) of the following symptoms occur:

Note: The abrupt surge can occur from a calm state or an anxious state.

1. Palpitations, pounding heart, or accelerated heart rate.
2. Sweating.
3. Trembling or shaking.
4. Sensations of shortness of breath or smothering.
5. Feelings of choking.
6. Chest pain or discomfort.
7. Nausea or abdominal distress.
8. Feeling dizzy, unsteady, light-headed, or faint.
9. Chills or heat sensations.
10. Paresthesias (numbness or tingling sensations).
11. Derealization (feelings of unreality) or depersonalization (being detached from oneself).
12. Fear of losing control or "going crazy."
13. Fear of dying.

Note: Culture-specific symptoms (e.g., tinnitus, neck soreness, headache, uncontrollable screaming or crying) may be seen. Such symptoms should not count as one of the four required symptoms.

Agoraphobia

F40.00

A. Marked fear or anxiety about two (or more) of the following five situations:

1. Using public transportation (e.g., automobiles, buses, trains, ships, planes).
2. Being in open spaces (e.g., parking lots, marketplaces, bridges).
3. Being in enclosed places (e.g., shops, theaters, cinemas).
4. Standing in line or being in a crowd.
5. Being outside of the home alone.

B. The individual fears or avoids these situations because of thoughts that escape might be difficult or help might not be available in the event of developing panic-like symptoms or other incapacitating or embarrassing symptoms (e.g., fear of falling in the elderly; fear of incontinence).

C. The agoraphobic situations almost always provoke fear or anxiety.

D. The agoraphobic situations are actively avoided, require the presence of a companion, or are endured with intense fear or anxiety.

E. The fear or anxiety is out of proportion to the actual danger posed by the agoraphobic situations and to the sociocultural context.

F. The fear, anxiety, or avoidance is persistent, typically lasting for 6 months or more.

G. The fear, anxiety, or avoidance causes clinically significant distress or impairment in social, occupational, or other important areas of functioning.

H. If another medical condition (e.g., inflammatory bowel disease, Parkinson's disease) is present, the fear, anxiety, or avoidance is clearly excessive.

I. The fear, anxiety, or avoidance is not better explained by the symptoms of another mental disorder—for example, the symptoms are not confined to specific phobia, situational type; do not involve only social situations (as in social anxiety disorder); and are not related exclusively to obsessions (as in obsessive-compulsive disorder), perceived defects or flaws in physical appearance (as in body dysmorphic disorder), reminders of traumatic events (as in posttraumatic stress disorder), or fear of separation (as in separation anxiety disorder).

Note: Agoraphobia is diagnosed irrespective of the presence of panic disorder. If an individual's presentation meets criteria for panic disorder and agoraphobia, both diagnoses should be assigned.

Generalized Anxiety Disorder

F41.1

A. Excessive anxiety and worry (apprehensive expectation), occurring more days than not for at least 6 months, about a number of events or activities (such as work or school performance).
B. The individual finds it difficult to control the worry.
C. The anxiety and worry are associated with three (or more) of the following six symptoms (with at least some symptoms having been present for more days than not for the past 6 months):

Note: Only one item is required in children.

1. Restlessness or feeling keyed up or on edge.
2. Being easily fatigued.
3. Difficulty concentrating or mind going blank.
4. Irritability.
5. Muscle tension.
6. Sleep disturbance (difficulty falling or staying asleep, or restless, unsatisfying sleep).

D. The anxiety, worry, or physical symptoms cause clinically significant distress or impairment in social, occupational, or other important areas of functioning.
E. The disturbance is not attributable to the physiological effects of a substance (e.g., a drug of abuse, a medication) or another medical condition (e.g., hyperthyroidism).
F. The disturbance is not better explained by another mental disorder (e.g., anxiety or worry about having panic attacks in panic disorder, negative evaluation in social anxiety disorder, contamination or other obsessions in obsessive-compulsive disorder, separation from attachment figures in separation anxiety disorder, reminders of traumatic events in posttraumatic stress disorder, gaining weight in anorexia nervosa, physical complaints in somatic symptom disorder, perceived appearance flaws in body dysmorphic disorder, having a serious illness in illness anxiety disorder, or the content of delusional beliefs in schizophrenia or delusional disorder).

Substance/Medication-Induced Anxiety Disorder

A. Panic attacks or anxiety is predominant in the clinical picture.
B. There is evidence from the history, physical examination, or laboratory findings of both (1) and (2):

1. The symptoms in Criterion A developed during or soon after substance intoxication or withdrawal or after exposure to or withdrawal from a medication.
2. The involved substance/medication is capable of producing the symptoms in Criterion A.

C. The disturbance is not better explained by an anxiety disorder that is not substance/medication-induced. Such evidence of an independent anxiety disorder could include the following:

>   The symptoms precede the onset of the substance/medication use; the symptoms persist for a substantial period of time (e.g., about 1 month) after the cessation of acute withdrawal or severe intoxication; or there is other evidence suggesting the existence of an independent non-substance/medication-induced anxiety disorder (e.g., a history of recurrent non-substance/medication-related episodes).

D. The disturbance does not occur exclusively during the course of a delirium.

E. The disturbance causes clinically significant distress or impairment in social, occupational, or other important areas of functioning.

Note: This diagnosis should be made instead of a diagnosis of substance intoxication or substance withdrawal only when the symptoms in Criterion A predominate in the clinical picture and they are sufficiently severe to warrant clinical attention.

Coding note: The ICD-10-CM codes for the [specific substance/medication]-induced anxiety disorders are indicated in the table below. Note that the ICD-10-CM code depends on whether or not there is a comorbid substance use disorder present for the same class of substance. In any case, an additional separate diagnosis of a substance use disorder is not given. If a mild substance use disorder is comorbid with the substance-induced anxiety disorder, the 4th position character is "1," and the clinician should record "mild [substance] use disorder" before the substance-induced anxiety disorder (e.g., "mild cocaine use disorder with cocaine-induced anxiety disorder"). If a moderate or severe substance use disorder is comorbid with the substance-induced anxiety disorder, the 4th position character is "2," and the clinician should record "moderate [substance] use disorder" or "severe [substance] use disorder," depending on the severity of the comorbid substance use disorder. If there is no comorbid substance use disorder (e.g., after a one-time heavy use of the substance), then the 4th position character is "9," and the clinician should record only the substance-induced anxiety disorder.

	ICD-10-CM		
	With mild use disorder	With moderate or severe use disorder	Without use disorder
Alcohol	F10.180	F10.280	F10.980
Caffeine	NA	NA	F15.980
Cannabis	F12.180	F12.280	F12.980

	ICD-10-CM		
	With mild use disorder	With moderate or severe use disorder	Without use disorder
Phencyclidine	F16.180	F16.280	F16.980
Other hallucinogen	F16.180	F16.280	F16.980
Inhalant	F18.180	F18.280	F18.980
Opioid	F11.188	F11.288	F11.988
Sedative, hypnotic, or anxiolytic	F13.180	F13.280	F13.980
Amphetamine-type substance (or other stimulant)	F15.180	F15.280	F15.980
Cocaine	F14.180	F14.280	F14.980
Other (or unknown) substance	F19.180	F19.280	F19.980

Specify (see Table 1 in the chapter "Substance-Related and Addictive Disorders," which indicates whether "with onset during intoxication" and/or "with onset during withdrawal" applies to a given substance class; or *specify* "with onset after medication use"):

With onset during intoxication: If criteria are met for intoxication with the substance and the symptoms develop during intoxication.

With onset during withdrawal: If criteria are met for withdrawal from the substance and the symptoms develop during, or shortly after, withdrawal.

With onset after medication use: If symptoms developed at initiation of medication, with a change in use of medication, or during withdrawal of medication.

Recording Procedures

The name of the substance/medication-induced anxiety disorder begins with the specific substance (e.g., cocaine, salbutamol) that is presumed to be causing the anxiety symptoms. The diagnostic code is selected from the table included in the criteria set, which is based on the drug class and presence or absence of a comorbid substance use disorder. For substances that do not fit into any of the classes (e.g., salbutamol), the code for "other (or unknown) substance" should be used; and in cases in which a substance is judged to be an etiological factor but the specific class of substance is unknown, the same code should also be used.

To record the name of the disorder, the comorbid substance use disorder (if any) is listed first, followed by "with substance/medication-

induced anxiety disorder" (incorporating the name of the specific etiological substance/medication), followed by the specification of onset
(i.e., onset during intoxication, onset during withdrawal, with onset
after medication use). For example, in the case of anxiety symptoms
occurring during withdrawal in a man with a severe lorazepam use
disorder, the diagnosis is F13.280 severe lorazepam use disorder with
lorazepam-induced anxiety disorder, with onset during withdrawal. A
separate diagnosis of the comorbid severe lorazepam use disorder is
not given. If the substance-induced anxiety disorder occurs without a
comorbid substance use disorder (e.g., after a one-time heavy use of
the substance), no accompanying substance use disorder is noted (e.g.,
F16.980 psilocybin-induced anxiety disorder, with onset during intoxication). When more than one substance is judged to play a significant
role in the development of anxiety symptoms, each should be listed separately (e.g., F15.280 severe methylphenidate use disorder with methylphenidate-induced anxiety disorder, with onset during intoxication;
F19.980 salbutamol-induced anxiety disorder, with onset after medication use).

Anxiety Disorder Due to Another Medical Condition

F06.4

A. Panic attacks or anxiety is predominant in the clinical picture.
B. There is evidence from the history, physical examination, or laboratory findings that the disturbance is the direct pathophysiological consequence of another medical condition.
C. The disturbance is not better explained by another mental disorder.
D. The disturbance does not occur exclusively during the course of
   a delirium.
E. The disturbance causes clinically significant distress or impairment
   in social, occupational, or other important areas of functioning.

Coding note: Include the name of the other medical condition within
the name of the mental disorder (e.g., F06.4 anxiety disorder due to
pheochromocytoma). The other medical condition should be coded and
listed separately immediately before the anxiety disorder due to the
medical condition (e.g., D35.00 pheochromocytoma; F06.4 anxiety disorder due to pheochromocytoma).

Other Specified Anxiety Disorder

F41.8

This category applies to presentations in which symptoms characteristic of an anxiety disorder that cause clinically significant distress or
impairment in social, occupational, or other important areas of functioning predominate but do not meet the full criteria for any of the disor-

ders in the anxiety disorders diagnostic class, and do not meet criteria for adjustment disorder with anxiety or adjustment disorder with mixed anxiety and depressed mood. The other specified anxiety disorder category is used in situations in which the clinician chooses to communicate the specific reason that the presentation does not meet the criteria for any specific anxiety disorder. This is done by recording "other specified anxiety disorder" followed by the specific reason (e.g., "generalized anxiety occurring less often than 'more days than not'").

Examples of presentations that can be specified using the "other specified" designation include the following:

1. **Limited-symptom attacks.**
2. **Generalized anxiety occurring less often than "more days than not."**
3. *Khyâl cap* **(wind attacks):** See "Culture and Psychiatric Diagnosis" in Section III of DSM-5-TR.
4. *Ataque de nervios* **(attack of nerves):** See "Culture and Psychiatric Diagnosis" in Section III of DSM-5-TR.

Unspecified Anxiety Disorder

F41.9

This category applies to presentations in which symptoms characteristic of an anxiety disorder that cause clinically significant distress or impairment in social, occupational, or other important areas of functioning predominate but do not meet the full criteria for any of the disorders in the anxiety disorders diagnostic class, and do not meet criteria for adjustment disorder with anxiety or adjustment disorder with mixed anxiety and depressed mood. The unspecified anxiety disorder category is used in situations in which the clinician chooses *not* to specify the reason that the criteria are not met for a specific anxiety disorder and includes presentations in which there is insufficient information to make a more specific diagnosis (e.g., in emergency room settings).

Obsessive-Compulsive and Related Disorders

Obsessive-Compulsive Disorder

F42.2

A. Presence of obsessions, compulsions, or both:

Obsessions are defined by (1) and (2):

1. Recurrent and persistent thoughts, urges, or images that are experienced, at some time during the disturbance, as intrusive and unwanted, and that in most individuals cause marked anxiety or distress.
2. The individual attempts to ignore or suppress such thoughts, urges, or images, or to neutralize them with some other thought or action (i.e., by performing a compulsion).

Compulsions are defined by (1) and (2):

1. Repetitive behaviors (e.g., hand washing, ordering, checking) or mental acts (e.g., praying, counting, repeating words silently) that the individual feels driven to perform in response to an obsession or according to rules that must be applied rigidly.
2. The behaviors or mental acts are aimed at preventing or reducing anxiety or distress, or preventing some dreaded event or situation; however, these behaviors or mental acts are not connected in a realistic way with what they are designed to neutralize or prevent, or are clearly excessive.

   Note: Young children may not be able to articulate the aims of these behaviors or mental acts.

B. The obsessions or compulsions are time-consuming (e.g., take more than 1 hour per day) or cause clinically significant distress or impairment in social, occupational, or other important areas of functioning.

C. The obsessive-compulsive symptoms are not attributable to the physiological effects of a substance (e.g., a drug of abuse, a medication) or another medical condition.

D. The disturbance is not better explained by the symptoms of another mental disorder (e.g., excessive worries, as in generalized anxiety disorder; preoccupation with appearance, as in body dysmorphic disorder; difficulty discarding or parting with possessions, as in hoarding disorder; hair pulling, as in trichotillomania [hair-pulling disorder]; skin picking, as in excoriation [skin-picking] disorder; stereotypies, as in stereotypic movement disorder; ritualized eating behavior, as in eating disorders; preoccupation with substances or gambling, as in substance-related and addictive disorders; preoccupation with having an illness, as in illness anxiety disorder; sexual urges or fantasies, as in paraphilic disorders; impulses, as in disruptive, impulse-control, and conduct disorders; guilty ruminations, as in major depressive disorder; thought insertion or delusional preoccupations, as in schizophrenia spectrum and other psychotic disorders; or repetitive patterns of behavior, as in autism spectrum disorder).

Specify if:

With good or fair insight: The individual recognizes that obsessive-compulsive disorder beliefs are definitely or probably not true or that they may or may not be true.
With poor insight: The individual thinks obsessive-compulsive disorder beliefs are probably true.
With absent insight/delusional beliefs: The individual is completely convinced that obsessive-compulsive disorder beliefs are true.

Specify if:

Tic-related: The individual has a current or past history of a tic disorder.

Body Dysmorphic Disorder

F45.22

A. Preoccupation with one or more perceived defects or flaws in physical appearance that are not observable or appear slight to others.
B. At some point during the course of the disorder, the individual has performed repetitive behaviors (e.g., mirror checking, excessive grooming, skin picking, reassurance seeking) or mental acts (e.g., comparing his or her appearance with that of others) in response to the appearance concerns.
C. The preoccupation causes clinically significant distress or impairment in social, occupational, or other important areas of functioning.
D. The appearance preoccupation is not better explained by concerns with body fat or weight in an individual whose symptoms meet diagnostic criteria for an eating disorder.

Specify if:

With muscle dysmorphia: The individual is preoccupied with the idea that his or her body build is too small or insufficiently muscular. This specifier is used even if the individual is preoccupied with other body areas, which is often the case.

Specify if:

Indicate degree of insight regarding body dysmorphic disorder beliefs (e.g., "I look ugly" or "I look deformed").

With good or fair insight: The individual recognizes that the body dysmorphic disorder beliefs are definitely or probably not true or that they may or may not be true.
With poor insight: The individual thinks that the body dysmorphic disorder beliefs are probably true.
With absent insight/delusional beliefs: The individual is completely convinced that the body dysmorphic disorder beliefs are true.

Hoarding Disorder

F42.3

A. Persistent difficulty discarding or parting with possessions, regardless of their actual value.
B. This difficulty is due to a perceived need to save the items and to distress associated with discarding them.
C. The difficulty discarding possessions results in the accumulation of possessions that congest and clutter active living areas and substantially compromises their intended use. If living areas are uncluttered, it is only because of the interventions of third parties (e.g., family members, cleaners, authorities).
D. The hoarding causes clinically significant distress or impairment in social, occupational, or other important areas of functioning (including maintaining a safe environment for self and others).
E. The hoarding is not attributable to another medical condition (e.g., brain injury, cerebrovascular disease, Prader-Willi syndrome).
F. The hoarding is not better explained by the symptoms of another mental disorder (e.g., obsessions in obsessive-compulsive disorder, decreased energy in major depressive disorder, delusions in schizophrenia or another psychotic disorder, cognitive deficits in major neurocognitive disorder, restricted interests in autism spectrum disorder).

Specify if:
With excessive acquisition: If difficulty discarding possessions is accompanied by excessive acquisition of items that are not needed or for which there is no available space.

Specify if:
With good or fair insight: The individual recognizes that hoarding-related beliefs and behaviors (pertaining to difficulty discarding items, clutter, or excessive acquisition) are problematic.
With poor insight: The individual is mostly convinced that hoarding-related beliefs and behaviors (pertaining to difficulty discarding items, clutter, or excessive acquisition) are not problematic despite evidence to the contrary.

With absent insight/delusional beliefs: The individual is completely convinced that hoarding-related beliefs and behaviors (pertaining to difficulty discarding items, clutter, or excessive acquisition) are not problematic despite evidence to the contrary.

Trichotillomania (Hair-Pulling Disorder)

F63.3

A. Recurrent pulling out of one's hair, resulting in hair loss.
B. Repeated attempts to decrease or stop hair pulling.
C. The hair pulling causes clinically significant distress or impairment in social, occupational, or other important areas of functioning.
D. The hair pulling or hair loss is not attributable to another medical condition (e.g., a dermatological condition).
E. The hair pulling is not better explained by the symptoms of another mental disorder (e.g., attempts to improve a perceived defect or flaw in appearance in body dysmorphic disorder).

Excoriation (Skin-Picking) Disorder

F42.4

A. Recurrent skin picking resulting in skin lesions.
B. Repeated attempts to decrease or stop skin picking.
C. The skin picking causes clinically significant distress or impairment in social, occupational, or other important areas of functioning.
D. The skin picking is not attributable to the physiological effects of a substance (e.g., cocaine) or another medical condition (e.g., scabies).
E. The skin picking is not better explained by symptoms of another mental disorder (e.g., delusions or tactile hallucinations in a psychotic disorder, attempts to improve a perceived defect or flaw in appearance in body dysmorphic disorder, stereotypies in stereotypic movement disorder, or intention to harm oneself in nonsuicidal self-injury).

Substance/Medication-Induced
Obsessive-Compulsive and Related Disorder

A. Obsessions, compulsions, skin picking, hair pulling, other body-focused repetitive behaviors, or other symptoms characteristic of the obsessive-compulsive and related disorders predominate in the clinical picture.
B. There is evidence from the history, physical examination, or laboratory findings of both (1) and (2):

1. The symptoms in Criterion A developed during or soon after substance intoxication or withdrawal or after exposure to or withdrawal from a medication.
2. The involved substance/medication is capable of producing the symptoms in Criterion A.

C. The disturbance is not better explained by an obsessive-compulsive and related disorder that is not substance/medication-induced. Such evidence of an independent obsessive-compulsive and related disorder could include the following:

> The symptoms precede the onset of the substance/medication use; the symptoms persist for a substantial period of time (e.g., about 1 month) after the cessation of acute withdrawal or severe intoxication; or there is other evidence suggesting the existence of an independent non-substance/medication-induced obsessive-compulsive and related disorder (e.g., a history of recurrent non-substance/medication-related episodes).

D. The disturbance does not occur exclusively during the course of a delirium.
E. The disturbance causes clinically significant distress or impairment in social, occupational, or other important areas of functioning.

Note: This diagnosis should be made in addition to a diagnosis of substance intoxication or substance withdrawal only when the symptoms in Criterion A predominate in the clinical picture and are sufficiently severe to warrant clinical attention.

Coding note: The ICD-10-CM codes for the [specific substance/medication]-induced obsessive-compulsive and related disorders are indicated in the table below. Note that the ICD-10-CM code depends on whether or not there is a comorbid substance use disorder present for the same class of substance. In any case, an additional separate diagnosis of a substance use disorder is not given. If a mild substance use disorder is comorbid with the substance-induced obsessive-compulsive and related disorder, the 4th position character is "1," and the clinician should record "mild [substance] use disorder" before the substance-induced obsessive-compulsive and related disorder (e.g., "mild cocaine use disorder with cocaine-induced obsessive-compulsive and related disorder"). If a moderate or severe substance use disorder is comorbid with the substance-induced obsessive-compulsive and related disorder, the 4th position character is "2," and the clinician should record "moderate [substance] use disorder" or "severe [substance] use disorder," depending on the severity of the comorbid substance use disorder. If there is no comorbid substance use disorder (e.g., after a one-time heavy use of the substance), then the 4th position character is "9," and the clinician should record only the substance-induced obsessive-compulsive and related disorder.

	ICD-10-CM		
	With mild use disorder	With moderate or severe use disorder	Without use disorder
Amphetamine-type substance (or other stimulant)	F15.188	F15.288	F15.988
Cocaine	F14.188	F14.288	F14.988
Other (or unknown) substance	F19.188	F19.288	F19.988

Specify (see Table 1 in the chapter "Substance-Related and Addictive Disorders," which indicates whether "with onset during intoxication" and/ or "with onset during withdrawal" applies to a given substance class; or *specify* "with onset after medication use"):

With onset during intoxication: If criteria are met for intoxication with the substance and the symptoms develop during intoxication.
With onset during withdrawal: If criteria are met for withdrawal from the substance and the symptoms develop during, or shortly after, withdrawal.
With onset after medication use: If symptoms developed at initiation of medication, with a change in use of medication, or during withdrawal of medication.

Recording Procedures

The name of the substance/medication-induced obsessive-compulsive and related disorder begins with the specific substance (e.g., cocaine) that is presumed to be causing the obsessive-compulsive and related symptoms. The diagnostic code is selected from the table included in the criteria set, which is based on the drug class and presence or absence of a comorbid substance use disorder. For substances that do not fit into any of the classes (e.g., ropinirole), the code for "other (or unknown) substance" should be used; and in cases in which a substance is judged to be an etiological factor but the specific class of substance is unknown, the same code should also be used.

To record the name of the disorder, the comorbid substance use disorder (if any) is listed first, followed by "with substance/medication-induced obsessive-compulsive and related disorder" (incorporating the name of the specific etiological substance/medication), followed by the specification of onset (i.e., onset during intoxication, onset during withdrawal, with onset after medication use). For example, in the case of repetitive skin-picking occurring during intoxication in a man with a severe cocaine use disorder, the diagnosis is F14.288 severe cocaine use disorder with cocaine-induced obsessive-compulsive and related disorder, with onset during intoxication. A separate diagnosis of the comorbid severe cocaine use disorder is not given. If the substance-induced obsessive-compulsive and related disorder occurs without a comorbid substance use disorder (e.g., after a one-time heavy use of the substance), no accompanying substance use disorder is noted (e.g., F15.988 amphetamine-induced obsessive-compulsive and related disorder, with onset during intoxication). When more than one substance is judged to play a significant role in the development of the obsessive-compulsive and related disorder, each should be listed separately.

Obsessive-Compulsive and Related Disorder Due to Another Medical Condition

F06.8

A. Obsessions, compulsions, preoccupations with appearance, hoarding, skin picking, hair pulling, other body-focused repetitive behaviors, or other symptoms characteristic of obsessive-compulsive and related disorder predominate in the clinical picture.

B. There is evidence from the history, physical examination, or laboratory findings that the disturbance is the direct pathophysiological consequence of another medical condition.

C. The disturbance is not better explained by another mental disorder.

D. The disturbance does not occur exclusively during the course of a delirium.

E. The disturbance causes clinically significant distress or impairment in social, occupational, or other important areas of functioning.

Specify if:

With obsessive-compulsive disorder–like symptoms: If obsessive-compulsive disorder–like symptoms predominate in the clinical presentation.

With appearance preoccupations: If preoccupation with perceived appearance defects or flaws predominates in the clinical presentation.

With hoarding symptoms: If hoarding predominates in the clinical presentation.

With hair-pulling symptoms: If hair pulling predominates in the clinical presentation.

With skin-picking symptoms: If skin picking predominates in the clinical presentation.

Coding note: Include the name of the other medical condition in the name of the mental disorder (e.g., F06.8 obsessive-compulsive and related disorder due to cerebral infarction). The other medical condition should be coded and listed separately immediately before the obsessive-compulsive and related disorder due to the medical condition (e.g., I69.398 cerebral infarction; F06.8 obsessive-compulsive and related disorder due to cerebral infarction).

Other Specified Obsessive-Compulsive and Related Disorder

F42.8

This category applies to presentations in which symptoms characteristic of an obsessive-compulsive and related disorder that cause clinically significant distress or impairment in social, occupational, or other important areas of functioning predominate but do not meet the full criteria for any of the disorders in the obsessive-compulsive and related disorders diagnostic class. The other specified obsessive-compulsive and related disorder category is used in situations in which the clinician chooses to communicate the specific reason that the presentation does not meet the criteria for any specific obsessive-compulsive and related disorder. This is done by recording "other specified obsessive-compulsive and related disorder" followed by the specific reason (e.g., "obsessional jealousy").

Examples of presentations that can be specified using the "other specified" designation include the following:

1. **Body dysmorphic–like disorder with actual flaws:** This is similar to body dysmorphic disorder except that the defects or flaws in physical appearance are clearly observable by others (i.e., they are more noticeable than "slight"). In such cases, the preoccupation with these flaws is clearly excessive and causes significant impairment or distress.

2. **Body dysmorphic–like disorder without repetitive behaviors:** Presentations that meet body dysmorphic disorder except that the individual has never performed repetitive behaviors or mental acts in response to the appearance concerns.

3. **Other body-focused repetitive behavior disorder:** Presentations involving recurrent body-focused repetitive behaviors other than hair pulling and skin picking (e.g., nail biting, lip biting, cheek chewing) that are accompanied by repeated attempts to decrease or stop the behaviors and that cause clinically significant distress or impairment in social, occupational, or other important areas of functioning.

4. **Obsessional jealousy:** This is characterized by nondelusional preoccupation with a partner's perceived infidelity. The preoccupations may lead to repetitive behaviors or mental acts in response to the infidelity concerns; they cause clinically significant distress or impairment in social, occupational, or other important areas of functioning; and they are not better explained by another mental disorder such as delusional disorder, jealous type, or paranoid personality disorder.

5. **Olfactory reference disorder (olfactory reference syndrome):** This is characterized by the individual's persistent preoccupation with the belief that he or she emits a foul or offensive body odor that is unnoticeable or only slightly noticeable to others; in response to this preoccupation, these individuals often engage in repetitive and excessive behaviors such as repeatedly checking for body odor,

excessive showering, or seeking reassurance, as well as excessive attempts to camouflage the perceived odor. These symptoms cause clinically significant distress or impairment in social, occupational, or other important areas of functioning. In traditional Japanese psychiatry, this disorder is known as *jikoshu-kyofu*, a variant of *taijin kyofusho* (see "Culture and Psychiatric Diagnosis" in Section III of DSM-5-TR).

6. ***Shubo-kyofu:*** A variant of *taijin kyofusho* (see "Culture and Psychiatric Diagnosis" in Section III of DSM-5-TR) that is similar to body dysmorphic disorder and is characterized by excessive fear of having a bodily deformity.

7. ***Koro:*** Related to *dhat syndrome* (see "Culture and Psychiatric Diagnosis" in Section III of DSM-5-TR), an episode of sudden and intense anxiety that the penis in males (or the vulva and nipples in females) will recede into the body, possibly leading to death.

Unspecified Obsessive-Compulsive and Related Disorder

F42.9

This category applies to presentations in which symptoms characteristic of an obsessive-compulsive and related disorder that cause clinically significant distress or impairment in social, occupational, or other important areas of functioning predominate but do not meet the full criteria for any of the disorders in the obsessive-compulsive and related disorders diagnostic class. The unspecified obsessive-compulsive and related disorder category is used in situations in which the clinician chooses *not* to specify the reason that the criteria are not met for a specific obsessive-compulsive and related disorder and includes presentations in which there is insufficient information to make a more specific diagnosis (e.g., in emergency room settings).

Trauma- and Stressor-Related Disorders

Reactive Attachment Disorder

F94.1

A. A consistent pattern of inhibited, emotionally withdrawn behavior toward adult caregivers, manifested by both of the following:

1. The child rarely or minimally seeks comfort when distressed.
2. The child rarely or minimally responds to comfort when distressed.

B. A persistent social and emotional disturbance characterized by at least two of the following:

1. Minimal social and emotional responsiveness to others.
2. Limited positive affect.
3. Episodes of unexplained irritability, sadness, or fearfulness that are evident even during nonthreatening interactions with adult caregivers.

C. The child has experienced a pattern of extremes of insufficient care as evidenced by at least one of the following:

1. Social neglect or deprivation in the form of persistent lack of having basic emotional needs for comfort, stimulation, and affection met by caregiving adults.
2. Repeated changes of primary caregivers that limit opportunities to form stable attachments (e.g., frequent changes in foster care).
3. Rearing in unusual settings that severely limit opportunities to form selective attachments (e.g., institutions with high child-to-caregiver ratios).

D. The care in Criterion C is presumed to be responsible for the disturbed behavior in Criterion A (e.g., the disturbances in Criterion A began following the lack of adequate care in Criterion C).

E. The criteria are not met for autism spectrum disorder.

F. The disturbance is evident before age 5 years.

G. The child has a developmental age of at least 9 months.

Specify if:

Persistent: The disorder has been present for more than 12 months.

Specify current severity:

Reactive attachment disorder is specified as **severe** when a child exhibits all symptoms of the disorder, with each symptom manifesting at relatively high levels.

Disinhibited Social Engagement Disorder

F94.2

A. A pattern of behavior in which a child actively approaches and interacts with unfamiliar adults and exhibits at least two of the following:

1. Reduced or absent reticence in approaching and interacting with unfamiliar adults.
2. Overly familiar verbal or physical behavior (that is not consistent with culturally sanctioned and with age-appropriate social boundaries).
3. Diminished or absent checking back with adult caregiver after venturing away, even in unfamiliar settings.
4. Willingness to go off with an unfamiliar adult with minimal or no hesitation.

B. The behaviors in Criterion A are not limited to impulsivity (as in attention-deficit/hyperactivity disorder) but include socially disinhibited behavior.

C. The child has experienced a pattern of extremes of insufficient care as evidenced by at least one of the following:

1. Social neglect or deprivation in the form of persistent lack of having basic emotional needs for comfort, stimulation, and affection met by caregiving adults.
2. Repeated changes of primary caregivers that limit opportunities to form stable attachments (e.g., frequent changes in foster care).
3. Rearing in unusual settings that severely limit opportunities to form selective attachments (e.g., institutions with high child-to-caregiver ratios).

D. The care in Criterion C is presumed to be responsible for the disturbed behavior in Criterion A (e.g., the disturbances in Criterion A began following the pathogenic care in Criterion C).

E. The child has a developmental age of at least 9 months.

Specify if:

Persistent: The disorder has been present for more than 12 months.

Specify current severity:

Disinhibited social engagement disorder is specified as **severe** when the child exhibits all symptoms of the disorder, with each symptom manifesting at relatively high levels.

Posttraumatic Stress Disorder

F43.10

Posttraumatic Stress Disorder in Individuals Older Than 6 Years

Note: The following criteria apply to adults, adolescents, and children older than 6 years. For children 6 years and younger, see corresponding criteria below.

A. Exposure to actual or threatened death, serious injury, or sexual violence in one (or more) of the following ways:

1. Directly experiencing the traumatic event(s).
2. Witnessing, in person, the event(s) as it occurred to others.
3. Learning that the traumatic event(s) occurred to a close family member or close friend. In cases of actual or threatened death of a family member or friend, the event(s) must have been violent or accidental.
4. Experiencing repeated or extreme exposure to aversive details of the traumatic event(s) (e.g., first responders collecting human remains; police officers repeatedly exposed to details of child abuse).

    Note: Criterion A4 does not apply to exposure through electronic media, television, movies, or pictures, unless this exposure is work related.

B. Presence of one (or more) of the following intrusion symptoms associated with the traumatic event(s), beginning after the traumatic event(s) occurred:

1. Recurrent, involuntary, and intrusive distressing memories of the traumatic event(s).

    Note: In children older than 6 years, repetitive play may occur in which themes or aspects of the traumatic event(s) are expressed.
2. Recurrent distressing dreams in which the content and/or affect of the dream are related to the traumatic event(s).

    Note: In children, there may be frightening dreams without recognizable content.
3. Dissociative reactions (e.g., flashbacks) in which the individual feels or acts as if the traumatic event(s) were recurring. (Such reactions may occur on a continuum, with the most extreme expression being a complete loss of awareness of present surroundings.)

    Note: In children, trauma-specific reenactment may occur in play.

4. Intense or prolonged psychological distress at exposure to internal or external cues that symbolize or resemble an aspect of the traumatic event(s).

5. Marked physiological reactions to internal or external cues that symbolize or resemble an aspect of the traumatic event(s).

C. Persistent avoidance of stimuli associated with the traumatic event(s), beginning after the traumatic event(s) occurred, as evidenced by one or both of the following:

1. Avoidance of or efforts to avoid distressing memories, thoughts, or feelings about or closely associated with the traumatic event(s).

2. Avoidance of or efforts to avoid external reminders (people, places, conversations, activities, objects, situations) that arouse distressing memories, thoughts, or feelings about or closely associated with the traumatic event(s).

D. Negative alterations in cognitions and mood associated with the traumatic event(s), beginning or worsening after the traumatic event(s) occurred, as evidenced by two (or more) of the following:

1. Inability to remember an important aspect of the traumatic event(s) (typically due to dissociative amnesia and not to other factors such as head injury, alcohol, or drugs).

2. Persistent and exaggerated negative beliefs or expectations about oneself, others, or the world (e.g., "I am bad," "No one can be trusted," "The world is completely dangerous," "My whole nervous system is permanently ruined").

3. Persistent, distorted cognitions about the cause or consequences of the traumatic event(s) that lead the individual to blame himself/herself or others.

4. Persistent negative emotional state (e.g., fear, horror, anger, guilt, or shame).

5. Markedly diminished interest or participation in significant activities.

6. Feelings of detachment or estrangement from others.

7. Persistent inability to experience positive emotions (e.g., inability to experience happiness, satisfaction, or loving feelings).

E. Marked alterations in arousal and reactivity associated with the traumatic event(s), beginning or worsening after the traumatic event(s) occurred, as evidenced by two (or more) of the following:

1. Irritable behavior and angry outbursts (with little or no provocation) typically expressed as verbal or physical aggression toward people or objects.

2. Reckless or self-destructive behavior.

3. Hypervigilance.

4. Exaggerated startle response.

5. Problems with concentration.

6. Sleep disturbance (e.g., difficulty falling or staying asleep or restless sleep).

F. Duration of the disturbance (Criteria B, C, D, and E) is more than 1 month.

G. The disturbance causes clinically significant distress or impairment in social, occupational, or other important areas of functioning.

H. The disturbance is not attributable to the physiological effects of a substance (e.g., medication, alcohol) or another medical condition.

Specify whether:

With dissociative symptoms: The individual's symptoms meet the criteria for posttraumatic stress disorder, and in addition, in response to the stressor, the individual experiences persistent or recurrent symptoms of either of the following:

1. **Depersonalization:** Persistent or recurrent experiences of feeling detached from, and as if one were an outside observer of, one's mental processes or body (e.g., feeling as though one were in a dream; feeling a sense of unreality of self or body or of time moving slowly).

2. **Derealization:** Persistent or recurrent experiences of unreality of surroundings (e.g., the world around the individual is experienced as unreal, dreamlike, distant, or distorted).

Note: To use this subtype, the dissociative symptoms must not be attributable to the physiological effects of a substance (e.g., blackouts, behavior during alcohol intoxication) or another medical condition (e.g., complex partial seizures).

Specify if:

With delayed expression: If the full diagnostic criteria are not met until at least 6 months after the event (although the onset and expression of some symptoms may be immediate).

Posttraumatic Stress Disorder in Children 6 Years and Younger

A. In children 6 years and younger, exposure to actual or threatened death, serious injury, or sexual violence in one (or more) of the following ways:

1. Directly experiencing the traumatic event(s).

2. Witnessing, in person, the event(s) as it occurred to others, especially primary caregivers.

3. Learning that the traumatic event(s) occurred to a parent or caregiving figure.

B. Presence of one (or more) of the following intrusion symptoms associated with the traumatic event(s), beginning after the traumatic event(s) occurred:

1. Recurrent, involuntary, and intrusive distressing memories of the traumatic event(s).

Note: Spontaneous and intrusive memories may not necessarily appear distressing and may be expressed as play reenactment.

2. Recurrent distressing dreams in which the content and/or affect of the dream are related to the traumatic event(s).

Note: It may not be possible to ascertain that the frightening content is related to the traumatic event.

3. Dissociative reactions (e.g., flashbacks) in which the child feels or acts as if the traumatic event(s) were recurring. (Such reactions may occur on a continuum, with the most extreme expression being a complete loss of awareness of present surroundings.) Such trauma-specific reenactment may occur in play.

4. Intense or prolonged psychological distress at exposure to internal or external cues that symbolize or resemble an aspect of the traumatic event(s).

5. Marked physiological reactions to reminders of the traumatic event(s).

C. One (or more) of the following symptoms, representing either persistent avoidance of stimuli associated with the traumatic event(s) or negative alterations in cognitions and mood associated with the traumatic event(s), must be present, beginning after the event(s) or worsening after the event(s):

Persistent Avoidance of Stimuli

1. Avoidance of or efforts to avoid activities, places, or physical reminders that arouse recollections of the traumatic event(s).

2. Avoidance of or efforts to avoid people, conversations, or interpersonal situations that arouse recollections of the traumatic event(s).

Negative Alterations in Cognitions

3. Substantially increased frequency of negative emotional states (e.g., fear, guilt, sadness, shame, confusion).

4. Markedly diminished interest or participation in significant activities, including constriction of play.

5. Socially withdrawn behavior.

6. Persistent reduction in expression of positive emotions.

D. Alterations in arousal and reactivity associated with the traumatic event(s), beginning or worsening after the traumatic event(s) occurred, as evidenced by two (or more) of the following:

1. Irritable behavior and angry outbursts (with little or no provocation) typically expressed as verbal or physical aggression toward people or objects (including extreme temper tantrums).

2. Hypervigilance.

3. Exaggerated startle response.

4. Problems with concentration.

5. Sleep disturbance (e.g., difficulty falling or staying asleep or restless sleep).

E. The duration of the disturbance is more than 1 month.

F. The disturbance causes clinically significant distress or impairment in relationships with parents, siblings, peers, or other caregivers or with school behavior.

G. The disturbance is not attributable to the physiological effects of a substance (e.g., medication or alcohol) or another medical condition.

Specify whether:

With dissociative symptoms: The individual's symptoms meet the criteria for posttraumatic stress disorder, and the individual experiences persistent or recurrent symptoms of either of the following:

1. **Depersonalization:** Persistent or recurrent experiences of feeling detached from, and as if one were an outside observer of, one's mental processes or body (e.g., feeling as though one were in a dream; feeling a sense of unreality of self or body or of time moving slowly).

2. **Derealization:** Persistent or recurrent experiences of unreality of surroundings (e.g., the world around the individual is experienced as unreal, dreamlike, distant, or distorted).

Note: To use this subtype, the dissociative symptoms must not be attributable to the physiological effects of a substance (e.g., blackouts) or another medical condition (e.g., complex partial seizures).

Specify if:

With delayed expression: If the full diagnostic criteria are not met until at least 6 months after the event (although the onset and expression of some symptoms may be immediate).

Acute Stress Disorder

F43.0

A. Exposure to actual or threatened death, serious injury, or sexual violence in one (or more) of the following ways:

1. Directly experiencing the traumatic event(s).

2. Witnessing, in person, the event(s) as it occurred to others.

3. Learning that the event(s) occurred to a close family member or close friend. **Note:** In cases of actual or threatened death of a family member or friend, the event(s) must have been violent or accidental.

4. Experiencing repeated or extreme exposure to aversive details of the traumatic event(s) (e.g., first responders collecting human remains, police officers repeatedly exposed to details of child abuse).

Note: This does not apply to exposure through electronic media, television, movies, or pictures, unless this exposure is work related.

B. Presence of nine (or more) of the following symptoms from any of the five categories of intrusion, negative mood, dissociation, avoidance, and arousal, beginning or worsening after the traumatic event(s) occurred:

Intrusion Symptoms

1. Recurrent, involuntary, and intrusive distressing memories of the traumatic event(s). **Note:** In children, repetitive play may occur in which themes or aspects of the traumatic event(s) are expressed.
2. Recurrent distressing dreams in which the content and/or affect of the dream are related to the event(s). **Note:** In children, there may be frightening dreams without recognizable content.
3. Dissociative reactions (e.g., flashbacks) in which the individual feels or acts as if the traumatic event(s) were recurring. (Such reactions may occur on a continuum, with the most extreme expression being a complete loss of awareness of present surroundings.) **Note:** In children, trauma-specific reenactment may occur in play.
4. Intense or prolonged psychological distress or marked physiological reactions in response to internal or external cues that symbolize or resemble an aspect of the traumatic event(s).

Negative Mood

5. Persistent inability to experience positive emotions (e.g., inability to experience happiness, satisfaction, or loving feelings).

Dissociative Symptoms

6. An altered sense of the reality of one's surroundings or oneself (e.g., seeing oneself from another's perspective, being in a daze, time slowing).
7. Inability to remember an important aspect of the traumatic event(s) (typically due to dissociative amnesia and not to other factors such as head injury, alcohol, or drugs).

Avoidance Symptoms

8. Efforts to avoid distressing memories, thoughts, or feelings about or closely associated with the traumatic event(s).
9. Efforts to avoid external reminders (people, places, conversations, activities, objects, situations) that arouse distressing memories, thoughts, or feelings about or closely associated with the traumatic event(s).

Arousal Symptoms

10. Sleep disturbance (e.g., difficulty falling or staying asleep, restless sleep).

11. Irritable behavior and angry outbursts (with little or no provocation), typically expressed as verbal or physical aggression toward people or objects.
12. Hypervigilance.
13. Problems with concentration.
14. Exaggerated startle response.

C. Duration of the disturbance (symptoms in Criterion B) is 3 days to 1 month after trauma exposure.

Note: Symptoms typically begin immediately after the trauma, but persistence for at least 3 days and up to a month is needed to meet disorder criteria.

D. The disturbance causes clinically significant distress or impairment in social, occupational, or other important areas of functioning.
E. The disturbance is not attributable to the physiological effects of a substance (e.g., medication or alcohol) or another medical condition (e.g., mild traumatic brain injury) and is not better explained by brief psychotic disorder.

Adjustment Disorders

A. The development of emotional or behavioral symptoms in response to an identifiable stressor(s) occurring within 3 months of the onset of the stressor(s).
B. These symptoms or behaviors are clinically significant, as evidenced by one or both of the following:

1. Marked distress that is out of proportion to the severity or intensity of the stressor, taking into account the external context and the cultural factors that might influence symptom severity and presentation.
2. Significant impairment in social, occupational, or other important areas of functioning.

C. The stress-related disturbance does not meet the criteria for another mental disorder and is not merely an exacerbation of a preexisting mental disorder.
D. The symptoms do not represent normal bereavement and are not better explained by prolonged grief disorder.
E. Once the stressor or its consequences have terminated, the symptoms do not persist for more than an additional 6 months.

Specify whether:

F43.21 With depressed mood: Low mood, tearfulness, or feelings of hopelessness are predominant.
F43.22 With anxiety: Nervousness, worry, jitteriness, or separation anxiety is predominant.
F43.23 With mixed anxiety and depressed mood: A combination of depression and anxiety is predominant.

F43.24 With disturbance of conduct: Disturbance of conduct is predominant.

F43.25   With mixed disturbance of emotions and conduct: Both emotional symptoms (e.g., depression, anxiety) and a disturbance of conduct are predominant.

F43.20 Unspecified: For maladaptive reactions that are not classifiable as one of the specific subtypes of adjustment disorder.

Specify if:

Acute: This specifier can be used to indicate persistence of symptoms for less than 6 months.

Persistent (chronic): This specifier can be used to indicate persistence of symptoms for 6 months or longer. By definition, symptoms cannot persist for more than 6 months after the termination of the stressor or its consequences. The persistent specifier therefore applies when the duration of the disturbance is longer than 6 months in response to a chronic stressor or to a stressor that has enduring consequences.

Prolonged Grief Disorder

F43.8

A. The death, at least 12 months ago, of a person who was close to the bereaved individual (for children and adolescents, at least 6 months ago).

B. Since the death, the development of a persistent grief response characterized by one or both of the following symptoms, which have been present most days to a clinically significant degree. In addition, the symptom(s) has occurred nearly every day for at least the last month:

   1. Intense yearning/longing for the deceased person.
   2. Preoccupation with thoughts or memories of the deceased person (in children and adolescents, preoccupation may focus on the circumstances of the death).

C. Since the death, at least three of the following symptoms have been present most days to a clinically significant degree. In addition, the symptoms have occurred nearly every day for at least the last month:

   1. Identity disruption (e.g., feeling as though part of oneself has died) since the death.
   2. Marked sense of disbelief about the death.
   3. Avoidance of reminders that the person is dead (in children and adolescents, may be characterized by efforts to avoid reminders).
   4. Intense emotional pain (e.g., anger, bitterness, sorrow) related to the death.
   5. Difficulty reintegrating into one's relationships and activities after the death (e.g., problems engaging with friends, pursuing interests, or planning for the future).

6. Emotional numbness (absence or marked reduction of emotional experience) as a result of the death.
7. Feeling that life is meaningless as a result of the death.
8. Intense loneliness as a result of the death.

D. The disturbance causes clinically significant distress or impairment in social, occupational, or other important areas of functioning.
E. The duration and severity of the bereavement reaction clearly exceed expected social, cultural, or religious norms for the individual's culture and context.
F. The symptoms are not better explained by another mental disorder, such as major depressive disorder or posttraumatic stress disorder, and are not attributable to the physiological effects of a substance (e.g., medication, alcohol) or another medical condition.

Other Specified Trauma- and Stressor-Related Disorder

F43.8

This category applies to presentations in which symptoms characteristic of a trauma- and stressor-related disorder that cause clinically significant distress or impairment in social, occupational, or other important areas of functioning predominate but do not meet the full criteria for any of the disorders in the trauma- and stressor-related disorders diagnostic class. The other specified trauma- and stressor-related disorder category is used in situations in which the clinician chooses to communicate the specific reason that the presentation does not meet the criteria for any specific trauma- and stressor-related disorder. This is done by recording "other specified trauma- and stressor-related disorder" followed by the specific reason (e.g., "persistent response to trauma with PTSD-like symptoms").

Examples of presentations that can be specified using the "other specified" designation include the following:

1. **Adjustment-like disorders with delayed onset of symptoms that occur more than 3 months after the stressor.**
2. **Adjustment-like disorders with prolonged duration of more than 6 months without prolonged duration of stressor.**
3. **Persistent response to trauma with PTSD-like symptoms** (i.e., symptoms occurring in response to a traumatic event that fall short of the diagnostic threshold for PTSD and that persist for longer than 6 months, sometimes referred to as "subthreshold/partial PTSD").
4. ***Ataque de nervios:*** See "Culture and Psychiatric Diagnosis" in Section III of DSM-5-TR.
5. **Other cultural syndromes:** See "Culture and Psychiatric Diagnosis" in Section III of DSM-5-TR.

Unspecified Trauma- and Stressor-Related Disorder

F43.9

This category applies to presentations in which symptoms characteristic of a trauma- and stressor-related disorder that cause clinically significant distress or impairment in social, occupational, or other important areas of functioning predominate but do not meet the full criteria for any of the disorders in the trauma- and stressor-related disorders diagnostic class. The unspecified trauma- and stressor-related disorder category is used in situations in which the clinician chooses *not* to specify the reason that the criteria are not met for a specific trauma- and stressor-related disorder and includes presentations in which there is insufficient information to make a more specific diagnosis (e.g., in emergency room settings).

Dissociative Identity Disorder

F44.81

A. Disruption of identity characterized by two or more distinct personality states, which may be described in some cultures as an experience of possession. The disruption in identity involves marked discontinuity in sense of self and sense of agency, accompanied by related alterations in affect, behavior, consciousness, memory, perception, cognition, and/or sensory-motor functioning. These signs and symptoms may be observed by others or reported by the individual.

B. Recurrent gaps in the recall of everyday events, important personal information, and/or traumatic events that are inconsistent with ordinary forgetting.

C. The symptoms cause clinically significant distress or impairment in social, occupational, or other important areas of functioning.

D. The disturbance is not a normal part of a broadly accepted cultural or religious practice.

Note: In children, the symptoms are not better explained by imaginary playmates or other fantasy play.

E. The symptoms are not attributable to the physiological effects of a substance (e.g., blackouts or chaotic behavior during alcohol intoxication) or another medical condition (e.g., complex partial seizures).

Dissociative Amnesia

F44.0

A. An inability to recall important autobiographical information, usually of a traumatic or stressful nature, that is inconsistent with ordinary forgetting.

Note: Dissociative amnesia most often consists of localized or selective amnesia for a specific event or events; or generalized amnesia for identity and life history.

B. The symptoms cause clinically significant distress or impairment in social, occupational, or other important areas of functioning.

C. The disturbance is not attributable to the physiological effects of a substance (e.g., alcohol or other drug of abuse, a medication) or a neurological or other medical condition (e.g., partial complex sei-

zures, transient global amnesia, sequelae of a closed head injury/
traumatic brain injury, other neurological condition).
D. The disturbance is not better explained by dissociative identity disorder, posttraumatic stress disorder, acute stress disorder, somatic
symptom disorder, or major or mild neurocognitive disorder.

Coding note: The code for dissociative amnesia without dissociative
fugue is **F44.0.** The code for dissociative amnesia with dissociative fugue
is **F44.1.**

Specify if:
  F44.1 With dissociative fugue: Apparently purposeful travel or
  bewildered wandering that is associated with amnesia for identity
  or for other important autobiographical information.

Depersonalization/Derealization Disorder

F48.1

A. The presence of persistent or recurrent experiences of depersonalization, derealization, or both:

  1. **Depersonalization:** Experiences of unreality, detachment, or
  being an outside observer with respect to one's thoughts, feelings, sensations, body, or actions (e.g., perceptual alterations,
  distorted sense of time, unreal or absent self, emotional and/
  or physical numbing).
  2. **Derealization:** Experiences of unreality or detachment with respect to surroundings (e.g., individuals or objects are experienced as unreal, dreamlike, foggy, lifeless, or visually distorted).

B. During the depersonalization or derealization experiences, reality
testing remains intact.
C. The symptoms cause clinically significant distress or impairment
in social, occupational, or other important areas of functioning.
D. The disturbance is not attributable to the physiological effects of
a substance (e.g., a drug of abuse, medication) or another medical
condition (e.g., seizures).
E. The disturbance is not better explained by another mental disorder,
such as schizophrenia, panic disorder, major depressive disorder,
acute stress disorder, posttraumatic stress disorder, or another
dissociative disorder.

Other Specified Dissociative Disorder

F44.89

This category applies to presentations in which symptoms characteristic
of a dissociative disorder that cause clinically significant distress or
impairment in social, occupational, or other important areas of function-

ing predominate but do not meet the full criteria for any of the disorders in the dissociative disorders diagnostic class. The other specified dissociative disorder category is used in situations in which the clinician chooses to communicate the specific reason that the presentation does not meet the criteria for any specific dissociative disorder. This is done by recording "other specified dissociative disorder" followed by the specific reason (e.g., "dissociative trance").

Examples of presentations that can be specified using the "other specified" designation include the following:

1. **Chronic and recurrent syndromes of mixed dissociative symptoms:** This category includes identity disturbance associated with less-than-marked discontinuities in sense of self and agency, or alterations of identity or episodes of possession in an individual who reports no dissociative amnesia.

2. **Identity disturbance due to prolonged and intense coercive persuasion:** Individuals who have been subjected to intense coercive persuasion (e.g., brainwashing, thought reform, indoctrination while captive, torture, long-term political imprisonment, recruitment by sects/cults or by terror organizations) may present with prolonged changes in, or conscious questioning of, their identity.

3. **Acute dissociative reactions to stressful events:** This category is for acute, transient conditions that typically last less than 1 month, and sometimes only a few hours or days. These conditions are characterized by constriction of consciousness; depersonalization; derealization; perceptual disturbances (e.g., time slowing, macropsia); micro-amnesias; transient stupor; and/or alterations in sensory-motor functioning (e.g., analgesia, paralysis).

4. **Dissociative trance:** This condition is characterized by an acute narrowing or complete loss of awareness of immediate surroundings that manifests as profound unresponsiveness or insensitivity to environmental stimuli. The unresponsiveness may be accompanied by minor stereotyped behaviors (e.g., finger movements) of which the individual is unaware and/or that he or she cannot control, as well as transient paralysis or loss of consciousness. The dissociative trance is not a normal part of a broadly accepted collective cultural or religious practice.

Unspecified Dissociative Disorder

F44.9

This category applies to presentations in which symptoms characteristic of a dissociative disorder that cause clinically significant distress or impairment in social, occupational, or other important areas of functioning predominate but do not meet the full criteria for any of the disorders in the dissociative disorders diagnostic class. The unspecified dissociative disorder category is used in situations in which the clinician chooses *not* to specify the reason that the criteria are not met for a specific dissociative disorder and includes presentations for which there is insufficient information to make a more specific diagnosis (e.g., in emergency room settings).

Somatic Symptom and Related Disorders

Somatic Symptom Disorder

F45.1

A. One or more somatic symptoms that are distressing or result in significant disruption of daily life.

B. Excessive thoughts, feelings, or behaviors related to the somatic symptoms or associated health concerns as manifested by at least one of the following:

1. Disproportionate and persistent thoughts about the seriousness of one's symptoms.
2. Persistently high level of anxiety about health or symptoms.
3. Excessive time and energy devoted to these symptoms or health concerns.

C. Although any one somatic symptom may not be continuously present, the state of being symptomatic is persistent (typically more than 6 months).

Specify if:

With predominant pain (previously pain disorder): This specifier is for individuals whose somatic symptoms predominantly involve pain.

Specify if:

Persistent: A persistent course is characterized by severe symptoms, marked impairment, and long duration (more than 6 months).

Specify current severity:

Mild: Only one of the symptoms specified in Criterion B is fulfilled.
Moderate: Two or more of the symptoms specified in Criterion B are fulfilled.
Severe: Two or more of the symptoms specified in Criterion B are fulfilled, plus there are multiple somatic complaints (or one very severe somatic symptom).

Illness Anxiety Disorder

F45.21

A. Preoccupation with having or acquiring a serious illness.

B. Somatic symptoms are not present or, if present, are only mild in intensity. If another medical condition is present or there is a high risk for developing a medical condition (e.g., strong family history is present), the preoccupation is clearly excessive or disproportionate.

C. There is a high level of anxiety about health, and the individual is easily alarmed about personal health status.

D. The individual performs excessive health-related behaviors (e.g., repeatedly checks his or her body for signs of illness) or exhibits maladaptive avoidance (e.g., avoids doctor appointments and hospitals).

E. Illness preoccupation has been present for at least 6 months, but the specific illness that is feared may change over that period of time.

F. The illness-related preoccupation is not better explained by another mental disorder, such as somatic symptom disorder, panic disorder, generalized anxiety disorder, body dysmorphic disorder, obsessive-compulsive disorder, or delusional disorder, somatic type.

Specify whether:

Care-seeking type: Medical care, including physician visits or undergoing tests and procedures, is frequently used.
Care-avoidant type: Medical care is rarely used.

Functional Neurological Symptom Disorder (Conversion Disorder)

A. One or more symptoms of altered voluntary motor or sensory function.

B. Clinical findings provide evidence of incompatibility between the symptom and recognized neurological or medical conditions.

C. The symptom or deficit is not better explained by another medical or mental disorder.

D. The symptom or deficit causes clinically significant distress or impairment in social, occupational, or other important areas of functioning or warrants medical evaluation.

Coding note: The ICD-10-CM code depends on the symptom type (see below).

Specify symptom type:

F44.4 With weakness or paralysis
F44.4 With abnormal movement (e.g., tremor, dystonia, myoclonus, gait disorder)
F44.4 With swallowing symptoms
F44.4 With speech symptom (e.g., dysphonia, slurred speech)
F44.5 With attacks or seizures
F44.6 With anesthesia or sensory loss
F44.6 With special sensory symptom (e.g., visual, olfactory, or hearing disturbance)
F44.7 With mixed symptoms

Specify if:
   Acute episode: Symptoms present for less than 6 months.
   Persistent: Symptoms occurring for 6 months or more.

Specify if:
   With psychological stressor *(specify stressor)*
   Without psychological stressor

Psychological Factors Affecting Other Medical Conditions

F54

A.   A medical symptom or condition (other than a mental disorder) is present.

B.   Psychological or behavioral factors adversely affect the medical condition in one of the following ways:

   1.   The factors have influenced the course of the medical condition as shown by a close temporal association between the psychological factors and the development or exacerbation of, or delayed recovery from, the medical condition.

   2.   The factors interfere with the treatment of the medical condition (e.g., poor adherence).

   3.   The factors constitute additional well-established health risks for the individual.

   4.   The factors influence the underlying pathophysiology, precipitating or exacerbating symptoms or necessitating medical attention.

C.   The psychological and behavioral factors in Criterion B are not better explained by another mental disorder (e.g., panic disorder, major depressive disorder, posttraumatic stress disorder).

Specify current severity:
   Mild: Increases medical risk (e.g., inconsistent adherence with antihypertension treatment).
   Moderate: Aggravates underlying medical condition (e.g., anxiety aggravating asthma).
   Severe: Results in medical hospitalization or emergency room visit.
   Extreme: Results in severe, life-threatening risk (e.g., ignoring heart attack symptoms).

Factitious Disorder

Factitious Disorder Imposed on Self   **F68.10**

A.   Falsification of physical or psychological signs or symptoms, or induction of injury or disease, associated with identified deception.

B. The individual presents himself or herself to others as ill, impaired, or injured.
C. The deceptive behavior is evident even in the absence of obvious external rewards.
D. The behavior is not better explained by another mental disorder, such as delusional disorder or another psychotic disorder.

Specify:

Single episode
Recurrent episodes (two or more events of falsification of illness and/or induction of injury)

Factitious Disorder Imposed on Another (Previously Factitious Disorder by Proxy)   F68.A

A. Falsification of physical or psychological signs or symptoms, or induction of injury or disease, in another, associated with identified deception.
B. The individual presents another individual (victim) to others as ill, impaired, or injured.
C. The deceptive behavior is evident even in the absence of obvious external rewards.
D. The behavior is not better explained by another mental disorder, such as delusional disorder or another psychotic disorder.

Note: The perpetrator, not the victim, receives this diagnosis.

Specify:

Single episode
Recurrent episodes (two or more events of falsification of illness and/or induction of injury)

Recording Procedures

When an individual falsifies illness in another (e.g., children, adults, pets), the diagnosis is factitious disorder imposed on another. The perpetrator, not the victim, is given the diagnosis. The victim may be given an abuse diagnosis (e.g., T74.12X; see the chapter "Other Conditions That May Be a Focus of Clinical Attention"). If an individual with factitious disorder imposed on another has also deceptively represented their own illness or injury, both factitious disorder imposed on self and on another can be diagnosed.

Other Specified Somatic Symptom and Related Disorder

F45.8

This category applies to presentations in which symptoms characteristic of a somatic symptom and related disorder that cause clinically significant distress or impairment in social, occupational, or other important areas of functioning predominate but do not meet the full criteria for any of the disorders in the somatic symptom and related disorders diagnostic class.

Examples of presentations that can be specified using the "other specified" designation include the following:

1. **Brief somatic symptom disorder:** Duration of symptoms is less than 6 months.
2. **Brief illness anxiety disorder:** Duration of symptoms is less than 6 months.
3. **Illness anxiety disorder without excessive health-related behaviors or maladaptive avoidance:** Criterion D for illness anxiety disorder is not met.
4. **Pseudocyesis:** A false belief of being pregnant that is associated with objective signs and reported symptoms of pregnancy.

Unspecified Somatic Symptom and Related Disorder

F45.9

This category applies to presentations in which symptoms characteristic of a somatic symptom and related disorder that cause clinically significant distress or impairment in social, occupational, or other important areas of functioning predominate but do not meet the full criteria for any of the disorders in the somatic symptom and related disorders diagnostic class. The unspecified somatic symptom and related disorder category should not be used unless there are decidedly unusual situations where there is insufficient information to make a more specific diagnosis.

Feeding and Eating Disorders

Pica

A. Persistent eating of nonnutritive, nonfood substances over a period of at least 1 month.

B. The eating of nonnutritive, nonfood substances is inappropriate to the developmental level of the individual.

C. The eating behavior is not part of a culturally supported or socially normative practice.

D. If the eating behavior occurs in the context of another mental disorder (e.g., intellectual developmental disorder [intellectual disability], autism spectrum disorder, schizophrenia) or medical condition (including pregnancy), it is sufficiently severe to warrant additional clinical attention.

Coding note: The ICD-10-CM codes for pica are **F98.3** in children and **F50.89** in adults.

Specify if:

In remission: After full criteria for pica were previously met, the criteria have not been met for a sustained period of time.

Rumination Disorder

F98.21

A. Repeated regurgitation of food over a period of at least 1 month. Regurgitated food may be re-chewed, re-swallowed, or spit out.

B. The repeated regurgitation is not attributable to an associated gastrointestinal or other medical condition (e.g., gastroesophageal reflux, pyloric stenosis).

C. The eating disturbance does not occur exclusively during the course of anorexia nervosa, bulimia nervosa, binge-eating disorder, or avoidant/restrictive food intake disorder.

D. If the symptoms occur in the context of another mental disorder (e.g., intellectual developmental disorder [intellectual disability] or another neurodevelopmental disorder), they are sufficiently severe to warrant additional clinical attention.

Specify if:

In remission: After full criteria for rumination disorder were previously met, the criteria have not been met for a sustained period of time.

Avoidant/Restrictive Food Intake Disorder
F50.82

A. An eating or feeding disturbance (e.g., apparent lack of interest in
    eating or food; avoidance based on the sensory characteristics of
    food; concern about aversive consequences of eating) associated
    with one (or more) of the following:

    1. Significant weight loss (or failure to achieve expected weight
        gain or faltering growth in children).
    2. Significant nutritional deficiency.
    3. Dependence on enteral feeding or oral nutritional supplements.
    4. Marked interference with psychosocial functioning.

B. The disturbance is not better explained by lack of available food or
    by an associated culturally sanctioned practice.
C. The eating disturbance does not occur exclusively during the course
    of anorexia nervosa or bulimia nervosa, and there is no evidence
    of a disturbance in the way in which one's body weight or shape is
    experienced.
D. The eating disturbance is not attributable to a concurrent medical
    condition or not better explained by another mental disorder. When
    the eating disturbance occurs in the context of another condition or
    disorder, the severity of the eating disturbance exceeds that rou-
    tinely associated with the condition or disorder and warrants ad-
    ditional clinical attention.

Specify if:

In remission: After full criteria for avoidant/restrictive food intake
disorder were previously met, the criteria have not been met for a
sustained period of time.

Anorexia Nervosa

A. Restriction of energy intake relative to requirements, leading to
    a significantly low body weight in the context of age, sex, develop-
    mental trajectory, and physical health. *Significantly low weight* is
    defined as a weight that is less than minimally normal or, for children
    and adolescents, less than that minimally expected.
B. Intense fear of gaining weight or of becoming fat, or persistent be-
    havior that interferes with weight gain, even though at a signifi-
    cantly low weight.
C. Disturbance in the way in which one's body weight or shape is
    experienced, undue influence of body weight or shape on self-
    evaluation, or persistent lack of recognition of the seriousness of
    the current low body weight.

Coding note: The ICD-10-CM code depends on the subtype (see below).

Specify whether:

F50.01 Restricting type: During the last 3 months, the individual has not engaged in recurrent episodes of binge-eating or purging behavior (i.e., self-induced vomiting or the misuse of laxatives, diuretics, or enemas). This subtype describes presentations in which weight loss is accomplished primarily through dieting, fasting, and/or excessive exercise.

F50.02 Binge-eating/purging type: During the last 3 months, the individual has engaged in recurrent episodes of binge-eating or purging behavior (i.e., self-induced vomiting or the misuse of laxatives, diuretics, or enemas).

Specify if:

In partial remission: After full criteria for anorexia nervosa were previously met, Criterion A (low body weight) has not been met for a sustained period, but either Criterion B (intense fear of gaining weight or becoming fat or behavior that interferes with weight gain) or Criterion C (disturbances in self-perception of weight and shape) is still met.

In full remission: After full criteria for anorexia nervosa were previously met, none of the criteria have been met for a sustained period of time.

Specify current severity:

The minimum level of severity is based, for adults, on current body mass index (BMI) (see below) or, for children and adolescents, on BMI percentile. The ranges below are derived from World Health Organization categories for thinness in adults; for children and adolescents, corresponding BMI percentiles should be used. The level of severity may be increased to reflect clinical symptoms, the degree of functional disability, and the need for supervision.

Mild: BMI ≥17 kg/m^2.
Moderate: BMI 16–16.99 kg/m^2.
Severe: BMI 15–15.99 kg/m^2.
Extreme: BMI <15 kg/m^2.

Bulimia Nervosa

F50.2

A. Recurrent episodes of binge eating. An episode of binge eating is characterized by both of the following:

1. Eating, in a discrete period of time (e.g., within any 2-hour period), an amount of food that is definitely larger than what most individuals would eat in a similar period of time under similar circumstances.

2. A sense of lack of control over eating during the episode (e.g.,
    a feeling that one cannot stop eating or control what or how
    much one is eating).

B. Recurrent inappropriate compensatory behaviors in order to prevent
    weight gain, such as self-induced vomiting; misuse of laxatives, di-
    uretics, or other medications; fasting; or excessive exercise.
C. The binge eating and inappropriate compensatory behaviors both
    occur, on average, at least once a week for 3 months.
D. Self-evaluation is unduly influenced by body shape and weight.
E. The disturbance does not occur exclusively during episodes of an-
    orexia nervosa.

Specify if:

In partial remission: After full criteria for bulimia nervosa were
previously met, some, but not all, of the criteria have been met for
a sustained period of time.
In full remission: After full criteria for bulimia nervosa were previously met, none of the criteria have been met for a sustained period of time.

Specify current severity:

The minimum level of severity is based on the frequency of inappropriate compensatory behaviors (see below). The level of severity may
be increased to reflect other symptoms and the degree of functional
disability.

Mild: An average of 1–3 episodes of inappropriate compensatory
behaviors per week.
Moderate: An average of 4–7 episodes of inappropriate compensatory behaviors per week.
Severe: An average of 8–13 episodes of inappropriate compensatory behaviors per week.
Extreme: An average of 14 or more episodes of inappropriate compensatory behaviors per week.

Binge-Eating Disorder

F50.81

A. Recurrent episodes of binge eating. An episode of binge eating is
    characterized by both of the following:

1. Eating, in a discrete period of time (e.g., within any 2-hour pe-
    riod), an amount of food that is definitely larger than what
    most people would eat in a similar period of time under similar
    circumstances.
2. A sense of lack of control over eating during the episode (e.g.,
    a feeling that one cannot stop eating or control what or how
    much one is eating).

B. The binge-eating episodes are associated with three (or more) of the following:

1. Eating much more rapidly than normal.
2. Eating until feeling uncomfortably full.
3. Eating large amounts of food when not feeling physically hungry.
4. Eating alone because of feeling embarrassed by how much one is eating.
5. Feeling disgusted with oneself, depressed, or very guilty afterward.

C. Marked distress regarding binge eating is present.

D. The binge eating occurs, on average, at least once a week for 3 months.

E. The binge eating is not associated with the recurrent use of inappropriate compensatory behavior as in bulimia nervosa and does not occur exclusively during the course of bulimia nervosa or anorexia nervosa.

Specify if:

In partial remission: After full criteria for binge-eating disorder were previously met, binge eating occurs at an average frequency of less than one episode per week for a sustained period of time.

In full remission: After full criteria for binge-eating disorder were previously met, none of the criteria have been met for a sustained period of time.

Specify current severity:

The minimum level of severity is based on the frequency of episodes of binge eating (see below). The level of severity may be increased to reflect other symptoms and the degree of functional disability.

Mild: 1–3 binge-eating episodes per week.
Moderate: 4–7 binge-eating episodes per week.
Severe: 8–13 binge-eating episodes per week.
Extreme: 14 or more binge-eating episodes per week.

Other Specified Feeding or Eating Disorder

F50.89

This category applies to presentations in which symptoms characteristic of a feeding and eating disorder that cause clinically significant distress or impairment in social, occupational, or other important areas of functioning predominate but do not meet the full criteria for any of the disorders in the feeding and eating disorders diagnostic class. The other specified feeding or eating disorder category is used in situations in which the clinician chooses to communicate the specific reason that the presentation does not meet the criteria for any specific feeding and eating disorder. This is done by recording "other specified feeding or eating disorder" followed by the specific reason (e.g., "bulimia nervosa of low frequency").

Examples of presentations that can be specified using the "other specified" designation include the following:

1. **Atypical anorexia nervosa:** All of the criteria for anorexia nervosa are met, except that despite significant weight loss, the individual's weight is within or above the normal range. Individuals with atypical anorexia nervosa may experience many of the physiological complications associated with anorexia nervosa.
2. **Bulimia nervosa (of low frequency and/or limited duration):** All of the criteria for bulimia nervosa are met, except that the binge eating and inappropriate compensatory behaviors occur, on average, less than once a week and/or for less than 3 months.
3. **Binge-eating disorder (of low frequency and/or limited duration):** All of the criteria for binge-eating disorder are met, except that the binge eating occurs, on average, less than once a week and/or for less than 3 months.
4. **Purging disorder:** Recurrent purging behavior to influence weight or shape (e.g., self-induced vomiting; misuse of laxatives, diuretics, or other medications) in the absence of binge eating.
5. **Night eating syndrome:** Recurrent episodes of night eating, as manifested by eating after awakening from sleep or by excessive food consumption after the evening meal. There is awareness and recall of the eating. The night eating is not better explained by external influences such as changes in the individual's sleep-wake cycle or by local social norms. The night eating causes significant distress and/or impairment in functioning. The disordered pattern of eating is not better explained by binge-eating disorder or another mental disorder, including substance use, and is not attributable to another medical condition or to an effect of medication.

Unspecified Feeding or Eating Disorder

F50.9

This category applies to presentations in which symptoms characteristic of a feeding and eating disorder that cause clinically significant distress or impairment in social, occupational, or other important areas of functioning predominate but do not meet the full criteria for any of the disorders in the feeding and eating disorders diagnostic class. The unspecified feeding or eating disorder category is used in situations in which the clinician chooses *not* to specify the reason that the criteria are not met for a specific feeding and eating disorder and includes presentations in which there is insufficient information to make a more specific diagnosis (e.g., in emergency room settings).

Enuresis

F98.0

A. Repeated voiding of urine into bed or clothes, whether involuntary or intentional.

B. The behavior is clinically significant as manifested by either a frequency of at least twice a week for at least 3 consecutive months or the presence of clinically significant distress or impairment in social, academic (occupational), or other important areas of functioning.

C. Chronological age is at least 5 years (or equivalent developmental level).

D. The behavior is not attributable to the physiological effects of a substance (e.g., a diuretic, an antipsychotic medication) or another medical condition (e.g., diabetes, spina bifida, a seizure disorder).

Specify whether:

Nocturnal only: Passage of urine only during nighttime sleep.

Diurnal only: Passage of urine during waking hours.

Nocturnal and diurnal: A combination of the two subtypes above.

Encopresis

F98.1

A. Repeated passage of feces into inappropriate places (e.g., clothing, floor), whether involuntary or intentional.

B. At least one such event occurs each month for at least 3 months.

C. Chronological age is at least 4 years (or equivalent developmental level).

D. The behavior is not attributable to the physiological effects of a substance (e.g., laxatives) or another medical condition except through a mechanism involving constipation.

Specify whether:

With constipation and overflow incontinence: There is evidence of constipation on physical examination or by history.

Without constipation and overflow incontinence: There is no evidence of constipation on physical examination or by history.

Other Specified Elimination Disorder

This category applies to presentations in which symptoms characteristic of an elimination disorder that cause clinically significant distress or impairment in social, occupational, or other important areas of functioning predominate but do not meet the full criteria for any of the disorders in the elimination disorders diagnostic class. The other specified elimination disorder category is used in situations in which the clinician chooses to communicate the specific reason that the presentation does not meet the criteria for any specific elimination disorder. This is done by recording "other specified elimination disorder" followed by the specific reason (e.g., "low-frequency enuresis").

Coding note: Code **N39.498** for other specified elimination disorder with urinary symptoms; **R15.9** for other specified elimination disorder with fecal symptoms.

Unspecified Elimination Disorder

This category applies to presentations in which symptoms characteristic of an elimination disorder that cause clinically significant distress or impairment in social, occupational, or other important areas of functioning predominate but do not meet the full criteria for any of the disorders in the elimination disorders diagnostic class. The unspecified elimination disorder category is used in situations in which the clinician chooses *not* to specify the reason that the criteria are not met for a specific elimination disorder and includes presentations in which there is insufficient information to make a more specific diagnosis (e.g., in emergency room settings).

Coding note: Code **R32** for unspecified elimination disorder with urinary symptoms; **R15.9** for unspecified elimination disorder with fecal symptoms.

Insomnia Disorder

F51.01

A. A predominant complaint of dissatisfaction with sleep quantity or quality, associated with one (or more) of the following symptoms:

1. Difficulty initiating sleep. (In children, this may manifest as difficulty initiating sleep without caregiver intervention.)
2. Difficulty maintaining sleep, characterized by frequent awakenings or problems returning to sleep after awakenings. (In children, this may manifest as difficulty returning to sleep without caregiver intervention.)
3. Early-morning awakening with inability to return to sleep.

B. The sleep disturbance causes clinically significant distress or impairment in social, occupational, educational, academic, behavioral, or other important areas of functioning.

C. The sleep difficulty occurs at least 3 nights per week.

D. The sleep difficulty is present for at least 3 months.

E. The sleep difficulty occurs despite adequate opportunity for sleep.

F. The insomnia is not better explained by and does not occur exclusively during the course of another sleep-wake disorder (e.g., narcolepsy, a breathing-related sleep disorder, a circadian rhythm sleep-wake disorder, a parasomnia).

G. The insomnia is not attributable to the physiological effects of a substance (e.g., a drug of abuse, a medication).

H. Coexisting mental disorders and medical conditions do not adequately explain the predominant complaint of insomnia.

Specify if:

With mental disorder, including substance use disorders
With medical condition
With another sleep disorder

Coding note: The code F51.01 applies to all three specifiers. Code also the relevant associated mental disorder, medical condition, or other sleep disorder immediately after the code for insomnia disorder in order to indicate the association.

Specify if:

Episodic: Symptoms last at least 1 month but less than 3 months.
Persistent: Symptoms last 3 months or longer.
Recurrent: Two (or more) episodes within the space of 1 year.

Note: Acute and short-term insomnia (i.e., symptoms lasting less than 3 months but otherwise meeting all criteria with regard to frequency, intensity, distress, and/or impairment) should be coded as an other specified insomnia disorder.

Recording Procedures

The specifiers "with mental disorder, including substance use disorders"; "with medical condition"; and "with another sleep disorder" are available to allow the clinician to note clinically relevant comorbidities. In such cases, record F51.01 insomnia disorder, with [name of comorbid condition(s) or disorder(s)] followed by the diagnostic code(s) for the comorbid conditions or disorders (e.g., F51.01 insomnia disorder, with moderate cocaine use disorder and trigeminal neuralagia; F14.20 moderate cocaine use disorder; G50.0 trigeminal neuralgia).

Hypersomnolence Disorder

F51.11

A. Self-reported excessive sleepiness (hypersomnolence) despite a main sleep period lasting at least 7 hours, with at least one of the following symptoms:

1. Recurrent periods of sleep or lapses into sleep within the same day.
2. A prolonged main sleep episode of more than 9 hours per day that is nonrestorative (i.e., unrefreshing).
3. Difficulty being fully awake after abrupt awakening.

B. The hypersomnolence occurs at least three times per week, for at least 3 months.

C. The hypersomnolence is accompanied by significant distress or impairment in cognitive, social, occupational, or other important areas of functioning.

D. The hypersomnolence is not better explained by and does not occur exclusively during the course of another sleep disorder (e.g., narcolepsy, breathing-related sleep disorder, circadian rhythm sleep-wake disorder, or a parasomnia).

E. The hypersomnolence is not attributable to the physiological effects of a substance (e.g., a drug of abuse, a medication).

F. Coexisting mental and medical disorders do not adequately explain the predominant complaint of hypersomnolence.

Specify if:

With mental disorder, including substance use disorders
With medical condition
With another sleep disorder

Coding note: The code F51.11 applies to all three specifiers. Code also the relevant associated mental disorder, medical condition, or other sleep disorder immediately after the code for hypersomnolence disorder in order to indicate the association.

Specify if:

Acute: Duration of less than 1 month.
Subacute: Duration of 1–3 months.
Persistent: Duration of more than 3 months.

Specify current severity:

Specify severity based on degree of difficulty maintaining daytime alertness as manifested by the occurrence of multiple attacks of irresistible sleepiness within any given day occurring, for example, while sedentary, driving, visiting with friends, or working.

Mild: Difficulty maintaining daytime alertness 1–2 days/week.
Moderate: Difficulty maintaining daytime alertness 3–4 days/week.
Severe: Difficulty maintaining daytime alertness 5–7 days/week.

Recording Procedures

The specifiers "with mental disorder, including substance use disorders"; "with medical condition"; and "with another sleep disorder" are available to allow the clinician to note clinically relevant comorbidities. In such cases, record F51.11 hypersomnolence disorder, with [name of comorbid condition(s) or disorder(s)] followed by the diagnostic code(s) for the comorbid conditions or disorders (e.g., F51.11 hypersomnolence disorder, with major depressive disorder; F33.1 major depressive disorder, recurrent, moderate).

Narcolepsy

A. Recurrent periods of an irrepressible need to sleep, lapsing into sleep, or napping occurring within the same day. These must have been occurring at least three times per week over the past 3 months.

B. The presence of at least one of the following:

1. Episodes of cataplexy, defined as either (a) or (b), occurring at least a few times per month:

    a. In individuals with long-standing disease, brief (seconds to minutes) episodes of sudden bilateral loss of muscle tone with maintained consciousness that are precipitated by laughter or joking.

    b. In children or in individuals within 6 months of onset, spontaneous grimaces or jaw-opening episodes with tongue thrusting or a global hypotonia, without any obvious emotional triggers.

2. Hypocretin deficiency, as measured using cerebrospinal fluid (CSF) hypocretin-1 immunoreactivity values (less than or equal to one-third of values obtained in healthy subjects tested using the same assay, or less than or equal to 110 pg/mL). Low CSF levels of hypocretin-1 must not be observed in the context of acute brain injury, inflammation, or infection.

3. Nocturnal sleep polysomnography showing rapid eye movement (REM) sleep latency less than or equal to 15 minutes, or

a multiple sleep latency test showing a mean sleep latency less than or equal to 8 minutes and two or more sleep-onset REM periods.

Specify whether:

G47.411 Narcolepsy with cataplexy or hypocretin deficiency (type 1): Criterion B1 (episodes of cataplexy) or Criterion B2 (low CSF hypocretin-1 levels) is met.

G47.419 Narcolepsy without cataplexy and either without hypocretin deficiency or hypocretin unmeasured (type 2): Criterion B3 (positive polysomnography/multiple sleep latency test) is met, but Criterion B1 is not met (i.e., no cataplexy is present) and Criterion B2 is not met (i.e., CSF hypocretin-1 levels are not low or have not been measured).

G47.421 Narcolepsy with cataplexy or hypocretin deficiency due to a medical condition

G47.429 Narcolepsy without cataplexy and without hypocretin deficiency due to a medical condition

Coding note: For the subtype narcolepsy with cataplexy or hypocretin deficiency due to a medical condition and the subtype narcolepsy without cataplexy and without hypocretin deficiency due to a medical condition, code first the underlying medical condition (e.g., G71.11 myotonic dystrophy; G47.429 narcolepsy without cataplexy and without hypocretin deficiency due to myotonic dystrophy).

Specify current severity:

Mild: Need for naps only once or twice per day. Sleep disturbance, if present, is mild. Cataplexy, when present, is infrequent (occurring less than once per week).

Moderate: Need for multiple naps daily. Sleep may be moderately disturbed. Cataplexy, when present, occurs daily or every few days.

Severe: Nearly constant sleepiness and, often, highly disturbed nocturnal sleep (which may include excessive body movement and vivid dreams). Cataplexy, when present, is drug-resistant, with multiple attacks daily.

Breathing-Related Sleep Disorders

Obstructive Sleep Apnea Hypopnea

G47.33

A. Either (1) or (2):

1. Evidence by polysomnography of at least five obstructive apneas or hypopneas per hour of sleep and either of the following sleep symptoms:

a. Nocturnal breathing disturbances: snoring, snorting/gasping, or breathing pauses during sleep.

b. Daytime sleepiness, fatigue, or unrefreshing sleep despite sufficient opportunities to sleep that is not better explained by another mental disorder (including a sleep disorder) and is not attributable to another medical condition.

2. Evidence by polysomnography of 15 or more obstructive apneas and/or hypopneas per hour of sleep regardless of accompanying symptoms.

Specify current severity:

Mild: Apnea hypopnea index is less than 15.

Moderate: Apnea hypopnea index is 15–30.

Severe: Apnea hypopnea index is greater than 30.

Central Sleep Apnea

A. Evidence by polysomnography of five or more central apneas per hour of sleep.

B. The disorder is not better explained by another current sleep disorder.

Specify whether:

G47.31 Idiopathic central sleep apnea: Characterized by repeated episodes of apneas and hypopneas during sleep caused by variability in respiratory effort but without evidence of airway obstruction.

R06.3   Cheyne-Stokes breathing: A pattern of periodic crescendo-decrescendo variation in tidal volume that results in central apneas and hypopneas at a frequency of at least five events per hour, accompanied by frequent arousal.

G47.37 Central sleep apnea comorbid with opioid use: The pathogenesis of this subtype is attributed to the effects of opioids on the respiratory rhythm generators in the medulla as well as the differential effects on hypoxic versus hypercapnic respiratory drive.

Coding note (for G47.37 code only): When an opioid use disorder is present, first code the opioid use disorder: F11.10 mild opioid use disorder or F11.20 moderate or severe opioid use disorder; then code G47.37 central sleep apnea comorbid with opioid use. When an opioid use disorder is not present (e.g., after a one-time heavy use of the substance), code only G47.37 central sleep apnea comorbid with opioid use.

Specify current severity:

Severity of central sleep apnea is graded according to the frequency of the breathing disturbances as well as the extent of associated oxygen desaturation and sleep fragmentation that occur as a consequence of repetitive respiratory disturbances.

Sleep-Related Hypoventilation

A. Polysomnograpy demonstrates episodes of decreased respiration associated with elevated CO_2 levels. (**Note:** In the absence of objective measurement of CO_2, persistent low levels of hemoglobin oxygen saturation unassociated with apneic/hypopneic events may indicate hypoventilation.)

B. The disturbance is not better explained by another current sleep disorder.

Specify whether:

G47.34 Idiopathic hypoventilation: This subtype is not attributable to any readily identified condition.

G47.35 Congenital central alveolar hypoventilation: This subtype is a rare congenital disorder in which the individual typically presents in the perinatal period with shallow breathing, or cyanosis and apnea during sleep.

G47.36 Comorbid sleep-related hypoventilation: This subtype occurs as a consequence of a medical condition, such as a pulmonary disorder (e.g., interstitial lung disease, chronic obstructive pulmonary disease) or a neuromuscular or chest wall disorder (e.g., muscular dystrophies, postpolio syndrome, cervical spinal cord injury, kyphoscoliosis), or medications (e.g., benzodiazepines, opiates). It also occurs with obesity (obesity hypoventilation disorder), where it reflects a combination of increased work of breathing due to reduced chest wall compliance and ventilation-perfusion mismatch and variably reduced ventilatory drive. Such individuals usually are characterized by body mass index of greater than 30 and hypercapnia during wakefulness (with a pCO_2 of greater than 45), without other evidence of hypoventilation.

Specify current severity:

Severity is graded according to the degree of hypoxemia and hypercarbia present during sleep and evidence of end organ impairment due to these abnormalities (e.g., right-sided heart failure). The presence of blood gas abnormalities during wakefulness is an indicator of greater severity.

Circadian Rhythm Sleep-Wake Disorders

A. A persistent or recurrent pattern of sleep disruption that is primarily due to an alteration of the circadian system or to a misalignment between the endogenous circadian rhythm and the sleep-wake schedule required by an individual's physical environment or social or professional schedule.

B. The sleep disruption leads to excessive sleepiness or insomnia, or both.

C. The sleep disturbance causes clinically significant distress or impairment in social. occupational, and other important areas of functioning.

Specify whether:

G47.21 Delayed sleep phase type: A pattern of delayed sleep onset and awakening times, with an inability to fall asleep and awaken at a desired or conventionally acceptable earlier time.

Specify if:

Familial: A family history of delayed sleep phase is present.

Specify if:

Overlapping with non-24-hour sleep-wake type: Delayed sleep phase type may overlap with another circadian rhythm sleep-wake disorder. non-24-hour sleep-wake type.

G47.22 Advanced sleep phase type: A pattern of advanced sleep onset and awakening times, with an inability to remain awake or asleep until the desired or conventionally acceptable later sleep or wake times.

Specify if:

Familial: A family history of advanced sleep phase is present.

G47.23 Irregular sleep-wake type: A temporally disorganized sleep-wake pattern, such that the timing of sleep and wake periods is variable throughout the 24-hour period.

G47.24 Non-24-hour sleep-wake type: A pattern of sleep-wake cycles that is not synchronized to the 24-hour environment, with a consistent daily drift (usually to later and later times) of sleep onset and wake times.

G47.26 Shift work type: Insomnia during the major sleep period and/or excessive sleepiness (including inadvertent sleep) during the major awake period associated with a shift work schedule (i.e., requiring unconventional work hours).

G47.20 Unspecified type

Specify if:

Episodic: Symptoms last at least 1 month but less than 3 months.
Persistent: Symptoms last 3 months or longer.
Recurrent: Two or more episodes occur within the space of 1 year.

Parasomnias

Non–Rapid Eye Movement Sleep Arousal Disorders

A. Recurrent episodes of incomplete awakening from sleep, usually occurring during the first third of the major sleep episode, accompanied by either one of the following:

1. **Sleepwalking:** Repeated episodes of rising from bed during sleep and walking about. While sleepwalking, the individual has a blank, staring face; is relatively unresponsive to the efforts of others to communicate with him or her; and can be awakened only with great difficulty.
2. **Sleep terrors:** Recurrent episodes of abrupt terror arousals from sleep, usually beginning with a panicky scream. There is intense fear and signs of autonomic arousal, such as mydriasis, tachycardia, rapid breathing, and sweating, during each episode. There is relative unresponsiveness to efforts of others to comfort the individual during the episodes.

B. No or little (e.g., only a single visual scene) dream imagery is recalled.
C. Amnesia for the episodes is present.
D. The episodes cause clinically significant distress or impairment in social, occupational, or other important areas of functioning.
E. The disturbance is not attributable to the physiological effects of a substance (e.g., a drug of abuse, a medication).
F. Coexisting mental and medical disorders do not explain the episodes of sleepwalking or sleep terrors.

Specify whether:

F51.3 Sleepwalking type

Specify if:

With sleep-related eating
With sleep-related sexual behavior (sexsomnia)

F51.4 Sleep terror type

Nightmare Disorder

F51.5

A. Repeated occurrences of extended, extremely dysphoric, and well-remembered dreams that usually involve efforts to avoid threats to survival, security, or physical integrity and that generally occur during the second half of the major sleep episode.
B. On awakening from the dysphoric dreams, the individual rapidly becomes oriented and alert.

C. The sleep disturbance causes clinically significant distress or impairment in social, occupational, or other important areas of functioning.

D. The nightmare symptoms are not attributable to the physiological effects of a substance (e.g., a drug of abuse, a medication).

E. Coexisting mental disorders and medical conditions do not adequately explain the predominant complaint of dysphoric dreams.

Specify if:

During sleep onset

Specify if:

With mental disorder, including substance use disorders
With medical condition
With another sleep disorder

Coding note: The code F51.5 applies to all three specifiers. Code also the relevant associated mental disorder, medical condition, or other sleep disorder immediately after the code for nightmare disorder in order to indicate the association.

Specify if:

Acute: Duration of period of nightmares is 1 month or less.
Subacute: Duration of period of nightmares is greater than 1 month but less than 6 months.
Persistent: Duration of period of nightmares is 6 months or greater.

Specify current severity:

Severity can be rated by the frequency with which the nightmares occur:

Mild: Less than one episode per week on average.
Moderate: One or more episodes per week but less than nightly.
Severe: Episodes nightly.

Recording Procedures

The specifiers "with mental disorder, including substance use disorders"; "with medical condition"; and "with another sleep disorder" are available to allow the clinician to note clinically relevant comorbidities. In such cases, record F51.5 nightmare disorder with [name of comorbid condition(s) or disorder(s)] followed by the diagnostic code(s) for the comorbid conditions or disorders (e.g., F51.5 nightmare disorder with moderate alcohol use disorder and rapid eye movement sleep behavior disorder; F10.20 moderate alcohol use disorder; G47.52 REM sleep behavior disorder).

Rapid Eye Movement Sleep Behavior Disorder

G47.52

A. Repeated episodes of arousal during sleep associated with vocalization and/or complex motor behaviors.

B. These behaviors arise during rapid eye movement (REM) sleep and therefore usually occur more than 90 minutes after sleep onset, are more frequent during the later portions of the sleep period, and uncommonly occur during daytime naps.

C. Upon awakening from these episodes, the individual is completely awake, alert, and not confused or disoriented.

D. Either of the following:

    1. REM sleep without atonia on polysomnographic recording.
    2. A history suggestive of REM sleep behavior disorder and an established synucleinopathy diagnosis (e.g., Parkinson's disease, multiple system atrophy).

E. The behaviors cause clinically significant distress or impairment in social, occupational, or other important areas of functioning (which may include injury to self or the bed partner).

F. The disturbance is not attributable to the physiological effects of a substance (e.g., a drug of abuse, a medication) or another medical condition.

G. Coexisting mental disorders and medical conditions do not explain the episodes.

Restless Legs Syndrome

G25.81

A. An urge to move the legs, usually accompanied by or in response to uncomfortable and unpleasant sensations in the legs, characterized by all of the following:

    1. The urge to move the legs begins or worsens during periods of rest or inactivity.
    2. The urge to move the legs is partially or totally relieved by movement.
    3. The urge to move the legs is worse in the evening or at night than during the day, or occurs only in the evening or at night.

B. The symptoms in Criterion A occur at least three times per week and have persisted for at least 3 months.

C. The symptoms in Criterion A are accompanied by significant distress or impairment in social, occupational, educational, academic, behavioral, or other important areas of functioning.

D. The symptoms in Criterion A are not attributable to another mental disorder or medical condition (e.g., arthritis, leg edema, peripheral ischemia, leg cramps) and are not better explained by a behavioral condition (e.g., positional discomfort, habitual foot tapping).

E. The symptoms are not attributable to the physiological effects of a drug of abuse or medication (e.g., akathisia).

Substance/Medication-Induced Sleep Disorder

A. A prominent and severe disturbance in sleep.

B. There is evidence from the history, physical examination, or laboratory findings of both (1) and (2):

1. The symptoms in Criterion A developed during or soon after substance intoxication or withdrawal or after exposure to or withdrawal from a medication.

2. The involved substance/medication is capable of producing the symptoms in Criterion A.

C. The disturbance is not better explained by a sleep disorder that is not substance/medication-induced. Such evidence of an independent sleep disorder could include the following:

The symptoms precede the onset of the substance/medication use; the symptoms persist for a substantial period of time (e.g., about 1 month) after the cessation of acute withdrawal or severe intoxication; or there is other evidence suggesting the existence of an independent non-substance/medication-induced sleep disorder (e.g., a history of recurrent non-substance/medication-related episodes).

D. The disturbance does not occur exclusively during the course of a delirium.

E. The disturbance causes clinically significant distress or impairment in social, occupational, or other important areas of functioning.

Note: This diagnosis should be made instead of a diagnosis of substance intoxication or substance withdrawal only when the symptoms in Criterion A predominate in the clinical picture and when they are sufficiently severe to warrant clinical attention.

Coding note: The ICD-10-CM codes for the [specific substance/medication]-induced sleep disorders are indicated in the table below. Note that the ICD-10-CM code depends on whether or not there is a comorbid substance use disorder present for the same class of substance. In any case, an additional separate diagnosis of a substance use disorder is not given. If a mild substance use disorder is comorbid with the substance-induced sleep disorder, the 4th position character is "1," and the clinician should record "mild [substance] use disorder" before the substance-induced sleep disorder (e.g., "mild cocaine use disorder with cocaine-induced sleep disorder"). If a moderate or severe substance use disorder is comorbid with the substance-induced sleep disorder, the 4th position character is "2," and the clinician should record "moderate [substance] use disorder" or "severe [substance] use disorder" depending on the severity of the comorbid substance use disorder. If there is no comorbid substance use disorder (e.g., after a one-time heavy use of the substance), then the 4th position character is "9," and the clinician should record only the substance-induced sleep disorder. There are two exceptions to this coding convention as it applies to caffeine- and tobacco-induced sleep disorders. Because caffeine use disorder is not an official DSM-5 category, there is only a single ICD-10-CM code for caffeine-induced sleep disorder: F15.982. Moreover, because ICD-10-CM assumes that tobacco-induced sleep disorder can only occur in the context of moderate or severe tobacco use disorder, the ICD-10-CM code for tobacco-induced sleep disorder is F17.208.

	ICD-10-CM		
	With mild use disorder	With moderate or severe use disorder	Without use disorder
Alcohol	F10.182	F10.282	F10.982
Caffeine	NA	NA	F15.982
Cannabis	F12.188	F12.288	F12.988
Opioid	F11.182	F11.282	F11.982
Sedative, hypnotic, or anxiolytic	F13.182	F13.282	F13.982
Amphetamine-type substance (or other stimulant)	F15.182	F15.282	F15.982
Cocaine	F14.182	F14.282	F14.982
Tobacco	NA	F17.208	NA
Other (or unknown) substance	F19.182	F19.282	F19.982

Specify whether:

Insomnia type: Characterized by difficulty falling asleep or maintaining sleep, frequent nocturnal awakenings, or nonrestorative sleep.

Daytime sleepiness type: Characterized by predominant complaint of excessive sleepiness/fatigue during waking hours or, less commonly, a long sleep period.

Parasomnia type: Characterized by abnormal behavioral events during sleep.

Mixed type: Characterized by a substance/medication-induced sleep problem characterized by multiple types of sleep symptoms, but no symptom clearly predominates.

Specify (see Table 1 in the chapter "Substance-Related and Addictive Disorders," which indicates whether "with onset during intoxication" and/or "with onset during withdrawal" applies to a given substance class; or *specify* "with onset after medication use"):

With onset during intoxication: If criteria are met for intoxication with the substance and the symptoms develop during intoxication.

With onset during withdrawal: If criteria are met for withdrawal from the substance and the symptoms develop during, or shortly after, withdrawal.

With onset after medication use: If symptoms developed at initiation of medication, with a change in use of medication, or during withdrawal of medication.

Recording Procedures

The name of the substance/medication-induced sleep disorder begins with the specific substance (e.g., alcohol) that is presumed to be causing the sleep disturbance. The ICD-10-CM code that corresponds to the applicable drug class is selected from the table included in the criteria set. For substances that do not fit into any of the classes (e.g., fluoxetine), the ICD-10-CM code for the other (or unknown) substance class should be used and the name of the specific substance recorded (e.g., F19.982 fluoxetine-induced sleep disorder, insomnia type). In cases in which a substance is judged to be an etiological factor but the specific substance is unknown, the ICD-10-CM code for the other (or unknown) substance class is used and the fact that the substance is unknown is recorded (e.g., F19.982 unknown substance-induced sleep disorder, hypersomnia type).

To record the name of the disorder, the comorbid substance use disorder (if any) is listed first, followed by "with substance/medication-induced sleep disorder" (incorporating the name of the specific etiological substance/medication), followed by the specification of onset (i.e., with onset during intoxication, with onset during withdrawal, with onset after medication use), followed by the subtype designation (i.e., insomnia type, daytime sleepiness type, parasomnia type, mixed type). For example, in the case of insomnia occurring during withdrawal in a man with a severe lorazepam use disorder, the diagnosis is F13.282 severe lorazepam use disorder with lorazepam-induced sleep disorder, with onset during withdrawal, insomnia type. A separate diagnosis of the comorbid severe lorazepam use disorder is not given. If the substance-induced sleep disorder occurs without a comorbid substance use disorder (e.g., with medication use as prescribed), no accompanying substance use disorder is noted (e.g., F19.982 bupropion-induced sleep disorder, with onset during medication use, insomnia type). When more than one substance is judged to play a significant role in the development of the sleep disturbance, each should be listed separately (e.g., F10.282 severe alcohol use disorder with alcohol-induced sleep disorder, with onset during intoxication, insomnia type; F14.282 severe cocaine use disorder with cocaine-induced sleep disorder, with onset during intoxication, insomnia type).

Other Specified Insomnia Disorder

G47.09

This category applies to presentations in which symptoms characteristic of insomnia disorder that cause clinically significant distress or impairment in social, occupational, or other important areas of functioning predominate but do not meet the full criteria for insomnia disorder or any of the disorders in the sleep-wake disorders diagnostic class. The other specified insomnia disorder category is used in situations in which the clinician chooses to communicate the specific reason that the presentation does not meet the criteria for insomnia disorder or any specific sleep-wake disorder. This is done by recording "other specified insomnia disorder" followed by the specific reason (e.g., "short-term insomnia disorder").

Examples of presentations that can be specified using the "other specified" designation include the following:

1. **Short-term insomnia disorder:** Duration is less than 3 months.
2. **Restricted to nonrestorative sleep:** Predominant complaint is nonrestorative sleep unaccompanied by other sleep symptoms such as difficulty falling asleep or remaining asleep.

Unspecified Insomnia Disorder

G47.00

This category applies to presentations in which symptoms characteristic of insomnia disorder that cause clinically significant distress or impairment in social, occupational, or other important areas of functioning predominate but do not meet the full criteria for insomnia disorder or any of the disorders in the sleep-wake disorders diagnostic class. The unspecified insomnia disorder category is used in situations in which the clinician chooses *not* to specify the reason that the criteria are not met for insomnia disorder or a specific sleep-wake disorder, and includes presentations in which there is insufficient information to make a more specific diagnosis.

Other Specified Hypersomnolence Disorder

G47.19

This category applies to presentations in which symptoms characteristic of hypersomnolence disorder that cause clinically significant distress or impairment in social, occupational, or other important areas of functioning predominate but do not meet the full criteria for hypersomnolence disorder or any of the disorders in the sleep-wake disorders diagnostic class. The other specified hypersomnolence disorder category is used in situations in which the clinician chooses to communicate the specific reason that the presentation does not meet the criteria for hypersomnolence disorder or any specific sleep-wake disorder. This is done by recording "other specified hypersomnolence disorder" followed by the specific reason (e.g., "brief-duration hypersomnolence," as in Kleine-Levin syndrome).

Unspecified Hypersomnolence Disorder

G47.10

This category applies to presentations in which symptoms characteristic of hypersomnolence disorder that cause clinically significant distress or impairment in social, occupational, or other important areas of functioning predominate but do not meet the full criteria for hypersomnolence disorder or any of the disorders in the sleep-wake disorders diagnostic class. The unspecified hypersomnolence disorder category is used in situations in which the clinician chooses *not* to specify the reason that the criteria are not met for hypersomnolence disorder or a specific sleep-wake disorder, and includes presentations in which there is insufficient information to make a more specific diagnosis.

Other Specified Sleep-Wake Disorder

G47.8

This category applies to presentations in which symptoms characteristic of a sleep-wake disorder that cause clinically significant distress or impairment in social, occupational, or other important areas of functioning predominate but do not meet the full criteria for any of the disorders in the sleep-wake disorders diagnostic class and do not qualify for a diagnosis of other specified insomnia disorder or other specified hypersomnolence disorder. The other specified sleep-wake disorder category is used in situations in which the clinician chooses to communicate the specific reason that the presentation does not meet the criteria for any specific sleep-wake disorder. This is done by recording "other specified sleep-wake disorder" followed by the specific reason (e.g., "repeated arousals during rapid eye movement sleep without polysomnography or history of Parkinson's disease or other synucleinopathy").

Unspecified Sleep-Wake Disorder

G47.9

This category applies to presentations in which symptoms characteristic of a sleep-wake disorder that cause clinically significant distress or impairment in social, occupational, or other important areas of functioning predominate but do not meet the full criteria for any of the disorders in the sleep-wake disorders diagnostic class and do not qualify for a diagnosis of unspecified insomnia disorder or unspecified hypersomnolence disorder. The unspecified sleep-wake disorder category is used in situations in which the clinician chooses *not* to specify the reason that the criteria are not met for a specific sleep-wake disorder, and includes presentations in which there is insufficient information to make a more specific diagnosis.

Delayed Ejaculation

F52.32

A. Either of the following symptoms must be experienced on almost all or all occasions (approximately 75%–100%) of partnered sexual activity (in identified situational contexts or, if generalized, in all contexts), and without the individual desiring delay:

1. Marked delay in ejaculation.
2. Marked infrequency or absence of ejaculation.

B. The symptoms in Criterion A have persisted for a minimum duration of approximately 6 months.

C. The symptoms in Criterion A cause clinically significant distress in the individual.

D. The sexual dysfunction is not better explained by a nonsexual mental disorder or as a consequence of severe relationship distress or other significant stressors and is not attributable to the effects of a substance/medication or another medical condition.

Specify whether:

Lifelong: The disturbance has been present since the individual became sexually active.

Acquired: The disturbance began after a period of relatively normal sexual function.

Specify whether:

Generalized: Not limited to certain types of stimulation, situations, or partners.

Situational: Only occurs with certain types of stimulation, situations, or partners.

Specify current severity:

Mild: Evidence of mild distress over the symptoms in Criterion A.

Moderate: Evidence of moderate distress over the symptoms in Criterion A.

Severe: Evidence of severe or extreme distress over the symptoms in Criterion A.

Erectile Disorder

F52.21

A. At least one of the three following symptoms must be experienced on almost all or all (approximately 75%–100%) occasions of sexual activity (in identified situational contexts or, if generalized, in all contexts):

1. Marked difficulty in obtaining an erection during sexual activity.
2. Marked difficulty in maintaining an erection until the completion of sexual activity.
3. Marked decrease in erectile rigidity.

B. The symptoms in Criterion A have persisted for a minimum duration of approximately 6 months.
C. The symptoms in Criterion A cause clinically significant distress in the individual.
D. The sexual dysfunction is not better explained by a nonsexual mental disorder or as a consequence of severe relationship distress or other significant stressors and is not attributable to the effects of a substance/medication or another medical condition.

Specify whether:
   Lifelong: The disturbance has been present since the individual became sexually active.
   Acquired: The disturbance began after a period of relatively normal sexual function.

Specify whether:
   Generalized: Not limited to certain types of stimulation, situations, or partners.
   Situational: Only occurs with certain types of stimulation, situations, or partners.

Specify current severity:
   Mild: Evidence of mild distress over the symptoms in Criterion A.
   Moderate: Evidence of moderate distress over the symptoms in Criterion A.
   Severe: Evidence of severe or extreme distress over the symptoms in Criterion A.

Female Orgasmic Disorder

F52.31

A. Presence of either of the following symptoms and experienced on almost all or all (approximately 75%–100%) occasions of sexual activity (in identified situational contexts or, if generalized, in all contexts):

1. Marked delay in, marked infrequency of, or absence of orgasm.
2. Markedly reduced intensity of orgasmic sensations.

B. The symptoms in Criterion A have persisted for a minimum duration of approximately 6 months.
C. The symptoms in Criterion A cause clinically significant distress in the individual.

D. The sexual dysfunction is not better explained by a nonsexual mental disorder or as a consequence of severe relationship distress (e.g., partner violence) or other significant stressors and is not attributable to the effects of a substance/medication or another medical condition.

Specify whether:

Lifelong: The disturbance has been present since the individual became sexually active.

Acquired: The disturbance began after a period of relatively normal sexual function.

Specify whether:

Generalized: Not limited to certain types of stimulation, situations, or partners.

Situational: Only occurs with certain types of stimulation, situations, or partners.

Specify if:

Never experienced an orgasm under any situation.

Specify current severity:

Mild: Evidence of mild distress over the symptoms in Criterion A.

Moderate: Evidence of moderate distress over the symptoms in Criterion A.

Severe: Evidence of severe or extreme distress over the symptoms in Criterion A.

Female Sexual Interest/Arousal Disorder

F52.22

A. Lack of, or significantly reduced, sexual interest/arousal, as manifested by at least three of the following:

1. Absent/reduced interest in sexual activity.
2. Absent/reduced sexual/erotic thoughts or fantasies.
3. No/reduced initiation of sexual activity, and typically unreceptive to a partner's attempts to initiate.
4. Absent/reduced sexual excitement/pleasure during sexual activity in almost all or all (approximately 75%–100%) sexual encounters (in identified situational contexts or, if generalized, in all contexts).
5. Absent/reduced sexual interest/arousal in response to any internal or external sexual/erotic cues (e.g., written, verbal, visual).
6. Absent/reduced genital or nongenital sensations during sexual activity in almost all or all (approximately 75%–100%) sexual encounters (in identified situational contexts or, if generalized, in all contexts).

B. The symptoms in Criterion A have persisted for a minimum duration of approximately 6 months.
C. The symptoms in Criterion A cause clinically significant distress in the individual.
D. The sexual dysfunction is not better explained by a nonsexual mental disorder or as a consequence of severe relationship distress (e.g., partner violence) or other significant stressors and is not attributable to the effects of a substance/medication or another medical condition.

Specify whether:

Lifelong: The disturbance has been present since the individual became sexually active.

Acquired: The disturbance began after a period of relatively normal sexual function.

Specify whether:

Generalized: Not limited to certain types of stimulation, situations, or partners.

Situational: Only occurs with certain types of stimulation, situations, or partners.

Specify current severity:

Mild: Evidence of mild distress over the symptoms in Criterion A.

Moderate: Evidence of moderate distress over the symptoms in Criterion A.

Severe: Evidence of severe or extreme distress over the symptoms in Criterion A.

Genito-Pelvic Pain/Penetration Disorder

F52.6

A. Persistent or recurrent difficulties with one (or more) of the following:

1. Vaginal penetration during intercourse.
2. Marked vulvovaginal or pelvic pain during vaginal intercourse or penetration attempts.
3. Marked fear or anxiety about vulvovaginal or pelvic pain in anticipation of, during, or as a result of vaginal penetration.
4. Marked tensing or tightening of the pelvic floor muscles during attempted vaginal penetration.

B. The symptoms in Criterion A have persisted for a minimum duration of approximately 6 months.
C. The symptoms in Criterion A cause clinically significant distress in the individual.
D. The sexual dysfunction is not better explained by a nonsexual mental disorder or as a consequence of a severe relationship distress (e.g., partner violence) or other significant stressors and is

not attributable to the effects of a substance/medication or another medical condition.

Specify whether:

Lifelong: The disturbance has been present since the individual became sexually active.

Acquired: The disturbance began after a period of relatively normal sexual function.

Specify current severity:

Mild: Evidence of mild distress over the symptoms in Criterion A.

Moderate: Evidence of moderate distress over the symptoms in Criterion A.

Severe: Evidence of severe or extreme distress over the symptoms in Criterion A.

Male Hypoactive Sexual Desire Disorder

F52.0

A. Persistently or recurrently deficient (or absent) sexual/erotic thoughts or fantasies and desire for sexual activity. The judgment of deficiency is made by the clinician, taking into account factors that affect sexual functioning, such as age and general and sociocultural contexts of the individual's life.

B. The symptoms in Criterion A have persisted for a minimum duration of approximately 6 months.

C. The symptoms in Criterion A cause clinically significant distress in the individual.

D. The sexual dysfunction is not better explained by a nonsexual mental disorder or as a consequence of severe relationship distress or other significant stressors and is not attributable to the effects of a substance/medication or another medical condition.

Specify whether:

Lifelong: The disturbance has been present since the individual became sexually active.

Acquired: The disturbance began after a period of relatively normal sexual function.

Specify whether:

Generalized: Not limited to certain types of stimulation, situations, or partners.

Situational: Only occurs with certain types of stimulation, situations, or partners.

Specify current severity:

Mild: Evidence of mild distress over the symptoms in Criterion A.

Moderate: Evidence of moderate distress over the symptoms in Criterion A.

Severe: Evidence of severe or extreme distress over the symptoms in Criterion A.

Premature (Early) Ejaculation

F52.4

A. A persistent or recurrent pattern of ejaculation occurring during partnered sexual activity within approximately 1 minute following vaginal penetration and before the individual wishes it.

Note: Although the diagnosis of premature (early) ejaculation may be applied to individuals engaged in nonvaginal sexual activities, specific duration criteria have not been established for these activities.

B. The symptom in Criterion A must have been present for at least 6 months and must be experienced on almost all or all (approximately 75%–100%) occasions of sexual activity (in identified situational contexts or, if generalized, in all contexts).

C. The symptom in Criterion A causes clinically significant distress in the individual.

D. The sexual dysfunction is not better explained by a nonsexual mental disorder or as a consequence of severe relationship distress or other significant stressors and is not attributable to the effects of a substance/medication or another medical condition.

Specify whether:

Lifelong: The disturbance has been present since the individual became sexually active.

Acquired: The disturbance began after a period of relatively normal sexual function.

Specify whether:

Generalized: Not limited to certain types of stimulation, situations, or partners.

Situational: Only occurs with certain types of stimulation, situations, or partners.

Specify current severity:

Mild: Ejaculation occurring within approximately 30 seconds to 1 minute of vaginal penetration.

Moderate: Ejaculation occurring within approximately 15–30 seconds of vaginal penetration.

Severe: Ejaculation occurring prior to sexual activity, at the start of sexual activity, or within approximately 15 seconds of vaginal penetration.

Substance/Medication-Induced
Sexual Dysfunction

A. A clinically significant disturbance in sexual function is predominant in the clinical picture.

B. There is evidence from the history, physical examination, or laboratory findings of both (1) and (2):

1. The symptoms in Criterion A developed during or soon after substance intoxication or withdrawal or after exposure to or withdrawal from a medication.
2. The involved substance/medication is capable of producing the symptoms in Criterion A.

C. The disturbance is not better explained by a sexual dysfunction that is not substance/medication-induced. Such evidence of an independent sexual dysfunction could include the following:

The symptoms precede the onset of the substance/medication use; the symptoms persist for a substantial period of time (e.g., about 1 month) after the cessation of acute withdrawal or severe intoxication; or there is other evidence suggesting the existence of an independent non-substance/medication-induced sexual dysfunction (e.g., a history of recurrent non-substance/medication-related episodes).

D. The disturbance does not occur exclusively during the course of a delirium.

E. The disturbance causes clinically significant distress in the individual.

Note: This diagnosis should be made instead of a diagnosis of substance intoxication or substance withdrawal only when the symptoms in Criterion A predominate in the clinical picture and are sufficiently severe to warrant clinical attention.

Coding note: The ICD-10-CM codes for the [specific substance/medication]-induced sexual dysfunctions are indicated in the table below. Note that the ICD-10-CM code depends on whether or not there is a comorbid substance use disorder present for the same class of substance. In any case, an additional separate diagnosis of a substance use disorder is not given. If a mild substance use disorder is comorbid with the substance-induced sexual dysfunction, the 4th position character is "1," and the clinician should record "mild [substance] use disorder" before the substance-induced sexual dysfunction (e.g., "mild cocaine use disorder with cocaine-induced sexual dysfunction"). If a moderate or severe substance use disorder is comorbid with the substance-induced sexual dysfunction, the 4th position character is "2," and the clinician should record "moderate [substance] use disorder" or "severe [substance] use disorder" depending on the severity of the comorbid substance use disorder. If there is no comorbid substance use disorder (e.g., after a one-time heavy use of the substance), then the 4th position character is "9," and the clinician should record only the substance-induced sexual dysfunction.

	ICD-10-CM		
	With mild use disorder	With moderate or severe use disorder	Without use disorder
Alcohol	F10.181	F10.281	F10.981
Opioid	F11.181	F11.281	F11.981
Sedative, hypnotic, or anxiolytic	F13.181	F13.281	F13.981
Amphetamine-type substance (or other stimulant)	F15.181	F15.281	F15.981
Cocaine	F14.181	F14.281	F14.981
Other (or unknown) substance	F19.181	F19.281	F19.981

Specify (see Table 1 in the chapter "Substance-Related and Addictive Disorders," which indicates whether "with onset during intoxication" and/or "with onset during withdrawal" applies to a given substance class; or *specify* "with onset after medication use"):

With onset during intoxication: If criteria are met for intoxication with the substance and the symptoms develop during intoxication.
With onset during withdrawal: If criteria are met for withdrawal from the substance and the symptoms develop during, or shortly after, withdrawal.
With onset after medication use: If symptoms developed at initiation of medication, with a change in use of medication, or during withdrawal of medication.

Specify current severity:

Mild: Occurs on 25%–50% of occasions of sexual activity.
Moderate: Occurs on 50%–75% of occasions of sexual activity.
Severe: Occurs on 75% or more of occasions of sexual activity.

Recording Procedures

The name of the substance/medication-induced sexual dysfunction begins with the specific substance (e.g., alcohol) that is presumed to be causing the sexual dysfunction. The ICD-10-CM code that corresponds to the applicable drug class is selected from the table included in the criteria set. For substances that do not fit into any of the classes (e.g., fluoxetine), the ICD-10-CM code for the other (or unknown) substance class should be used and the name of the specific substance recorded (e.g., F19.981 fluoxetine-induced sexual dysfunction). In cases in which a substance is judged to be an etiological factor but the specific substance is unknown, the ICD-10-CM code for the other (or unknown) substance class is used and the fact that the substance is unknown is recorded (e.g., F19.981 unknown substance-induced sexual dysfunction).

When recording the name of the disorder, the comorbid substance use disorder (if any) is listed first, followed by the word "with," followed by the name of the substance-induced sexual dysfunction, followed by the specification of onset (i.e., onset during intoxication, onset during withdrawal, with onset after medication use), followed by the severity specifier (e.g., mild, moderate, severe). For example, in the case of erectile dysfunction occurring during intoxication in a man with a severe alcohol use disorder, the diagnosis is F10.281 moderate alcohol use disorder with alcohol-induced sexual dysfunction, with onset during intoxication, moderate. A separate diagnosis of the comorbid severe alcohol use disorder is not given. If the substance-induced sexual dysfunction occurs without a comorbid substance use disorder (e.g., after a one-time heavy use of the substance), no accompanying substance use disorder is noted (e.g., F15.981 amphetamine-induced sexual dysfunction, with onset during intoxication). When more than one substance is judged to play a significant role in the development of the sexual dysfunction, each should be listed separately (e.g., F14.181 mild cocaine use disorder with cocaine-induced sexual dysfunction, with onset during intoxication, moderate; F19.981 fluoxetine-induced sexual dysfunction, with onset after medication use, moderate).

Other Specified Sexual Dysfunction

F52.8

This category applies to presentations in which symptoms characteristic of a sexual dysfunction that cause clinically significant distress in the individual predominate but do not meet the full criteria for any of the disorders in the sexual dysfunctions diagnostic class. The other specified sexual dysfunction category is used in situations in which the clinician chooses to communicate the specific reason that the presentation does not meet the criteria for any specific sexual dysfunction. This is done by recording "other specified sexual dysfunction" followed by the specific reason (e.g., "sexual aversion").

Unspecified Sexual Dysfunction

F52.9

This category applies to presentations in which symptoms characteristic of a sexual dysfunction that cause clinically significant distress in the individual predominate but do not meet the full criteria for any of the disorders in the sexual dysfunctions diagnostic class. The unspecified sexual dysfunction category is used in situations in which the clinician chooses *not* to specify the reason that the criteria are not met for a specific sexual dysfunction, and includes presentations for which there is insufficient information to make a more specific diagnosis.

Gender Dysphoria

Gender Dysphoria in Children   F64.2

A. A marked incongruence between one's experienced/expressed gender and assigned gender, of at least 6 months' duration, as manifested by at least six of the following (one of which must be Criterion A1):

1. A strong desire to be of the other gender or an insistence that he or she is the other gender (or some alternative gender different from one's assigned gender).
2. In boys (assigned gender), a strong preference for cross-dressing or simulating female attire; or in girls (assigned gender), a strong preference for wearing only typical masculine clothing and a strong resistance to the wearing of typical feminine clothing.
3. A strong preference for cross-gender roles in make-believe play or fantasy play.
4. A strong preference for the toys, games, or activities stereotypically used or engaged in by the other gender.
5. A strong preference for playmates of the other gender.
6. In boys (assigned gender), a strong rejection of typically masculine toys, games, and activities and a strong avoidance of rough-and-tumble play; or in girls (assigned gender), a strong rejection of typically feminine toys, games, and activities.
7. A strong dislike of one's sexual anatomy.
8. A strong desire for the primary and/or secondary sex characteristics that match one's experienced gender.

B. The condition is associated with clinically significant distress or impairment in social, school, or other important areas of functioning.

Specify if:

With a disorder/difference of sex development (e.g., a congenital adrenogenital disorder such as E25.0 congenital adrenal hyperplasia or E34.50 androgen insensitivity syndrome).

Coding note: Code the disorder/difference of sex development as well as gender dysphoria.

Gender Dysphoria in Adolescents and Adults   F64.0

A. A marked incongruence between one's experienced/expressed gender and assigned gender, of at least 6 months' duration, as manifested by at least two of the following:

1. A marked incongruence between one's experienced/expressed gender and primary and/or secondary sex characteristics (or in young adolescents, the anticipated secondary sex characteristics).
2. A strong desire to be rid of one's primary and/or secondary sex characteristics because of a marked incongruence with one's experienced/expressed gender (or in young adolescents, a desire to prevent the development of the anticipated secondary sex characteristics).
3. A strong desire for the primary and/or secondary sex characteristics of the other gender.
4. A strong desire to be of the other gender (or some alternative gender different from one's assigned gender).
5. A strong desire to be treated as the other gender (or some alternative gender different from one's assigned gender).
6. A strong conviction that one has the typical feelings and reactions of the other gender (or some alternative gender different from one's assigned gender).

B. The condition is associated with clinically significant distress or impairment in social, occupational, or other important areas of functioning.

Specify if:

With a disorder/difference of sex development (e.g., a congenital adrenogenital disorder such as E25.0 congenital adrenal hyperplasia or E34.50 androgen insensitivity syndrome).

Coding note: Code the disorder/difference of sex development as well as gender dysphoria.

Specify if:

Posttransition: The individual has transitioned to full-time living in the experienced gender (with or without legalization of gender change) and has undergone (or is preparing to have) at least one gender-affirming medical procedure or treatment regimen—namely, regular gender-affirming hormone treatment or gender reassignment surgery confirming the experienced gender (e.g., breast augmentation surgery and/or vulvovaginoplasty in an individual assigned male at birth; transmasculine chest surgery and/or phalloplasty or metoidioplasty in an individual assigned female at birth).

Other Specified Gender Dysphoria

F64.8

This category applies to presentations in which symptoms characteristic of gender dysphoria that cause clinically significant distress or impairment in social, occupational, or other important areas of functioning predominate but do not meet the full criteria for gender dysphoria. The other specified gender dysphoria category is used in situations in which the clinician chooses to communicate the specific reason that the pre-sentation does not meet the criteria for gender dysphoria. This is done by recording "other specified gender dysphoria" followed by the spe-cific reason (e.g., "brief gender dysphoria," in which symptoms meet full criteria for gender dysphoria but the duration is less than the required 6 months).

Unspecified Gender Dysphoria

F64.9

This category applies to presentations in which symptoms characteristic of gender dysphoria that cause clinically significant distress or impair-ment in social, occupational, or other important areas of functioning predominate but do not meet the full criteria for gender dysphoria. The unspecified gender dysphoria category is used in situations in which the clinician chooses *not* to specify the reason that the criteria are not met for gender dysphoria, and includes presentations in which there is insufficient information to make a more specific diagnosis.

Disruptive, Impulse-Control, and Conduct Disorders

Oppositional Defiant Disorder

F91.3

A. A pattern of angry/irritable mood, argumentative/defiant behavior, or vindictiveness lasting at least 6 months as evidenced by at least four symptoms from any of the following categories, and exhibited during interaction with at least one individual who is not a sibling.

Angry/Irritable Mood

1. Often loses temper.
2. Is often touchy or easily annoyed.
3. Is often angry and resentful.

Argumentative/Defiant Behavior

4. Often argues with authority figures or, for children and adolescents, with adults.
5. Often actively defies or refuses to comply with requests from authority figures or with rules.
6. Often deliberately annoys others.
7. Often blames others for his or her mistakes or misbehavior.

Vindictiveness

8. Has been spiteful or vindictive at least twice within the past 6 months.

Note: The persistence and frequency of these behaviors should be used to distinguish a behavior that is within normal limits from a behavior that is symptomatic. For children younger than 5 years, the behavior should occur on most days for a period of at least 6 months, unless otherwise noted (Criterion A8). For individuals 5 years or older, the behavior should occur at least once per week for at least 6 months, unless otherwise noted (Criterion A8). While these frequency criteria provide guidance on a minimal level of frequency to define symptoms, other factors should also be considered, such as whether the frequency and intensity of the behaviors are outside a range that is normative for the individual's developmental level, gender, and culture.

B. The disturbance in behavior is associated with distress in the individual or others in his or her immediate social context (e.g., family, peer group, work colleagues), or it impacts negatively on social, educational, occupational, or other important areas of functioning.

C. The behaviors do not occur exclusively during the course of a psychotic, substance use, depressive, or bipolar disorder. Also, the criteria are not met for disruptive mood dysregulation disorder.

Specify current severity:

Mild: Symptoms are confined to only one setting (e.g., at home, at school, at work, with peers).
Moderate: Some symptoms are present in at least two settings.
Severe: Some symptoms are present in three or more settings.

Intermittent Explosive Disorder

F63.81

A. Recurrent behavioral outbursts representing a failure to control aggressive impulses as manifested by either of the following:

1. Verbal aggression (e.g., temper tantrums, tirades, verbal arguments or fights) or physical aggression toward property, animals, or other individuals, occurring twice weekly, on average, for a period of 3 months. The physical aggression does not result in damage or destruction of property and does not result in physical injury to animals or other individuals.
2. Three behavioral outbursts involving damage or destruction of property and/or physical assault involving physical injury against animals or other individuals occurring within a 12-month period.

B. The magnitude of aggressiveness expressed during the recurrent outbursts is grossly out of proportion to the provocation or to any precipitating psychosocial stressors.
C. The recurrent aggressive outbursts are not premeditated (i.e., they are impulsive and/or anger-based) and are not committed to achieve some tangible objective (e.g., money, power, intimidation).
D. The recurrent aggressive outbursts cause either marked distress in the individual or impairment in occupational or interpersonal functioning, or are associated with financial or legal consequences.
E. Chronological age is at least 6 years (or equivalent developmental level).
F. The recurrent aggressive outbursts are not better explained by another mental disorder (e.g., major depressive disorder, bipolar disorder, disruptive mood dysregulation disorder, a psychotic disorder, antisocial personality disorder, borderline personality disorder) and are not attributable to another medical condition (e.g., head trauma, Alzheimer's disease) or to the physiological effects of a substance (e.g., a drug of abuse, a medication). For children ages 6–18 years, aggressive behavior that occurs as part of an adjustment disorder should not be considered for this diagnosis.

Note: This diagnosis can be made in addition to the diagnosis of attention-deficit/hyperactivity disorder, conduct disorder, oppositional defiant disorder, or autism spectrum disorder when recurrent impulsive aggressive outbursts are in excess of those usually seen in these disorders and warrant independent clinical attention.

Conduct Disorder

A. A repetitive and persistent pattern of behavior in which the basic rights of others or major age-appropriate societal norms or rules are violated, as manifested by the presence of at least three of the following 15 criteria in the past 12 months from any of the categories below, with at least one criterion present in the past 6 months:

Aggression to People and Animals

1. Often bullies, threatens, or intimidates others.
2. Often initiates physical fights.
3. Has used a weapon that can cause serious physical harm to others (e.g., a bat, brick, broken bottle, knife, gun).
4. Has been physically cruel to people.
5. Has been physically cruel to animals.
6. Has stolen while confronting a victim (e.g., mugging, purse snatching, extortion, armed robbery).
7. Has forced someone into sexual activity.

Destruction of Property

8. Has deliberately engaged in fire setting with the intention of causing serious damage.
9. Has deliberately destroyed others' property (other than by fire setting).

Deceitfulness or Theft

10. Has broken into someone else's house, building, or car.
11. Often lies to obtain goods or favors or to avoid obligations (i.e., "cons" others).
12. Has stolen items of nontrivial value without confronting a victim (e.g., shoplifting, but without breaking and entering; forgery).

Serious Violations of Rules

13. Often stays out at night despite parental prohibitions, beginning before age 13 years.
14. Has run away from home overnight at least twice while living in the parental or parental surrogate home, or once without returning for a lengthy period.
15. Is often truant from school, beginning before age 13 years.

B. The disturbance in behavior causes clinically significant impairment in social, academic, or occupational functioning.
C. If the individual is age 18 years or older, criteria are not met for antisocial personality disorder.

Specify whether:

F91.1 Childhood-onset type: Individuals show at least one symptom characteristic of conduct disorder prior to age 10 years.
F91.2 Adolescent-onset type: Individuals show no symptom characteristic of conduct disorder prior to age 10 years.

F91.9 Unspecified onset: Criteria for a diagnosis of conduct disorder are met, but there is not enough information available to determine whether the onset of the first symptom was before or after age 10 years.

Specify if:

With limited prosocial emotions: To qualify for this specifier, an individual must have displayed at least two of the following characteristics persistently over at least 12 months and in multiple relationships and settings. These characteristics reflect the individual's typical pattern of interpersonal and emotional functioning over this period and not just occasional occurrences in some situations. Thus, to assess the criteria for the specifier, multiple information sources are necessary. In addition to the individual's self-report, it is necessary to consider reports by others who have known the individual for extended periods of time (e.g., parents, teachers, co-workers, extended family members, peers).

Lack of remorse or guilt: Does not feel bad or guilty when he or she does something wrong (exclude remorse when expressed only when caught and/or facing punishment). The individual shows a general lack of concern about the negative consequences of his or her actions. For example, the individual is not remorseful after hurting someone or does not care about the consequences of breaking rules.

Callous—lack of empathy: Disregards and is unconcerned about the feelings of others. The individual is described as cold and uncaring. The individual appears more concerned about the effects of his or her actions on himself or herself, rather than their effects on others, even when they result in substantial harm to others.

Unconcerned about performance: Does not show concern about poor/problematic performance at school, at work, or in other important activities. The individual does not put forth the effort necessary to perform well, even when expectations are clear, and typically blames others for his or her poor performance.

Shallow or deficient affect: Does not express feelings or show emotions to others, except in ways that seem shallow, insincere, or superficial (e.g., actions contradict the emotion displayed; can turn emotions "on" or "off" quickly) or when emotional expressions are used for gain (e.g., emotions displayed to manipulate or intimidate others).

Specify current severity:

Mild: Few if any conduct problems in excess of those required to make the diagnosis are present, and conduct problems cause relatively minor harm to others (e.g., lying, truancy, staying out after dark without permission, other rule breaking).

Moderate: The number of conduct problems and the effect on others are intermediate between those specified in "mild" and those in "severe" (e.g., stealing without confronting a victim, vandalism).
Severe: Many conduct problems in excess of those required to make the diagnosis are present, or conduct problems cause considerable harm to others (e.g., forced sex, physical cruelty, use of a weapon, stealing while confronting a victim, breaking and entering).

Antisocial Personality Disorder

Criteria for antisocial personality disorder can be found in the chapter "Personality Disorders." Because this disorder is closely connected to the spectrum of "externalizing" conduct disorders in this chapter, as well as to the disorders in the adjoining chapter "Substance-Related and Addictive Disorders," it is listed here, and the criteria are presented in the chapter "Personality Disorders."

Pyromania

F63.1

A. Deliberate and purposeful fire setting on more than one occasion.
B. Tension or affective arousal before the act.
C. Fascination with, interest in, curiosity about, or attraction to fire and its situational contexts (e.g., paraphernalia, uses, consequences).
D. Pleasure, gratification, or relief when setting fires or when witnessing or participating in their aftermath.
E. The fire setting is not done for monetary gain, as an expression of sociopolitical ideology, to conceal criminal activity, to express anger or vengeance, to improve one's living circumstances, in response to a delusion or hallucination, or as a result of impaired judgment (e.g., in major neurocognitive disorder, intellectual developmental disorder [intellectual disability], substance intoxication).
F. The fire setting is not better explained by conduct disorder, a manic episode, or antisocial personality disorder.

Kleptomania

F63.2

A. Recurrent failure to resist impulses to steal objects that are not needed for personal use or for their monetary value.
B. Increasing sense of tension immediately before committing the theft.
C. Pleasure, gratification, or relief at the time of committing the theft.
D. The stealing is not committed to express anger or vengeance and is not in response to a delusion or a hallucination.
E. The stealing is not better explained by conduct disorder, a manic episode, or antisocial personality disorder.

Other Specified Disruptive, Impulse-Control, and Conduct Disorder

F91.8

This category applies to presentations in which symptoms characteristic of a disruptive, impulse-control, and conduct disorder that cause clinically significant distress or impairment in social, occupational, or other important areas of functioning predominate but do not meet the full criteria for any of the disorders in the disruptive, impulse-control, and conduct disorders diagnostic class. The other specified disruptive, impulse-control, and conduct disorder category is used in situations in which the clinician chooses to communicate the specific reason that the presentation does not meet the criteria for any specific disruptive, impulse-control, and conduct disorder. This is done by recording "other specified disruptive, impulse-control, and conduct disorder" followed by the specific reason (e.g., "recurrent behavioral outbursts of insufficient frequency").

Unspecified Disruptive, Impulse-Control, and Conduct Disorder

F91.9

This category applies to presentations in which symptoms characteristic of a disruptive, impulse-control, and conduct disorder that cause clinically significant distress or impairment in social, occupational, or other important areas of functioning predominate but do not meet the full criteria for any of the disorders in the disruptive, impulse-control, and conduct disorders diagnostic class. The unspecified disruptive, impulse-control, and conduct disorder category is used in situations in which the clinician chooses *not* to specify the reason that the criteria are not met for a specific disruptive, impulse-control, and conduct disorder, and includes presentations in which there is insufficient information to make a more specific diagnosis (e.g., in emergency room settings).

Substance-Related and Addictive Disorders

The substance-related disorders encompass 10 separate classes of drugs: alcohol; caffeine; cannabis; hallucinogens (with separate categories for phencyclidine [or similarly acting arylcyclohexylamines] and other hallucinogens); inhalants; opioids; sedatives, hypnotics, and anxiolytics; stimulants (amphetamine-type substances, cocaine, and other stimulants); tobacco; and other (or unknown) substances (e.g., nitrous oxide). This chapter also includes gambling disorder, reflecting evidence that gambling behaviors activate reward systems similar to those activated by drugs of abuse and that produce behavioral symptoms comparable to those in the criteria for substance use disorders.

Substance-related disorders are divided into two groups: substance use disorders (problematic pattern of substance use leading to clinically significant impairment) and substance-induced disorders, which include substance intoxication, substance withdrawal, and substance/medication-induced mental disorders (substance/medication-induced psychotic disorder, bipolar and related disorder, depressive disorder, anxiety disorder, obsessive-compulsive and related disorder, sleep disorder, sexual dysfunction, delirium, and neurocognitive disorders). The term *substance/medication-induced mental disorder* refers to symptomatic presentations that are due to the physiological effects of an exogenous substance on the central nervous system and includes typical intoxicants (e.g., alcohol, inhalants, cocaine), psychotropic medications (e.g., stimulants, sedative-hypnotics), other medications (e.g., steroids), and environmental toxins (e.g., organophosphate insecticides). To facilitate differential diagnosis, the diagnostic criteria for substance/medication-induced mental disorders are not included in this chapter but have been placed in other chapters of the manual with disorders with which they share phenomenology (e.g., substance/medication-induced depressive disorder is in the chapter "Depressive Disorders"). Note that only certain classes of drugs are capable of causing particular types of substance-induced disorders. The substance-related diagnostic categories associated with specific drug classes are shown in Table 1.

TABLE 1   Diagnoses associated with substance class

	Psychotic disorders	Bipolar and related disorders	Depressive disorders	Anxiety disorders	Obsessive-compulsive and related disorders	Sleep disorders	Sexual dysfunctions	Delirium	Neurocognitive disorders	Substance use disorders	Substance intoxication	Substance withdrawal
Alcohol	I/W	I/W	I/W	I/W		I/W	I/W	I/W	X (mild; major)	X	X	X
Caffeine				I		I/W					X	X
Cannabis	I			I		I/W		I		X	X	X
Hallucinogens												
Phencyclidine	I	I	I	I				I		X	X	
Other hallucinogens	I*	I	I	I				I		X	X	
Inhalants	I		I	I				I	X (mild; major)	X	X	
Opioids			I/W	W		I/W	I/W	I/W		X	X	X

TABLE 1 Diagnoses associated with substance class (continued)

	Psychotic disorders	Bipolar and related disorders	Depressive disorders	Anxiety disorders	Obsessive-compulsive and related disorders	Sleep disorders	Sexual dysfunctions	Delirium	Neurocognitive disorders	Substance use disorders	Substance intoxication	Substance withdrawal
Sedatives, hypnotics, or anxiolytics	I/W	I/W	I/W	W		I/W	I/W	I/W	X (mild; major)	X	X	X
Stimulants**	I	I/W	I/W	I/W	I/W	I/W	I	I	X (mild)	X	X	X
Tobacco						W				X		X
Other (or unknown)	I/W	I/W	I/W	I/W	I/W	I/W	I/W	I/W	X (mild; major)	X	X	X

Note. X = The category is recognized in DSM-5.
I = The specifier "with onset during intoxication" may be noted for the category.
W = The specifier "with onset during withdrawal" may be noted for the category.
I/W = Either "with onset during intoxication" or "with onset during withdrawal" may be noted for the category.
Major = major neurocognitive disorder; mild = mild neurocognitive disorder.
*Also hallucinogen persisting perception disorder (flashbacks).
**Includes amphetamine-type substances, cocaine, and other or unspecified stimulants.

Substance-Related Disorders

Substance Use Disorders

Recording Procedures for Substance Use Disorders

The clinician should use the code that applies to the substance class but record the name of the *specific substance*. For example, the clinician should record F13.20 moderate alprazolam use disorder (rather than moderate sedative, hypnotic, or anxiolytic use disorder) or F15.10 mild methamphetamine use disorder (rather than mild amphetamine-type substance use disorder). For substances that do not fit into any of the classes (e.g., anabolic steroids), the ICD-10-CM code for other (or unknown) substance use disorder should be used and the specific substance indicated (e.g., F19.10 mild anabolic steroid use disorder). If the substance taken by the individual is unknown, the same ICD-10-CM code (i.e., for "other [or unknown] substance use disorder") should be used (e.g., F19.20 severe unknown substance use disorder). If criteria are met for more than one substance use disorder, each should be diagnosed (e.g., F11.20 severe heroin use disorder; F14.20 moderate cocaine use disorder).

The appropriate ICD-10-CM code for a substance use disorder depends on whether there is a comorbid substance-induced disorder (including substance intoxication and substance withdrawal). In the first example in the paragraph above, the diagnostic code for moderate alprazolam use disorder, F13.20, reflects the absence of a comorbid alprazolam-induced mental disorder. Because ICD-10-CM codes for substance-induced disorders indicate both the presence (or absence) and the severity of the substance use disorder, ICD-10-CM codes for substance use disorders can be used only in the absence of a substance-induced disorder. See the individual substance-specific sections for additional coding information.

Substance-Induced Disorders

Recording Procedures for Substance Intoxication and Substance Withdrawal

The clinician should use the code that applies to the class of substances but record the name of the *specific substance*. For example, the clinician should record F13.230 secobarbital withdrawal (rather than sedative, hypnotic, or anxiolytic withdrawal) or F15.120 methamphetamine intoxication (rather than amphetamine-type substance intoxication). Note that the appropriate ICD-10-CM diagnostic codes for substance intoxication and substance withdrawal depend on whether there is a comorbid substance use disorder. In this case, the F15.120 code for methamphetamine intoxication indicates the presence of a comorbid mild methamphetamine use disorder. If there had been no comorbid methamphetamine use disorder (and no perceptual disturbances), the diagnostic code would have been F15.920. See the coding note for the substance-specific intoxication and withdrawal syndromes for the actual coding options.

For substances that do not fit into any of the classes (e.g., anabolic steroids), the ICD-10-CM code for other (or unknown) substance intoxication or other (or unknown) substance withdrawal should be used and the specific substance indicated (e.g., F19.920 anabolic steroid intoxication). If the substance taken by the individual is unknown, the same code (i.e., for the class "other [or unknown] substance") should be used (e.g., F19.920 unknown substance intoxication). If there are symptoms or problems associated with a particular substance but criteria are not met for any of the substance-specific disorders, the unspecified category can be used (e.g., F12.99 unspecified cannabis-related disorder).

As noted above, the substance-related codes in ICD-10-CM combine the substance use disorder aspect of the clinical picture and the substance-induced aspect into a single combined code. Thus, if both heroin withdrawal and moderate heroin use disorder are present, the single code F11.23 for heroin withdrawal is given to cover both presentations. See the individual substance-specific sections for additional coding information.

Recording Procedures for Substance/Medication-Induced Mental Disorders

Diagnostic criteria, coding notes, and recording procedures for the specific substance/medication-induced mental disorders are provided in chapters of the manual corresponding with disorders of shared phenomenology (see the substance/medication-induced mental disorders in these chapters: "Schizophrenia Spectrum and Other Psychotic Disorders," "Bipolar and Related Disorders," "Depressive Disorders," "Anxiety Disorders," "Obsessive-Compulsive and Related Disorders," "Sleep-Wake Disorders," "Sexual Dysfunctions," and "Neurocognitive Disorders"). When recording a substance/medication-induced mental disorder that is comorbid with a substance use disorder, only a single diagnosis is given that reflects both the type of substance and the type of mental disorder induced by the substance, as well as the severity of the comorbid substance use disorder (e.g., cocaine-induced psychotic disorder with severe cocaine use disorder). For a substance-induced mental disorder occurring in the absence of comorbid substance use disorder (e.g., when the disorder is induced by one-time use of a substance or medication), only the substance/medication-induced mental disorder is recorded (e.g., corticosteroid-induced depressive disorder). Additional information needed to record the diagnostic name of the substance/medication-induced mental disorder is provided in the section "Recording Procedures" for each substance/medication-induced mental disorder in its respective chapter.

Alcohol-Related Disorders

Alcohol Use Disorder

A. A problematic pattern of alcohol use leading to clinically significant impairment or distress, as manifested by at least two of the following, occurring within a 12-month period:

1. Alcohol is often taken in larger amounts or over a longer period than was intended.
2. There is a persistent desire or unsuccessful efforts to cut down or control alcohol use.
3. A great deal of time is spent in activities necessary to obtain alcohol, use alcohol, or recover from its effects.
4. Craving, or a strong desire or urge to use alcohol.
5. Recurrent alcohol use resulting in a failure to fulfill major role obligations at work, school, or home.
6. Continued alcohol use despite having persistent or recurrent social or interpersonal problems caused or exacerbated by the effects of alcohol.
7. Important social, occupational, or recreational activities are given up or reduced because of alcohol use.
8. Recurrent alcohol use in situations in which it is physically hazardous.
9. Alcohol use is continued despite knowledge of having a persistent or recurrent physical or psychological problem that is likely to have been caused or exacerbated by alcohol.
10. Tolerance, as defined by either of the following:

    a. A need for markedly increased amounts of alcohol to achieve intoxication or desired effect.
    b. A markedly diminished effect with continued use of the same amount of alcohol.

11. Withdrawal, as manifested by either of the following:

    a. The characteristic withdrawal syndrome for alcohol (refer to Criteria A and B of the criteria set for alcohol withdrawal).
    b. Alcohol (or a closely related substance, such as a benzodiazepine) is taken to relieve or avoid withdrawal symptoms.

Specify if:

In early remission: After full criteria for alcohol use disorder were previously met, none of the criteria for alcohol use disorder have been met for at least 3 months but for less than 12 months (with the exception that Criterion A4, "Craving, or a strong desire or urge to use alcohol," may be met).

In sustained remission: After full criteria for alcohol use disorder were previously met, none of the criteria for alcohol use disorder have been met at any time during a period of 12 months or longer (with the exception that Criterion A4, "Craving, or a strong desire or urge to use alcohol," may be met).

Specify if:

In a controlled environment: This additional specifier is used if the individual is in an environment where access to alcohol is restricted.

Code based on current severity/remission: If an alcohol intoxication, alcohol withdrawal, or another alcohol-induced mental disorder is also present, do not use the codes below for alcohol use disorder. Instead, the comorbid alcohol use disorder is indicated in the 4th character of the alcohol-induced disorder code (see the coding note for alcohol intoxication, alcohol withdrawal, or a specific alcohol-induced mental disorder). For example, if there is comorbid alcohol intoxication and alcohol use disorder, only the alcohol intoxication code is given, with the 4th character indicating whether the comorbid alcohol use disorder is mild, moderate, or severe: F10.129 for mild alcohol use disorder with alcohol intoxication or F10.229 for a moderate or severe alcohol use disorder with alcohol intoxication.

Specify current severity/remission:

F10.10 Mild: Presence of 2–3 symptoms.
F10.11 Mild, In early remission
F10.11 Mild, In sustained remission

F10.20 Moderate: Presence of 4–5 symptoms.
F10.21 Moderate, In early remission
F10.21 Moderate, In sustained remission

F10.20 Severe: Presence of 6 or more symptoms.
F10.21 Severe, In early remission
F10.21 Severe, In sustained remission

Alcohol Intoxication

A. Recent ingestion of alcohol.

B. Clinically significant problematic behavioral or psychological changes (e.g., inappropriate sexual or aggressive behavior, mood lability, impaired judgment) that developed during, or shortly after, alcohol ingestion.

C. One (or more) of the following signs or symptoms developing during, or shortly after, alcohol use:

1. Slurred speech.
2. Incoordination.
3. Unsteady gait.
4. Nystagmus.
5. Impairment in attention or memory.
6. Stupor or coma.

D. The signs or symptoms are not attributable to another medical condition and are not better explained by another mental disorder, including intoxication with another substance.

Coding note: The ICD-10-CM code depends on whether there is a co-morbid alcohol use disorder. If a mild alcohol use disorder is comorbid, the ICD-10-CM code is **F10.120,** and if a moderate or severe alcohol use disorder is comorbid, the ICD-10-CM code is **F10.220.** If there is no comorbid alcohol use disorder, then the ICD-10-CM code is **F10.920.**

Alcohol Withdrawal

A. Cessation of (or reduction in) alcohol use that has been heavy and prolonged.

B. Two (or more) of the following, developing within several hours to a few days after the cessation of (or reduction in) alcohol use described in Criterion A:

1. Autonomic hyperactivity (e.g., sweating or pulse rate greater than 100 bpm).
2. Increased hand tremor.
3. Insomnia.
4. Nausea or vomiting.
5. Transient visual, tactile, or auditory hallucinations or illusions.
6. Psychomotor agitation.
7. Anxiety.
8. Generalized tonic-clonic seizures.

C. The signs or symptoms in Criterion B cause clinically significant distress or impairment in social, occupational, or other important areas of functioning.

D. The signs or symptoms are not attributable to another medical condition and are not better explained by another mental disorder, including intoxication or withdrawal from another substance.

Specify if:

With perceptual disturbances: This specifier applies in the rare instance when hallucinations (usually visual or tactile) occur with intact reality testing, or auditory, visual, or tactile illusions occur in the absence of a delirium.

Coding note: The ICD-10-CM code depends on whether or not there is a comorbid alcohol use disorder and whether or not there are perceptual disturbances.

For alcohol withdrawal, without perceptual disturbances: If a mild alcohol use disorder is comorbid, the ICD-10-CM code is **F10.130**, and if a moderate or severe alcohol use disorder is comorbid, the ICD-10-CM code is **F10.230**. If there is no comorbid alcohol use disorder, then the ICD-10-CM code is **F10.930**.

For alcohol withdrawal, with perceptual disturbances: If a mild alcohol use disorder is comorbid, the ICD-10-CM code is **F10.132**, and if a moderate or severe alcohol use disorder is comorbid, the ICD-10-CM code is **F10.232**. If there is no comorbid alcohol use disorder, then the ICD-10-CM code is **F10.932**.

Alcohol-Induced Mental Disorders

The following alcohol-induced mental disorders are described in other chapters of the book with disorders with which they share phenomenology (see the substance/medication-induced mental disorders in these chapters): alcohol-induced psychotic disorder ("Schizophrenia Spectrum and Other Psychotic Disorders"); alcohol-induced bipolar and related disorder ("Bipolar and Related Disorders"); alcohol-induced depressive disorder ("Depressive Disorders"); alcohol-induced anxiety disorder ("Anxiety Disorders"); alcohol-induced sleep disorder ("Sleep-Wake Disorders"); alcohol-induced sexual dysfunction ("Sexual Dysfunctions"); and alcohol-induced major or mild neurocognitive disorder ("Neurocognitive Disorders"). For alcohol intoxication delirium and alcohol withdrawal delirium, see the criteria and discussion of delirium in the chapter "Neurocognitive Disorders." These alcohol-induced mental disorders are diagnosed instead of alcohol intoxication or alcohol withdrawal only when the symptoms are sufficiently severe to warrant independent clinical attention.

Unspecified Alcohol-Related Disorder

F10.99

This category applies to presentations in which symptoms characteristic of an alcohol-related disorder that cause clinically significant distress or impairment in social, occupational, or other important areas of functioning predominate but do not meet the full criteria for any specific alcohol-related disorder or any of the disorders in the substance-related and addictive disorders diagnostic class.

Caffeine-Related Disorders

Caffeine Intoxication

F15.920

A. Recent consumption of caffeine (typically a high dose well in excess of 250 mg).
B. Five (or more) of the following signs or symptoms developing during, or shortly after, caffeine use:

1. Restlessness.
2. Nervousness.
3. Excitement.
4. Insomnia.

5. Flushed face.
6. Diuresis.
7. Gastrointestinal disturbance.
8. Muscle twitching.
9. Rambling flow of thought and speech.
10. Tachycardia or cardiac arrhythmia.
11. Periods of inexhaustibility.
12. Psychomotor agitation.

C. The signs or symptoms in Criterion B cause clinically significant distress or impairment in social, occupational, or other important areas of functioning.
D. The signs or symptoms are not attributable to another medical condition and are not better explained by another mental disorder, including intoxication with another substance.

Caffeine Withdrawal

F15.93

A. Prolonged daily use of caffeine.
B. Abrupt cessation of or reduction in caffeine use, followed within 24 hours by three (or more) of the following signs or symptoms:

1. Headache.
2. Marked fatigue or drowsiness.
3. Dysphoric mood, depressed mood, or irritability.
4. Difficulty concentrating.
5. Flu-like symptoms (nausea, vomiting, or muscle pain/stiffness).

C. The signs or symptoms in Criterion B cause clinically significant distress or impairment in social, occupational, or other important areas of functioning.
D. The signs or symptoms are not associated with the physiological effects of another medical condition (e.g., migraine, viral illness) and are not better explained by another mental disorder, including intoxication or withdrawal from another substance.

Caffeine-Induced Mental Disorders

The following caffeine-induced mental disorders are described in other chapters of the book with disorders with which they share phenomenology (see the substance/medication-induced mental disorders in these chapters): caffeine-induced anxiety disorder ("Anxiety Disorders") and caffeine-induced sleep disorder ("Sleep-Wake Disorders"). These caffeine-induced mental disorders are diagnosed instead of caffeine intoxication or caffeine withdrawal only when the symptoms are sufficiently severe to warrant independent clinical attention.

Unspecified Caffeine-Related Disorder

F15.99

This category applies to presentations in which symptoms characteristic of a caffeine-related disorder that cause clinically significant distress or impairment in social, occupational, or other important areas of functioning predominate but do not meet the full criteria for any specific caffeine-related disorder or any of the disorders in the substance-related and addictive disorders diagnostic class.

Cannabis-Related Disorders

Cannabis Use Disorder

A. A problematic pattern of cannabis use leading to clinically significant impairment or distress, as manifested by at least two of the following, occurring within a 12-month period:

1. Cannabis is often taken in larger amounts or over a longer period than was intended.
2. There is a persistent desire or unsuccessful efforts to cut down or control cannabis use.
3. A great deal of time is spent in activities necessary to obtain cannabis, use cannabis, or recover from its effects.
4. Craving, or a strong desire or urge to use cannabis.
5. Recurrent cannabis use resulting in a failure to fulfill major role obligations at work, school, or home.
6. Continued cannabis use despite having persistent or recurrent social or interpersonal problems caused or exacerbated by the effects of cannabis.
7. Important social, occupational, or recreational activities are given up or reduced because of cannabis use.
8. Recurrent cannabis use in situations in which it is physically hazardous.
9. Cannabis use is continued despite knowledge of having a persistent or recurrent physical or psychological problem that is likely to have been caused or exacerbated by cannabis.
10. Tolerance, as defined by either of the following:
    a. A need for markedly increased amounts of cannabis to achieve intoxication or desired effect.
    b. Markedly diminished effect with continued use of the same amount of cannabis.

11. Withdrawal, as manifested by either of the following:

a. The characteristic withdrawal syndrome for cannabis (refer to Criteria A and B of the criteria set for cannabis withdrawal).

b. Cannabis (or a closely related substance) is taken to relieve or avoid withdrawal symptoms.

Specify if:

In early remission: After full criteria for cannabis use disorder were previously met, none of the criteria for cannabis use disorder have been met for at least 3 months but for less than 12 months (with the exception that Criterion A4, "Craving, or a strong desire or urge to use cannabis," may be met).

In sustained remission: After full criteria for cannabis use disorder were previously met, none of the criteria for cannabis use disorder have been met at any time during a period of 12 months or longer (with the exception that Criterion A4, "Craving, or a strong desire or urge to use cannabis," may be present).

Specify if:

In a controlled environment: This additional specifier is used if the individual is in an environment where access to cannabis is restricted.

Code based on current severity/remission: If a cannabis intoxication, cannabis withdrawal, or another cannabis-induced mental disorder is also present, do not use the codes below for cannabis use disorder. Instead, the comorbid cannabis use disorder is indicated in the 4th character of the cannabis-induced disorder code (see the coding note for cannabis intoxication, cannabis withdrawal, or a specific cannabis-induced mental disorder). For example, if there is comorbid cannabis-induced anxiety disorder and cannabis use disorder, only the cannabis-induced anxiety disorder code is given, with the 4th character indicating whether the comorbid cannabis use disorder is mild, moderate, or severe: F12.180 for mild cannabis use disorder with cannabis-induced anxiety disorder or F12.280 for a moderate or severe cannabis use disorder with cannabis-induced anxiety disorder.

Specify current severity/remission:

F12.10 Mild: Presence of 2–3 symptoms.
F12.11 Mild, In early remission
F12.11 Mild, In sustained remission

F12.20 Moderate: Presence of 4–5 symptoms.
F12.21 Moderate, In early remission
F12.21 Moderate, In sustained remission

F12.20 Severe: Presence of 6 or more symptoms.
F12.21 Severe, In early remission
F12.21 Severe, In sustained remission

Cannabis Intoxication

A. Recent use of cannabis.
B. Clinically significant problematic behavioral or psychological changes (e.g., impaired motor coordination, euphoria, anxiety, sensation of slowed time, impaired judgment, social withdrawal) that developed during, or shortly after, cannabis use.
C. Two (or more) of the following signs or symptoms developing within 2 hours of cannabis use:

    1. Conjunctival injection.
    2. Increased appetite.
    3. Dry mouth.
    4. Tachycardia.

D. The signs or symptoms are not attributable to another medical condition and are not better explained by another mental disorder, including intoxication with another substance.

Specify if:

   With perceptual disturbances: Hallucinations with intact reality testing or auditory, visual, or tactile illusions occur in the absence of a delirium.

Coding note: The ICD-10-CM code depends on whether or not there is a comorbid cannabis use disorder and whether or not there are perceptual disturbances.

   For cannabis intoxication, without perceptual disturbances: If a mild cannabis use disorder is comorbid, the ICD-10-CM code is **F12.120,** and if a moderate or severe cannabis use disorder is comorbid, the ICD-10-CM code is **F12.220.** If there is no comorbid cannabis use disorder, then the ICD-10-CM code is **F12.920.**

   For cannabis intoxication, with perceptual disturbances: If a mild cannabis use disorder is comorbid, the ICD-10-CM code is **F12.122,** and if a moderate or severe cannabis use disorder is comorbid, the ICD-10-CM code is **F12.222.** If there is no comorbid cannabis use disorder, then the ICD-10-CM code is **F12.922.**

Cannabis Withdrawal

A. Cessation of cannabis use that has been heavy and prolonged (i.e., usually daily or almost daily use over a period of at least a few months).
B. Three (or more) of the following signs and symptoms develop within approximately 1 week after Criterion A:

    1. Irritability, anger, or aggression.
    2. Nervousness or anxiety.
    3. Sleep difficulty (e.g., insomnia, disturbing dreams).
    4. Decreased appetite or weight loss.

5. Restlessness.
6. Depressed mood.
7. At least one of the following physical symptoms causing significant discomfort: abdominal pain, shakiness/tremors, sweating, fever, chills, or headache.

C. The signs or symptoms in Criterion B cause clinically significant distress or impairment in social, occupational, or other important areas of functioning.

D. The signs or symptoms are not attributable to another medical condition and are not better explained by another mental disorder, including intoxication or withdrawal from another substance.

Coding note: The ICD-10-CM code depends on whether or not there is a comorbid cannabis use disorder. If a mild cannabis use disorder is comorbid, the ICD-10-CM code is **F12.13**, and if a moderate or severe cannabis use disorder is comorbid, the ICD-10-CM code is **F12.23**. For cannabis withdrawal occurring in the absence of a cannabis use disorder (e.g., in a patient taking cannabis solely under appropriate medical supervision), the ICD-10-CM code is **F12.93**.

Cannabis-Induced Mental Disorders

The following cannabis-induced mental disorders are described in other chapters of the book with disorders with which they share phenomenology (see the substance/medication-induced mental disorders in these chapters): cannabis-induced psychotic disorder ("Schizophrenia Spectrum and Other Psychotic Disorders"); cannabis-induced anxiety disorder ("Anxiety Disorders"); and cannabis-induced sleep disorder ("Sleep-Wake Disorders"). For cannabis intoxication delirium and delirium induced by pharmaceutical cannabis receptor agonist taken as prescribed, see the criteria and discussion of delirium in the chapter "Neurocognitive Disorders." These cannabis-induced mental disorders are diagnosed instead of cannabis intoxication or cannabis withdrawal when the symptoms are sufficiently severe to warrant independent clinical attention.

Unspecified Cannabis-Related Disorder

F12.99

This category applies to presentations in which symptoms characteristic of a cannabis-related disorder that cause clinically significant distress or impairment in social, occupational, or other important areas of functioning predominate but do not meet the full criteria for any specific cannabis-related disorder or any of the disorders in the substance-related and addictive disorders diagnostic class.

Hallucinogen-Related Disorders

Phencyclidine Use Disorder

A. A pattern of phencyclidine (or a pharmacologically similar substance) use leading to clinically significant impairment or distress, as manifested by at least two of the following, occurring within a 12-month period:

1. Phencyclidine is often taken in larger amounts or over a longer period than was intended.
2. There is a persistent desire or unsuccessful efforts to cut down or control phencyclidine use.
3. A great deal of time is spent in activities necessary to obtain phencyclidine, use the phencyclidine, or recover from its effects.
4. Craving, or a strong desire or urge to use phencyclidine.
5. Recurrent phencyclidine use resulting in a failure to fulfill major role obligations at work, school, or home (e.g., repeated absences from work or poor work performance related to phencyclidine use; phencyclidine-related absences, suspensions, or expulsions from school; neglect of children or household).
6. Continued phencyclidine use despite having persistent or recurrent social or interpersonal problems caused or exacerbated by the effects of the phencyclidine (e.g., arguments with a spouse about consequences of intoxication; physical fights).
7. Important social, occupational, or recreational activities are given up or reduced because of phencyclidine use.
8. Recurrent phencyclidine use in situations in which it is physically hazardous (e.g., driving an automobile or operating a machine when impaired by a phencyclidine).
9. Phencyclidine use is continued despite knowledge of having a persistent or recurrent physical or psychological problem that is likely to have been caused or exacerbated by the phencyclidine.
10. Tolerance, as defined by either of the following:

    a. A need for markedly increased amounts of the phencyclidine to achieve intoxication or desired effect.
    b. A markedly diminished effect with continued use of the same amount of the phencyclidine.

Note: Withdrawal symptoms and signs are not established for phencyclidines, and so this criterion does not apply. (Withdrawal from phencyclidines has been reported in animals but not documented in human users.)

Specify if:

> **In early remission:** After full criteria for phencyclidine use disorder were previously met, none of the criteria for phencyclidine use disorder have been met for at least 3 months but for less than 12 months (with the exception that Criterion A4, "Craving, or a strong desire or urge to use the phencyclidine," may be met).
>
> **In sustained remission:** After full criteria for phencyclidine use disorder were previously met, none of the criteria for phencyclidine use disorder have been met at any time during a period of 12 months or longer (with the exception that Criterion A4, "Craving, or a strong desire or urge to use the phencyclidine," may be met).

Specify if:

> **In a controlled environment:** This additional specifier is used if the individual is in an environment where access to phencyclidines is restricted.

Code based on current severity/remission: If a phencyclidine intoxication or another phencyclidine-induced mental disorder is also present, do not use the codes below for phencyclidine use disorder. Instead, the co-morbid phencyclidine use disorder is indicated in the 4th character of the phencyclidine-induced disorder code (see the coding note for phencyclidine intoxication or a specific phencyclidine-induced mental disorder). For example, if there is comorbid phencyclidine-induced psychotic disorder, only the phencyclidine-induced psychotic disorder code is given, with the 4th character indicating whether the comorbid phencyclidine use disorder is mild, moderate, or severe: F16.159 for mild phencyclidine use disorder with phencyclidine-induced psychotic disorder or F16.259 for a moderate or severe phencyclidine use disorder with phencyclidine-induced psychotic disorder.

Specify current severity/remission:

> **F16.10 Mild:** Presence of 2–3 symptoms.
> **F16.11 Mild, In early remission**
> **F16.11 Mild, In sustained remission**
>
> **F16.20 Moderate:** Presence of 4–5 symptoms.
> **F16.21 Moderate, In early remission**
> **F16.21 Moderate, In sustained remission**
>
> **F16.20 Severe:** Presence of 6 or more symptoms.
> **F16.21 Severe, In early remission**
> **F16.21 Severe, In sustained remission**

Other Hallucinogen Use Disorder

A. A problematic pattern of hallucinogen (other than phencyclidine) use leading to clinically significant impairment or distress, as manifested by at least two of the following, occurring within a 12-month period:

1. The hallucinogen is often taken in larger amounts or over a longer period than was intended.
2. There is a persistent desire or unsuccessful efforts to cut down or control hallucinogen use.
3. A great deal of time is spent in activities necessary to obtain the hallucinogen, use the hallucinogen, or recover from its effects.
4. Craving, or a strong desire or urge to use the hallucinogen.
5. Recurrent hallucinogen use resulting in a failure to fulfill major role obligations at work, school, or home (e.g., repeated absences from work or poor work performance related to hallucinogen use; hallucinogen-related absences, suspensions, or expulsions from school; neglect of children or household).
6. Continued hallucinogen use despite having persistent or recurrent social or interpersonal problems caused or exacerbated by the effects of the hallucinogen (e.g., arguments with a spouse about consequences of intoxication; physical fights).
7. Important social, occupational, or recreational activities are given up or reduced because of hallucinogen use.
8. Recurrent hallucinogen use in situations in which it is physically hazardous (e.g., driving an automobile or operating a machine when impaired by the hallucinogen).
9. Hallucinogen use is continued despite knowledge of having a persistent or recurrent physical or psychological problem that is likely to have been caused or exacerbated by the hallucinogen.
10. Tolerance, as defined by either of the following:

    a. A need for markedly increased amounts of the hallucinogen to achieve intoxication or desired effect.
    b. A markedly diminished effect with continued use of the same amount of the hallucinogen.

Note: Withdrawal symptoms and signs are not established for hallucinogens, and so this criterion does not apply.

Specify **the particular hallucinogen.**

Specify if:

> **In early remission:** After full criteria for other hallucinogen use disorder were previously met, none of the criteria for other hallucinogen use disorder have been met for at least 3 months but for less than 12 months (with the exception that Criterion A4, "Craving, or a strong desire or urge to use the hallucinogen," may be met).
> **In sustained remission:** After full criteria for other hallucinogen use disorder were previously met, none of the criteria for other hallucinogen use disorder have been met at any time during a period of 12 months or longer (with the exception that Criterion A4, "Craving, or a strong desire or urge to use the hallucinogen," may be met).

Specify if:

> **In a controlled environment:** This additional specifier is used if the individual is in an environment where access to hallucinogens is restricted.

Code based on current severity/remission: If a hallucinogen intoxication or another hallucinogen-induced mental disorder is also present, do not use the codes below for hallucinogen use disorder. Instead, the comorbid hallucinogen use disorder is indicated in the 4th character of the hallucinogen-induced disorder code (see the coding note for hallucinogen intoxication or a specific hallucinogen-induced mental disorder). For example, if there is comorbid hallucinogen-induced psychotic disorder and hallucinogen use disorder, only the hallucinogen-induced psychotic disorder code is given, with the 4th character indicating whether the comorbid hallucinogen use disorder is mild, moderate, or severe: F16.159 for mild hallucinogen use disorder with hallucinogen-induced psychotic disorder or F16.259 for a moderate or severe hallucinogen use disorder with hallucinogen-induced psychotic disorder.

Specify current severity/remission:

F16.10 Mild: Presence of 2–3 symptoms.
F16.11 Mild, In early remission
F16.11 Mild, In sustained remission

F16.20 Moderate: Presence of 4–5 symptoms.
F16.21 Moderate, In early remission
F16.21 Moderate, In sustained remission

F16.20 Severe: Presence of 6 or more symptoms.
F16.21 Severe, In early remission
F16.21 Severe, In sustained remission

Phencyclidine Intoxication

A. Recent use of phencyclidine (or a pharmacologically similar substance).
B. Clinically significant problematic behavioral changes (e.g., belligerence, assaultiveness, impulsiveness, unpredictability, psychomotor agitation, impaired judgment) that developed during, or shortly after, phencyclidine use.
C. Within 1 hour, two (or more) of the following signs or symptoms:
   Note: When the drug is smoked, "snorted," or used intravenously, the onset may be particularly rapid.

   1. Vertical or horizontal nystagmus.
   2. Hypertension or tachycardia.
   3. Numbness or diminished responsiveness to pain.
   4. Ataxia.
   5. Dysarthria.
   6. Muscle rigidity.

    7. Seizures or coma.

    8. Hyperacusis.

D. The signs or symptoms are not attributable to another medical condition and are not better explained by another mental disorder, including intoxication with another substance.

Coding note: The ICD-10-CM code depends on whether there is a co-morbid phencyclidine use disorder. If a mild phencyclidine use disorder is comorbid, the ICD-10-CM code is **F16.120,** and if a moderate or severe phencyclidine use disorder is comorbid, the ICD-10-CM code is **F16.220.** If there is no comorbid phencyclidine use disorder, then the ICD-10-CM code is **F16.920.**

Other Hallucinogen Intoxication

A. Recent use of a hallucinogen (other than phencyclidine).

B. Clinically significant problematic behavioral or psychological changes (e.g., marked anxiety or depression, ideas of reference, fear of "losing one's mind," paranoid ideation, impaired judgment) that developed during, or shortly after, hallucinogen use.

C. Perceptual changes occurring in a state of full wakefulness and alertness (e.g., subjective intensification of perceptions, depersonalization, derealization, illusions, hallucinations, synesthesias) that developed during, or shortly after, hallucinogen use.

D. Two (or more) of the following signs developing during, or shortly after, hallucinogen use:

    1. Pupillary dilation.

    2. Tachycardia.

    3. Sweating.

    4. Palpitations.

    5. Blurring of vision.

    6. Tremors.

    7. Incoordination.

E. The signs or symptoms are not attributable to another medical condition and are not better explained by another mental disorder, including intoxication with another substance.

Coding note: The ICD-10-CM code depends on whether there is a comorbid hallucinogen use disorder. If a mild hallucinogen use disorder is comorbid, the ICD-10-CM code is **F16.120,** and if a moderate or severe hallucinogen use disorder is comorbid, the ICD-10-CM code is **F16.220.** If there is no comorbid hallucinogen use disorder, then the ICD-10-CM code is **F16.920.**

Hallucinogen Persisting Perception Disorder

F16.983

A. Following cessation of use of a hallucinogen, the reexperiencing of one or more of the perceptual symptoms that were experienced while intoxicated with the hallucinogen (e.g., geometric hallucinations, false perceptions of movement in the peripheral visual fields, flashes of color, intensified colors, trails of images of moving objects, positive afterimages, halos around objects, macropsia and micropsia).

B. The symptoms in Criterion A cause clinically significant distress or impairment in social, occupational, or other important areas of functioning.

C. The symptoms are not attributable to another medical condition (e.g., anatomical lesions and infections of the brain, visual epilepsies) and are not better explained by another mental disorder (e.g., delirium, major neurocognitive disorder, schizophrenia) or hypnopompic hallucinations.

Phencyclidine-Induced Mental Disorders

Other phencyclidine-induced mental disorders are described in other chapters of the book with disorders with which they share phenomenology (see the substance/medication-induced mental disorders in these chapters): phencyclidine-induced psychotic disorder ("Schizophrenia Spectrum and Other Psychotic Disorders"); phencyclidine-induced bipolar and related disorder ("Bipolar and Related Disorders"); phencyclidine-induced depressive disorder ("Depressive Disorders"); and phencyclidine-induced anxiety disorder ("Anxiety Disorders"). For phencyclidine-induced intoxication delirium and delirium induced by ketamine taken as prescribed, see the criteria and discussion of delirium in the chapter "Neurocognitive Disorders." These phencyclidine-induced mental disorders are diagnosed instead of phencyclidine intoxication only when the symptoms are sufficiently severe to warrant independent clinical attention.

Hallucinogen-Induced Mental Disorders

The following other hallucinogen-induced mental disorders are described in other chapters of the book with disorders with which they share phenomenology (see the substance/medication-induced mental disorders in these chapters): other hallucinogen-induced psychotic disorder ("Schizophrenia Spectrum and Other Psychotic Disorders"); other hallucinogen-induced bipolar and related disorder ("Bipolar and Related Disorders"); other hallucinogen-induced depressive disorder

("Depressive Disorders"); and other hallucinogen-induced anxiety disorder ("Anxiety Disorders"). For other hallucinogen intoxication delirium and delirium induced by other hallucinogens taken as prescribed, see the criteria and discussion of delirium in the chapter "Neurocognitive Disorders." These hallucinogen-induced mental disorders are diagnosed instead of other hallucinogen intoxication only when the symptoms are sufficiently severe to warrant independent clinical attention.

Unspecified Phencyclidine-Related Disorder

F16.99

This category applies to presentations in which symptoms characteristic of a phencyclidine-related disorder that cause clinically significant distress or impairment in social, occupational, or other important areas of functioning predominate but do not meet the full criteria for any specific phencyclidine-related disorder or any of the disorders in the substance-related and addictive disorders diagnostic class.

Unspecified Hallucinogen-Related Disorder

F16.99

This category applies to presentations in which symptoms characteristic of a hallucinogen-related disorder that cause clinically significant distress or impairment in social, occupational, or other important areas of functioning predominate but do not meet the full criteria for any specific hallucinogen-related disorder or any of the disorders in the substance-related and addictive disorders diagnostic class.

Inhalant-Related Disorders

Inhalant Use Disorder

A. A problematic pattern of use of a hydrocarbon-based inhalant substance leading to clinically significant impairment or distress, as manifested by at least two of the following, occurring within a 12-month period:

1. The inhalant substance is often taken in larger amounts or over a longer period than was intended.
2. There is a persistent desire or unsuccessful efforts to cut down or control use of the inhalant substance.

3. A great deal of time is spent in activities necessary to obtain the inhalant substance, use it, or recover from its effects.
4. Craving, or a strong desire or urge to use the inhalant substance.
5. Recurrent use of the inhalant substance resulting in a failure to fulfill major role obligations at work, school, or home.
6. Continued use of the inhalant substance despite having persistent or recurrent social or interpersonal problems caused or exacerbated by the effects of its use.
7. Important social, occupational, or recreational activities are given up or reduced because of use of the inhalant substance.
8. Recurrent use of the inhalant substance in situations in which it is physically hazardous.
9. Use of the inhalant substance is continued despite knowledge of having a persistent or recurrent physical or psychological problem that is likely to have been caused or exacerbated by the substance.
10. Tolerance, as defined by either of the following:

    a. A need for markedly increased amounts of the inhalant substance to achieve intoxication or desired effect.
    b. A markedly diminished effect with continued use of the same amount of the inhalant substance.

Specify **the particular inhalant:** When possible, the particular substance involved should be named (e.g., "solvent use disorder").

Specify if:

In early remission: After full criteria for inhalant use disorder were previously met, none of the criteria for inhalant use disorder have been met for at least 3 months but for less than 12 months (with the exception that Criterion A4, "Craving, or a strong desire or urge to use the inhalant substance," may be met).

In sustained remission: After full criteria for inhalant use disorder were previously met, none of the criteria for inhalant use disorder have been met at any time during a period of 12 months or longer (with the exception that Criterion A4, "Craving, or a strong desire or urge to use the inhalant substance," may be met).

Specify if:

In a controlled environment: This additional specifier is used if the individual is in an environment where access to inhalant substances is restricted.

Code based on current severity/remission: If an inhalant intoxication or another inhalant-induced mental disorder is also present, do not use the codes below for inhalant use disorder. Instead, the comorbid inhalant use disorder is indicated in the 4th character of the inhalant-induced disorder code (see the coding note for inhalant intoxication or a specific inhalant-induced mental disorder). For example, if there is comorbid inhalant-induced depressive disorder and inhalant use disorder, only the inhalant-induced depressive disorder code is given, with the 4th character indicating whether the comorbid inhalant use disorder is mild, moderate, or severe: F18.14 for mild inhalant use disorder with inhalant-induced depressive disorder or F18.24 for a moderate or severe inhalant use disorder with inhalant-induced depressive disorder.

Specify current severity/remission:

F18.10 Mild: Presence of 2–3 symptoms.
F18.11 Mild, In early remission
F18.11 Mild, In sustained remission

F18.20 Moderate: Presence of 4–5 symptoms.
F18.21 Moderate, In early remission
F18.21 Moderate, In sustained remission

F18.20 Severe: Presence of 6 or more symptoms.
F18.21 Severe, In early remission
F18.21 Severe, In sustained remission

Inhalant Intoxication

A. Recent intended or unintended short-term, high-dose exposure to inhalant substances, including volatile hydrocarbons such as toluene or gasoline.

B. Clinically significant problematic behavioral or psychological changes (e.g., belligerence, assaultiveness, apathy, impaired judgment) that developed during, or shortly after, exposure to inhalants.

C. Two (or more) of the following signs or symptoms developing during, or shortly after, inhalant use or exposure:

1. Dizziness.
2. Nystagmus.
3. Incoordination.
4. Slurred speech.
5. Unsteady gait.
6. Lethargy.
7. Depressed reflexes.
8. Psychomotor retardation.
9. Tremor.
10. Generalized muscle weakness.
11. Blurred vision or diplopia.
12. Stupor or coma.
13. Euphoria.

D. The signs or symptoms are not attributable to another medical condition and are not better explained by another mental disorder, including intoxication with another substance.

Coding note: The ICD-10-CM code depends on whether there is a co-morbid inhalant use disorder. If a mild inhalant use disorder is comorbid, the ICD-10-CM code is **F18.120,** and if a moderate or severe inhalant use disorder is comorbid, the ICD-10-CM code is **F18.220.** If there is no comorbid inhalant use disorder, then the ICD-10-CM code is **F18.920.**

Inhalant-Induced Mental Disorders

The following inhalant-induced mental disorders are described in other chapters of the book with disorders with which they share phenomenology (see the substance/medication-induced mental disorders in these chapters): inhalant-induced psychotic disorder ("Schizophrenia Spectrum and Other Psychotic Disorders"); inhalant-induced depressive disorder ("Depressive Disorders"); inhalant-induced anxiety disorder ("Anxiety Disorders"); and inhalant-induced major or mild neurocognitive disorder ("Neurocognitive Disorders"). For inhalant intoxication delirium, see the criteria and discussion of delirium in the chapter "Neurocognitive Disorders." These inhalant-induced mental disorders are diagnosed instead of inhalant intoxication only when symptoms are sufficiently severe to warrant independent clinical attention.

Unspecified Inhalant-Related Disorder

F18.99

This category applies to presentations in which symptoms characteristic of an inhalant-related disorder that cause clinically significant distress or impairment in social, occupational, or other important areas of functioning predominate but do not meet the full criteria for any specific inhalant-related disorder or any of the disorders in the substance-related and addictive disorders diagnostic class.

Opioid-Related Disorders

Opioid Use Disorder

A. A problematic pattern of opioid use leading to clinically significant impairment or distress, as manifested by at least two of the following, occurring within a 12-month period:

    1. Opioids are often taken in larger amounts or over a longer period than was intended.

    2. There is a persistent desire or unsuccessful efforts to cut down or control opioid use.

3. A great deal of time is spent in activities necessary to obtain the opioid, use the opioid, or recover from its effects.
4. Craving, or a strong desire or urge to use opioids.
5. Recurrent opioid use resulting in a failure to fulfill major role obligations at work, school, or home.
6. Continued opioid use despite having persistent or recurrent social or interpersonal problems caused or exacerbated by the effects of opioids.
7. Important social, occupational, or recreational activities are given up or reduced because of opioid use.
8. Recurrent opioid use in situations in which it is physically hazardous.
9. Continued opioid use despite knowledge of having a persistent or recurrent physical or psychological problem that is likely to have been caused or exacerbated by the substance.
10. Tolerance, as defined by either of the following:

   a. A need for markedly increased amounts of opioids to achieve intoxication or desired effect.
   b. A markedly diminished effect with continued use of the same amount of an opioid.

   Note: This criterion is not considered to be met for those taking opioids solely under appropriate medical supervision.

11. Withdrawal, as manifested by either of the following:

   a. The characteristic opioid withdrawal syndrome (refer to Criteria A and B of the criteria set for opioid withdrawal).
   b. Opioids (or a closely related substance) are taken to relieve or avoid withdrawal symptoms.

   Note: This criterion is not considered to be met for those individuals taking opioids solely under appropriate medical supervision.

Specify if:

   In early remission: After full criteria for opioid use disorder were previously met, none of the criteria for opioid use disorder have been met for at least 3 months but for less than 12 months (with the exception that Criterion A4, "Craving, or a strong desire or urge to use opioids," may be met).

   In sustained remission: After full criteria for opioid use disorder were previously met, none of the criteria for opioid use disorder have been met at any time during a period of 12 months or longer (with the exception that Criterion A4, "Craving, or a strong desire or urge to use opioids," may be met).

Specify if:

   On maintenance therapy: This additional specifier is used if the individual is taking a prescribed agonist medication such as methadone or buprenorphine and none of the criteria for opioid use disorder have been met for that class of medication (except tolerance to, or withdrawal from, the agonist). This category also applies to those individuals being maintained on a partial agonist, an agonist/ antagonist, or a full antagonist such as oral naltrexone or depot naltrexone.

In a controlled environment: This additional specifier is used if the individual is in an environment where access to opioids is restricted.

Code based on current severity/remission: If an opioid intoxication, opioid withdrawal, or another opioid-induced mental disorder is also present, do not use the codes below for opioid use disorder. Instead, the comorbid opioid use disorder is indicated in the 4th character of the opioid-induced disorder code (see the coding note for opioid intoxication, opioid withdrawal, or a specific opioid-induced mental disorder). For example, if there is comorbid opioid-induced depressive disorder and opioid use disorder, only the opioid-induced depressive disorder code is given, with the 4th character indicating whether the comorbid opioid use disorder is mild, moderate, or severe: F11.14 for mild opioid use disorder with opioid-induced depressive disorder or F11.24 for a moderate or severe opioid use disorder with opioid-induced depressive disorder.

Specify current severity/remission:

F11.10 Mild: Presence of 2–3 symptoms.
F11.11 Mild, In early remission
F11.11 Mild, In sustained remission

F11.20 Moderate: Presence of 4–5 symptoms.
F11.21 Moderate, In early remission
F11.21 Moderate, In sustained remission

F11.20 Severe: Presence of 6 or more symptoms.
F11.21 Severe, In early remission
F11.21 Severe, In sustained remission

Opioid Intoxication

A. Recent use of an opioid.
B. Clinically significant problematic behavioral or psychological changes (e.g., initial euphoria followed by apathy, dysphoria, psychomotor agitation or retardation, impaired judgment) that developed during, or shortly after, opioid use.
C. Pupillary constriction (or pupillary dilation due to anoxia from severe overdose) and one (or more) of the following signs or symptoms developing during, or shortly after, opioid use:

1. Drowsiness or coma.
2. Slurred speech.
3. Impairment in attention or memory.

D. The signs or symptoms are not attributable to another medical condition and are not better explained by another mental disorder, including intoxication with another substance.

Specify if:

With perceptual disturbances: This specifier may be noted in the rare instance in which hallucinations with intact reality testing or auditory, visual, or tactile illusions occur in the absence of a delirium.

Coding note: The ICD-10-CM code depends on whether or not there is a comorbid opioid use disorder and whether or not there are perceptual disturbances.

For opioid intoxication, without perceptual disturbances: If a mild opioid use disorder is comorbid, the ICD-10-CM code is **F11.120,** and if a moderate or severe opioid use disorder is comorbid, the ICD-10-CM code is **F11.220.** If there is no comorbid opioid use disorder, then the ICD-10-CM code is **F11.920.**

For opioid intoxication, with perceptual disturbances: If a mild opioid use disorder is comorbid, the ICD-10-CM code is **F11.122,** and if a moderate or severe opioid use disorder is comorbid, the ICD-10-CM code is **F11.222.** If there is no comorbid opioid use disorder, then the ICD-10-CM code is **F11.922.**

Opioid Withdrawal

A. Presence of either of the following:

1. Cessation of (or reduction in) opioid use that has been heavy and prolonged (i.e., several weeks or longer).
2. Administration of an opioid antagonist after a period of opioid use.

B. Three (or more) of the following developing within minutes to several days after Criterion A:

1. Dysphoric mood.
2. Nausea or vomiting.
3. Muscle aches.
4. Lacrimation or rhinorrhea.
5. Pupillary dilation, piloerection, or sweating.
6. Diarrhea.
7. Yawning.
8. Fever.
9. Insomnia.

C. The signs or symptoms in Criterion B cause clinically significant distress or impairment in social, occupational, or other important areas of functioning.

D. The signs or symptoms are not attributable to another medical condition and are not better explained by another mental disorder, including intoxication or withdrawal from another substance.

Coding note: The ICD-10-CM code depends on whether or not there is a comorbid opioid use disorder. If a mild opioid use disorder is comorbid, the ICD-10-CM code is **F11.13**, and if a moderate or severe opioid use disorder is comorbid, the ICD-10-CM code is **F11.23**. For opioid withdrawal occurring in the absence of an opioid use disorder (e.g., in a patient taking opioids solely under appropriate medical supervision), the ICD-10-CM code is **F11.93**.

Opioid-Induced Mental Disorders

The following opioid-induced mental disorders are described in other chapters of the book with disorders with which they share phenomenology (see the substance/medication-induced mental disorders in these chapters): opioid-induced depressive disorder ("Depressive Disorders"); opioid-induced anxiety disorder ("Anxiety Disorders"); opioid-induced sleep disorder ("Sleep-Wake Disorders"); and opioid-induced sexual dysfunction ("Sexual Dysfunctions"). For opioid intoxication delirium, opioid withdrawal delirium, and delirium induced by opioids taken as prescribed, see the criteria and discussion of delirium in the chapter "Neurocognitive Disorders." These opioid-induced mental disorders are diagnosed instead of opioid intoxication or opioid withdrawal only when the symptoms are sufficiently severe to warrant independent clinical attention.

Unspecified Opioid-Related Disorder

F11.99

This category applies to presentations in which symptoms characteristic of an opioid-related disorder that cause clinically significant distress or impairment in social, occupational, or other important areas of functioning predominate but do not meet the full criteria for any specific opioid-related disorder or any of the disorders in the substance-related and addictive disorders diagnostic class.

Sedative-, Hypnotic-, or Anxiolytic-Related Disorders

Sedative, Hypnotic, or Anxiolytic Use Disorder

A. A problematic pattern of sedative, hypnotic, or anxiolytic use leading to clinically significant impairment or distress, as manifested by at least two of the following, occurring within a 12-month period:

1. Sedatives, hypnotics, or anxiolytics are often taken in larger amounts or over a longer period than was intended.

2. There is a persistent desire or unsuccessful efforts to cut down or control sedative, hypnotic, or anxiolytic use.

3. A great deal of time is spent in activities necessary to obtain the sedative, hypnotic, or anxiolytic; use the sedative, hypnotic, or anxiolytic; or recover from its effects.

4. Craving, or a strong desire or urge to use the sedative, hypnotic, or anxiolytic.

5. Recurrent sedative, hypnotic, or anxiolytic use resulting in a failure to fulfill major role obligations at work, school, or home (e.g., repeated absences from work or poor work performance related to sedative, hypnotic, or anxiolytic use; sedative-, hypnotic-, or anxiolytic-related absences, suspensions, or expulsions from school; neglect of children or household).

6. Continued sedative, hypnotic, or anxiolytic use despite having persistent or recurrent social or interpersonal problems caused or exacerbated by the effects of sedatives, hypnotics, or anxiolytics (e.g., arguments with a spouse about consequences of intoxication; physical fights).

7. Important social, occupational, or recreational activities are given up or reduced because of sedative, hypnotic, or anxiolytic use.

8. Recurrent sedative, hypnotic, or anxiolytic use in situations in which it is physically hazardous (e.g., driving an automobile or operating a machine when impaired by sedative, hypnotic, or anxiolytic use).

9. Sedative, hypnotic, or anxiolytic use is continued despite knowledge of having a persistent or recurrent physical or psychological problem that is likely to have been caused or exacerbated by the sedative, hypnotic, or anxiolytic.

10. Tolerance, as defined by either of the following:

    a. A need for markedly increased amounts of the sedative, hypnotic, or anxiolytic to achieve intoxication or desired effect.

    b. A markedly diminished effect with continued use of the same amount of the sedative, hypnotic, or anxiolytic.

Note: This criterion is not considered to be met for individuals taking sedatives, hypnotics, or anxiolytics under medical supervision.

11. Withdrawal, as manifested by either of the following:

   a. The characteristic withdrawal syndrome for sedatives, hypnotics, or anxiolytics (refer to Criteria A and B of the criteria set for sedative, hypnotic, or anxiolytic withdrawal).

   b. Sedatives, hypnotics, or anxiolytics (or a closely related substance, such as alcohol) are taken to relieve or avoid withdrawal symptoms.

   Note: This criterion is not considered to be met for individuals taking sedatives, hypnotics, or anxiolytics under medical supervision.

Specify if:

   In early remission: After full criteria for sedative, hypnotic, or anxiolytic use disorder were previously met, none of the criteria for sedative, hypnotic, or anxiolytic use disorder have been met for at least 3 months but for less than 12 months (with the exception that Criterion A4, "Craving, or a strong desire or urge to use the sedative, hypnotic, or anxiolytic," may be met).

   In sustained remission: After full criteria for sedative, hypnotic, or anxiolytic use disorder were previously met, none of the criteria for sedative, hypnotic, or anxiolytic use disorder have been met at any time during a period of 12 months or longer (with the exception that Criterion A4, "Craving, or a strong desire or urge to use the sedative, hypnotic, or anxiolytic," may be met).

Specify if:

   In a controlled environment: This additional specifier is used if the individual is in an environment where access to sedatives, hypnotics, or anxiolytics is restricted.

Code based on current severity/remission: If a sedative, hypnotic, or anxiolytic intoxication; sedative, hypnotic, or anxiolytic withdrawal; or another sedative-, hypnotic-, or anxiolytic-induced mental disorder is also present, do not use the codes below for sedative, hypnotic, or anxiolytic use disorder. Instead, the comorbid sedative, hypnotic, or anxiolytic use disorder is indicated in the 4th character of the sedative-hypnotic-, or anxiolytic-induced disorder (see the coding note for sedative, hypnotic, or anxiolytic intoxication; sedative, hypnotic, or anxiolytic withdrawal; or specific sedative-, hypnotic-, or anxiolytic-induced mental disorder). For example, if there is comorbid sedative-, hypnotic-, or anxiolytic-induced depressive disorder and sedative, hypnotic, or anxiolytic use disorder, only the sedative-, hypnotic-, or anxiolytic-induced depressive disorder code is given, with the 4th character indicating whether the comorbid sedative, hypnotic, or anxiolytic use disorder is mild, moderate, or severe: F13.14 for mild sedative, hypnotic, or anxiolytic use disorder with sedative-, hypnotic-, or anxiolytic-induced depressive disorder or F13.24 for a moderate or severe sedative, hypnotic, or anxiolytic use disorder with sedative-, hypnotic-, or anxiolytic-induced depressive disorder.

Specify current severity/remission:

F13.10 Mild: Presence of 2–3 symptoms.
F13.11 Mild, In early remission
F13.11 Mild, In sustained remission

F13.20 Moderate: Presence of 4–5 symptoms.
F13.21 Moderate, In early remission
F13.21 Moderate, In sustained remission

F13.20 Severe: Presence of 6 or more symptoms.
F13.21 Severe, In early remission
F13.21 Severe, In sustained remission

Sedative, Hypnotic, or Anxiolytic Intoxication

A. Recent use of a sedative, hypnotic, or anxiolytic.
B. Clinically significant maladaptive behavioral or psychological changes (e.g., inappropriate sexual or aggressive behavior, mood lability, impaired judgment) that developed during, or shortly after, sedative, hypnotic, or anxiolytic use.
C. One (or more) of the following signs or symptoms developing during, or shortly after, sedative, hypnotic, or anxiolytic use:

1. Slurred speech.
2. Incoordination.
3. Unsteady gait.
4. Nystagmus.
5. Impairment in cognition (e.g., attention, memory).
6. Stupor or coma.

D. The signs or symptoms are not attributable to another medical condition and are not better explained by another mental disorder, including intoxication with another substance.

Coding note: The ICD-10-CM code depends on whether there is a comorbid sedative, hypnotic, or anxiolytic use disorder. If a mild sedative, hypnotic, or anxiolytic use disorder is comorbid, the ICD-10-CM code is **F13.120,** and if a moderate or severe sedative, hypnotic, or anxiolytic use disorder is comorbid, the ICD-10-CM code is **F13.220.** If there is no comorbid sedative, hypnotic, or anxiolytic use disorder, then the ICD-10-CM code is **F13.920.**

Sedative, Hypnotic, or Anxiolytic Withdrawal

A. Cessation of (or reduction in) sedative, hypnotic, or anxiolytic use that has been prolonged.

B. Two (or more) of the following, developing within several hours to a few days after the cessation of (or reduction in) sedative, hypnotic, or anxiolytic use described in Criterion A:

1. Autonomic hyperactivity (e.g., sweating or pulse rate greater than 100 bpm).
2. Hand tremor.
3. Insomnia.
4. Nausea or vomiting.
5. Transient visual, tactile, or auditory hallucinations or illusions.
6. Psychomotor agitation.
7. Anxiety.
8. Grand mal seizures.

C. The signs or symptoms in Criterion B cause clinically significant distress or impairment in social, occupational, or other important areas of functioning.

D. The signs or symptoms are not attributable to another medical condition and are not better explained by another mental disorder, including intoxication or withdrawal from another substance.

Specify if:

With perceptual disturbances: This specifier may be noted when hallucinations with intact reality testing or auditory, visual, or tactile illusions occur in the absence of a delirium.

Coding note: The ICD-10-CM code depends on whether or not there is a comorbid sedative, hypnotic, or anxiolytic use disorder and whether or not there are perceptual disturbances.

For sedative, hypnotic, or anxiolytic withdrawal, without perceptual disturbances: If a mild sedative, hypnotic, or anxiolytic use disorder is comorbid, the ICD-10-CM code is **F13.130**, and if a moderate or severe sedative, hypnotic, or anxiolytic use disorder is comorbid, the ICD-10-CM code is **F13.230**. If there is no comorbid sedative, hypnotic, or anxiolytic use disorder (e.g., in a patient taking sedatives, hypnotics, or anxiolytics solely under appropriate medical supervision), then the ICD-10-CM code is **F13.930**.

For sedative, hypnotic, or anxiolytic withdrawal, with perceptual disturbances: If a mild sedative, hypnotic, or anxiolytic use disorder is comorbid, the ICD-10-CM code is **F13.132**, and if a moderate or severe sedative, hypnotic, or anxiolytic use disorder is comorbid, the ICD-10-CM code is **F13.232**. If there is no comorbid sedative, hypnotic, or anxiolytic use disorder (e.g., in a patient taking sedatives, hypnotics, or anxiolytics solely under appropriate medical supervision), then the ICD-10-CM code is **F13.932**.

Sedative-, Hypnotic-, or Anxiolytic-Induced Mental Disorders

The following sedative-, hypnotic-, or anxiolytic-induced mental disorders are described in other chapters of the book with disorders with which they share phenomenology (see the substance/medication-induced mental disorders in these chapters): sedative-, hypnotic-, or anxiolytic-induced psychotic disorder ("Schizophrenia Spectrum and Other Psychotic Disorders"); sedative-, hypnotic-, or anxiolytic-induced bipolar and related disorder ("Bipolar and Related Disorders"); sedative-, hypnotic-, or anxiolytic-induced depressive disorder ("Depressive Disorders"); sedative-, hypnotic-, or anxiolytic-induced anxiety disorder ("Anxiety Disorders"); sedative-, hypnotic-, or anxiolytic-induced sleep disorder ("Sleep-Wake Disorders"); sedative-, hypnotic-, or anxiolytic-induced sexual dysfunction ("Sexual Dysfunctions"); and sedative-, hypnotic-, or anxiolytic-induced major or mild neurocognitive disorder ("Neurocognitive Disorders"). For sedative, hypnotic, or anxiolytic intoxication delirium; sedative, hypnotic, or anxiolytic withdrawal delirium; and delirium induced by sedatives, hypnotics, or anxiolytics taken as prescribed, see the criteria and discussion of delirium in the chapter "Neurocognitive Disorders." These sedative-, hypnotic-, or anxiolytic-induced mental disorders are diagnosed instead of sedative, hypnotic, or anxiolytic intoxication or sedative, hypnotic, or anxiolytic withdrawal only when the symptoms are sufficiently severe to warrant independent clinical attention.

Unspecified Sedative-, Hypnotic-, or Anxiolytic-Related Disorder

F13.99

This category applies to presentations in which symptoms characteristic of a sedative-, hypnotic-, or anxiolytic-related disorder that cause clinically significant distress or impairment in social, occupational, or other important areas of functioning predominate but do not meet the full criteria for any specific sedative-, hypnotic-, or anxiolytic-related disorder or any of the disorders in the substance-related and addictive disorders diagnostic class.

Stimulant-Related Disorders

Stimulant Use Disorder

A. A pattern of amphetamine-type substance, cocaine, or other stimulant use leading to clinically significant impairment or distress, as manifested by at least two of the following, occurring within a 12-month period:

1. The stimulant is often taken in larger amounts or over a longer period than was intended.
2. There is a persistent desire or unsuccessful efforts to cut down or control stimulant use.
3. A great deal of time is spent in activities necessary to obtain the stimulant, use the stimulant, or recover from its effects.
4. Craving, or a strong desire or urge to use the stimulant.
5. Recurrent stimulant use resulting in a failure to fulfill major role obligations at work, school, or home.
6. Continued stimulant use despite having persistent or recurrent social or interpersonal problems caused or exacerbated by the effects of the stimulant.
7. Important social, occupational, or recreational activities are given up or reduced because of stimulant use.
8. Recurrent stimulant use in situations in which it is physically hazardous.
9. Stimulant use is continued despite knowledge of having a persistent or recurrent physical or psychological problem that is likely to have been caused or exacerbated by the stimulant.
10. Tolerance, as defined by either of the following:
    a. A need for markedly increased amounts of the stimulant to achieve intoxication or desired effect.
    b. A markedly diminished effect with continued use of the same amount of the stimulant.

    Note: This criterion is not considered to be met for those taking stimulant medications solely under appropriate medical supervision, such as medications for attention-deficit/hyperactivity disorder or narcolepsy.

11. Withdrawal, as manifested by either of the following:

    a. The characteristic withdrawal syndrome for the stimulant (refer to Criteria A and B of the criteria set for stimulant withdrawal).
    b. The stimulant (or a closely related substance) is taken to relieve or avoid withdrawal symptoms.

    Note: This criterion is not considered to be met for those taking stimulant medications solely under appropriate medical supervision, such as medications for attention-deficit/hyperactivity disorder or narcolepsy.

Specify if:

In early remission: After full criteria for stimulant use disorder were previously met, none of the criteria for stimulant use disorder have been met for at least 3 months but for less than 12 months (with the exception that Criterion A4, "Craving, or a strong desire or urge to use the stimulant," may be met).

In sustained remission: After full criteria for stimulant use disorder were previously met, none of the criteria for stimulant use disorder have been met at any time during a period of 12 months or longer (with the exception that Criterion A4, "Craving, or a strong desire or urge to use the stimulant," may be met).

Specify if:

In a controlled environment: This additional specifier is used if the individual is in an environment where access to stimulants is restricted.

Code based on current severity/remission: If an amphetamine-type substance intoxication, amphetamine-type substance withdrawal, or amphetamine-type substance-induced mental disorder is also present, do not use the codes below for amphetamine-type substance use disorder. Instead, the comorbid amphetamine-type substance use disorder is indicated in the 4th character of the amphetamine-type substance-induced disorder code (see the coding note for amphetamine-type substance intoxication, amphetamine-type substance withdrawal, or a specific amphetamine-type substance-induced mental disorder). For example, if there is comorbid amphetamine-induced depressive disorder and amphetamine use disorder, only the amphetamine-induced depressive disorder code is given, with the 4th character indicating whether the comorbid amphetamine use disorder is mild, moderate, or severe: F15.14 for mild amphetamine use disorder with amphetamine-induced depressive disorder or F15.24 for a moderate or severe amphetamine use disorder with amphetamine-induced depressive disorder. (The instructions for amphetamine-type substance also apply to other or unspecified stimulant intoxication, other or unspecified stimulant withdrawal, and other or unspecified stimulant-induced mental disorder.) Similarly, if there is comorbid cocaine-induced depressive disorder and cocaine use disorder, only the cocaine-induced depressive disorder code is given, with the 4th character indicating whether the comorbid cocaine use disorder is mild, moderate, or severe: F14.14 for a mild cocaine use disorder with cocaine-induced depressive disorder or F14.24 for a moderate or severe cocaine use disorder with cocaine-induced depressive disorder.

Specify current severity/remission:

Mild: Presence of 2–3 symptoms.

    F15.10 Amphetamine-type substance

    F14.10 Cocaine

    F15.10 Other or unspecified stimulant

Mild, In early remission

    F15.11 Amphetamine-type substance
    F14.11 Cocaine
    F15.11 Other or unspecified stimulant

Mild, In sustained remission

    F15.11 Amphetamine-type substance
    F14.11 Cocaine
    F15.11 Other or unspecified stimulant

Moderate: Presence of 4–5 symptoms.

    F15.20 Amphetamine-type substance
    F14.20 Cocaine
    F15.20 Other or unspecified stimulant

Moderate, In early remission

    F15.21 Amphetamine-type substance
    F14.21 Cocaine
    F15.21 Other or unspecified stimulant

Moderate, In sustained remission

    F15.21 Amphetamine-type substance
    F14.21 Cocaine
    F15.21 Other or unspecified stimulant

Severe: Presence of 6 or more symptoms.

    F15.20 Amphetamine-type substance
    F14.20 Cocaine
    F15.20 Other or unspecified stimulant

Severe, In early remission

    F15.21 Amphetamine-type substance
    F14.21 Cocaine
    F15.21 Other or unspecified stimulant

Severe, In sustained remission

    F15.21 Amphetamine-type substance
    F14.21 Cocaine
    F15.21 Other or unspecified stimulant

Stimulant Intoxication

A. Recent use of an amphetamine-type substance, cocaine, or other stimulant.

B. Clinically significant problematic behavioral or psychological changes (e.g., euphoria or affective blunting; changes in sociability; hypervigilance; interpersonal sensitivity; anxiety, tension, or anger; stereotyped behaviors; impaired judgment) that developed during, or shortly after, use of a stimulant.

C. Two (or more) of the following signs or symptoms, developing during, or shortly after, stimulant use:

1. Tachycardia or bradycardia.
2. Pupillary dilation.

3. Elevated or lowered blood pressure.
4. Perspiration or chills.
5. Nausea or vomiting.
6. Evidence of weight loss.
7. Psychomotor agitation or retardation.
8. Muscular weakness, respiratory depression, chest pain, or cardiac arrhythmias.
9. Confusion, seizures, dyskinesias, dystonias, or coma.

D. The signs or symptoms are not attributable to another medical condition and are not better explained by another mental disorder, including intoxication with another substance.

Specify **the particular intoxicant** (i.e., amphetamine-type substance, cocaine, or other stimulant).

Specify if:

> **With perceptual disturbances:** This specifier may be noted when hallucinations with intact reality testing or auditory, visual, or tactile illusions occur in the absence of a delirium.

Coding note: The ICD-10-CM code depends on whether the stimulant is an amphetamine-type substance, cocaine, or other stimulant; whether there is a comorbid amphetamine-type substance, cocaine, or other stimulant use disorder; and whether or not there are perceptual disturbances.

> **For amphetamine-type substance, cocaine, or other stimulant intoxication, without perceptual disturbances:** If a mild amphetamine-type substance or other stimulant use disorder is comorbid, the ICD-10-CM code is **F15.120,** and if a moderate or severe amphetamine-type substance or other stimulant use disorder is comorbid, the ICD-10-CM code is **F15.220.** If there is no comorbid amphetamine-type substance or other stimulant use disorder, then the ICD-10-CM code is **F15.920.** Similarly, if a mild cocaine use disorder is comorbid, the ICD-10-CM code is **F14.120,** and if a moderate or severe cocaine use disorder is comorbid, the ICD-10-CM code is **F14.220.** If there is no comorbid cocaine use disorder, then the ICD-10-CM code is **F14.920.**

> **For amphetamine-type substance, cocaine, or other stimulant intoxication, with perceptual disturbances:** If a mild amphetamine-type substance or other stimulant use disorder is comorbid, the ICD-10-CM code is **F15.122,** and if a moderate or severe amphetamine-type substance or other stimulant use disorder is comorbid, the ICD-10-CM code is **F15.222.** If there is no comorbid amphetamine-type substance or other stimulant use disorder, then the ICD-10-CM code is **F15.922.** Similarly, if a mild cocaine use disorder is comorbid, the ICD-10-CM code is **F14.122,** and if a moderate or severe cocaine use disorder is comorbid, the ICD-10-CM code is **F14.222.** If there is no comorbid cocaine use disorder, then the ICD-10-CM code is **F14.922.**

Stimulant Withdrawal

A. Cessation of (or reduction in) prolonged amphetamine-type substance, cocaine, or other stimulant use.

B. Dysphoric mood and two (or more) of the following physiological changes, developing within a few hours to several days after Criterion A:

1. Fatigue.
2. Vivid, unpleasant dreams.
3. Insomnia or hypersomnia.
4. Increased appetite.
5. Psychomotor retardation or agitation.

C. The signs or symptoms in Criterion B cause clinically significant distress or impairment in social, occupational, or other important areas of functioning.

D. The signs or symptoms are not attributable to another medical condition and are not better explained by another mental disorder, including intoxication or withdrawal from another substance.

Specify **the particular substance that causes the withdrawal syndrome** (i.e., amphetamine-type substance, cocaine, or other stimulant).

Coding note: The ICD-10-CM code depends on whether the stimulant is an amphetamine-type substance, cocaine, or other stimulant and on whether or not there is a comorbid amphetamine-type substance, cocaine, or other stimulant use disorder. If mild amphetamine-type substance or other stimulant use disorder is comorbid, the ICD-10-CM code is **F15.13**. If moderate or severe amphetamine-type substance or other stimulant use disorder is comorbid, the ICD-10-CM code is **F15.23**. For amphetamine-type substance or other stimulant withdrawal occurring in the absence of amphetamine-type substance or other stimulant use disorder (e.g., in a patient taking amphetamine solely under appropriate medical supervision), the ICD-10-CM code is **F15.93**. If mild cocaine use disorder is comorbid, the ICD-10-CM code is **F14.13**. If moderate or severe cocaine use disorder is comorbid, the ICD-10-CM code is **F14.23**. For cocaine withdrawal occurring in the absence of a cocaine use disorder, the ICD-10-CM code is **F14.93**.

Stimulant-Induced Mental Disorders

The following stimulant-induced mental disorders (which include amphetamine-type substance–, cocaine-, and other stimulant–induced mental disorders) are described in other chapters of the book with disorders with which they share phenomenology (see the substance/medication-induced mental disorders in these chapters): stimulant-induced psychotic disorder ("Schizophrenia Spectrum and Other Psychotic Disorders"); stimulant-induced bipolar and related disorder ("Bipolar and Related Disorders"); stimulant-induced depressive disorder ("Depressive Disorders"); stimulant-induced anxiety disorder

("Anxiety Disorders"); stimulant-induced obsessive-compulsive disorder ("Obsessive-Compulsive and Related Disorders"); stimulant-induced sleep disorder ("Sleep-Wake Disorders"); stimulant-induced sexual dysfunction ("Sexual Dysfunctions"); and stimulant-induced mild neurocognitive disorder ("Neurocognitive Disorders"). For stimulant intoxication delirium and delirium induced by stimulants taken as prescribed, see the criteria and discussion of delirium in the chapter "Neurocognitive Disorders." These stimulant-induced mental disorders are diagnosed instead of stimulant intoxication or stimulant withdrawal only when the symptoms are sufficiently severe to warrant independent clinical attention.

Unspecified Stimulant-Related Disorder

This category applies to presentations in which symptoms characteristic of a stimulant-related disorder that cause clinically significant distress or impairment in social, occupational, or other important areas of functioning predominate but do not meet the full criteria for any specific stimulant-related disorder or any of the disorders in the substance-related and addictive disorders diagnostic class.

Coding note: The ICD-10-CM code depends on whether the stimulant is an amphetamine-type substance, cocaine, or other stimulant. The ICD-10-CM code for an unspecified amphetamine-type substance or other stimulant–related disorder is **F15.99**. The ICD-10-CM code for an unspecified cocaine-related disorder is **F14.99**.

Tobacco-Related Disorders

Tobacco Use Disorder

A. A problematic pattern of tobacco use leading to clinically significant impairment or distress, as manifested by at least two of the following, occurring within a 12-month period:

1. Tobacco is often taken in larger amounts or over a longer period than was intended.
2. There is a persistent desire or unsuccessful efforts to cut down or control tobacco use.
3. A great deal of time is spent in activities necessary to obtain or use tobacco.
4. Craving, or a strong desire or urge to use tobacco.
5. Recurrent tobacco use resulting in a failure to fulfill major role obligations at work, school, or home (e.g., interference with work).

6. Continued tobacco use despite having persistent or recurrent social or interpersonal problems caused or exacerbated by the effects of tobacco (e.g., arguments with others about tobacco use).
7. Important social, occupational, or recreational activities are given up or reduced because of tobacco use.
8. Recurrent tobacco use in situations in which it is physically hazardous (e.g., smoking in bed).
9. Tobacco use is continued despite knowledge of having a persistent or recurrent physical or psychological problem that is likely to have been caused or exacerbated by tobacco.
10. Tolerance, as defined by either of the following:
    a. A need for markedly increased amounts of tobacco to achieve the desired effect.
    b. A markedly diminished effect with continued use of the same amount of tobacco.
11. Withdrawal, as manifested by either of the following:
    a. The characteristic withdrawal syndrome for tobacco (refer to Criteria A and B of the criteria set for tobacco withdrawal).
    b. Tobacco (or a closely related substance, such as nicotine) is taken to relieve or avoid withdrawal symptoms.

Specify if:

In early remission: After full criteria for tobacco use disorder were previously met, none of the criteria for tobacco use disorder have been met for at least 3 months but for less than 12 months (with the exception that Criterion A4, "Craving, or a strong desire or urge to use tobacco," may be met).

In sustained remission: After full criteria for tobacco use disorder were previously met, none of the criteria for tobacco use disorder have been met at any time during a period of 12 months or longer (with the exception that Criterion A4, "Craving, or a strong desire or urge to use tobacco," may be met).

Specify if:

On maintenance therapy: The individual is taking a long-term maintenance medication, such as nicotine replacement medication, and no criteria for tobacco use disorder have been met for that class of medication (except tolerance to, or withdrawal from, the nicotine replacement medication).

In a controlled environment: This additional specifier is used if the individual is in an environment where access to tobacco is restricted.

Code based on current severity/remission: If a tobacco withdrawal or tobacco-induced sleep disorder is also present, do not use the codes below for tobacco use disorder. Instead, the comorbid tobacco use disorder is indicated in the 4th character of the tobacco-induced disorder code (see the coding note for tobacco withdrawal or tobacco-induced sleep disorder). For example, if there is comorbid tobacco-induced sleep disorder and tobacco use disorder, only the tobacco-induced sleep disorder code is given, with the 4th character indicating whether the comorbid tobacco use disorder is moderate or severe: F17.208 for moderate or severe tobacco use disorder with tobacco-induced sleep disorder. It is not permissible to code a comorbid mild tobacco use disorder with a tobacco-induced sleep disorder.

Specify current severity/remission:

Z72.0 Mild: Presence of 2–3 symptoms.

F17.200 Moderate: Presence of 4–5 symptoms.
F17.201 Moderate, In early remission
F17.201 Moderate, In sustained remission

F17.200 Severe: Presence of 6 or more symptoms.
F17.201 Severe, In early remission
F17.201 Severe, In sustained remission

Tobacco Withdrawal

F17.203

A. Daily use of tobacco for at least several weeks.
B. Abrupt cessation of tobacco use, or reduction in the amount of tobacco used, followed within 24 hours by four (or more) of the following signs or symptoms:

1. Irritability, frustration, or anger.
2. Anxiety.
3. Difficulty concentrating.
4. Increased appetite.
5. Restlessness.
6. Depressed mood.
7. Insomnia.

C. The signs or symptoms in Criterion B cause clinically significant distress or impairment in social, occupational, or other important areas of functioning.
D. The signs or symptoms are not attributable to another medical condition and are not better explained by another mental disorder, including intoxication or withdrawal from another substance.

Coding note: The ICD-10-CM code for tobacco withdrawal is **F17.203**. Note that the ICD-10-CM code indicates the comorbid presence of a moderate or severe tobacco use disorder, reflecting the fact that tobacco withdrawal can only occur in the presence of a moderate or severe tobacco use disorder.

Tobacco-Induced Mental Disorders

Tobacco-induced sleep disorder is discussed in the chapter "Sleep-Wake Disorders" (see "Substance/Medication-Induced Sleep Disorder").

Unspecified Tobacco-Related Disorder

F17.209

This category applies to presentations in which symptoms characteristic of a tobacco-related disorder that cause clinically significant distress or impairment in social, occupational, or other important areas of functioning predominate but do not meet the full criteria for any specific tobacco-related disorder or any of the disorders in the substance-related and addictive disorders diagnostic class.

Other (or Unknown) Substance–Related Disorders

Other (or Unknown) Substance Use Disorder

A. A problematic pattern of use of an intoxicating substance not able to be classified within the alcohol; caffeine; cannabis; hallucinogen (phencyclidine and others); inhalant; opioid; sedative, hypnotic, or anxiolytic; stimulant; or tobacco categories and leading to clinically significant impairment or distress, as manifested by at least two of the following, occurring within a 12-month period:

1. The substance is often taken in larger amounts or over a longer period than was intended.
2. There is a persistent desire or unsuccessful efforts to cut down or control use of the substance.
3. A great deal of time is spent in activities necessary to obtain the substance, use the substance, or recover from its effects.
4. Craving, or a strong desire or urge to use the substance.
5. Recurrent use of the substance resulting in a failure to fulfill major role obligations at work, school, or home.
6. Continued use of the substance despite having persistent or recurrent social or interpersonal problems caused or exacerbated by the effects of its use.
7. Important social, occupational, or recreational activities are given up or reduced because of use of the substance.
8. Recurrent use of the substance in situations in which it is physically hazardous.

9. Use of the substance is continued despite knowledge of having a persistent or recurrent physical or psychological problem that is likely to have been caused or exacerbated by the substance.

10. Tolerance, as defined by either of the following:

 a. A need for markedly increased amounts of the substance to achieve intoxication or desired effect.

 b. A markedly diminished effect with continued use of the same amount of the substance.

11. Withdrawal, as manifested by either of the following:

 a. The characteristic withdrawal syndrome for other (or unknown) substance (refer to Criteria A and B of the criteria sets for other [or unknown] substance withdrawal).

 b. The substance (or a closely related substance) is taken to relieve or avoid withdrawal symptoms.

Specify if:

In early remission: After full criteria for other (or unknown) substance use disorder were previously met, none of the criteria for other (or unknown) substance use disorder have been met for at least 3 months but for less than 12 months (with the exception that Criterion A4, "Craving, or a strong desire or urge to use the substance," may be met).

In sustained remission: After full criteria for other (or unknown) substance use disorder were previously met, none of the criteria for other (or unknown) substance use disorder have been met at any time during a period of 12 months or longer (with the exception that Criterion A4, "Craving, or a strong desire or urge to use the substance," may be met).

Specify if:

In a controlled environment: This additional specifier is used if the individual is in an environment where access to the substance is restricted.

Code based on current severity/remission: If an other (or unknown) substance intoxication, other (or unknown) substance withdrawal, or other (or unknown) substance–induced mental disorder is present, do not use the codes below for other (or unknown) substance use disorder. Instead, the comorbid other (or unknown) substance use disorder is indicated in the 4th character of the other (or unknown) substance–induced disorder code (see the coding note for other [or unknown] substance intoxication, other [or unknown] substance withdrawal, or specific other [or unknown] substance–induced mental disorder). For example, if there is comorbid other (or unknown) substance–induced depressive disorder and other (or unknown) substance use disorder, only the other (or unknown) substance–induced depressive disorder code is given with the 4th character indicating whether the comorbid other (or unknown) substance use disorder is mild, moderate, or severe: F19.14 for other (or unknown) substance use disorder with other (or unknown) substance–induced depressive disorder or F19.24 for a moderate or severe other (or unknown) substance use disorder with other (or unknown) substance–induced depressive disorder.

Specify current severity/remission:

F19.10 Mild: Presence of 2–3 symptoms.
F19.11 Mild, In early remission
F19.11 Mild, In sustained remission

F19.20 Moderate: Presence of 4–5 symptoms.
F19.21 Moderate, In early remission
F19.21 Moderate, In sustained remission

F19.20 Severe: Presence of 6 or more symptoms.
F19.21 Severe, In early remission
F19.21 Severe, In sustained remission

Other (or Unknown) Substance Intoxication

A. The development of a reversible substance-specific syndrome attributable to recent ingestion of (or exposure to) a substance that is not listed elsewhere or is unknown.

B. Clinically significant problematic behavioral or psychological changes that are attributable to the effect of the substance on the central nervous system (e.g., impaired motor coordination, psychomotor agitation or retardation, euphoria, anxiety, belligerence, mood lability, cognitive impairment, impaired judgment, social withdrawal) and develop during, or shortly after, use of the substance.

C. The signs or symptoms are not attributable to another medical condition and are not better explained by another mental disorder, including intoxication with another substance.

Specify if:

With perceptual disturbances: This specifier may be noted when hallucinations with intact reality testing or auditory, visual, or tactile illusions occur in the absence of a delirium.

Coding note: The ICD-10-CM code depends on whether there is a comorbid other (or unknown) substance use disorder involving the same substance and whether or not there are perceptual disturbances.

For other (or unknown) substance intoxication, without perceptual disturbances: If a mild other (or unknown) substance use disorder is comorbid, the ICD-10-CM code is **F19.120**, and if a moderate or severe other (or unknown) substance use disorder is comorbid, the ICD-10-CM code is **F19.220**. If there is no comorbid other (or unknown) substance use disorder, then the ICD-10-CM code is **F19.920**.

For other (or unknown) substance intoxication, with perceptual disturbances: If a mild other (or unknown) substance use disorder is comorbid, the ICD-10-CM code is **F19.122**, and if a moderate or severe other (or unknown) substance use disorder is comorbid, the ICD-10-CM code is **F19.222**. If there is no comorbid other (or unknown) substance use disorder, then the ICD-10-CM code is **F19.922**.

Other (or Unknown) Substance Withdrawal

A. Cessation of (or reduction in) use of a substance that has been heavy and prolonged.

B. The development of a substance-specific syndrome shortly after the cessation of (or reduction in) substance use.

C. The substance-specific syndrome causes clinically significant distress or impairment in social, occupational, or other important areas of functioning.

D. The symptoms are not attributable to another medical condition and are not better explained by another mental disorder, including withdrawal from another substance.

E. The substance involved cannot be classified under any of the other substance categories (alcohol; caffeine; cannabis; opioids; sedatives, hypnotics, or anxiolytics; stimulants; or tobacco) or is unknown.

Specify if:

With perceptual disturbances: This specifier may be noted when hallucinations with intact reality testing or auditory, visual, or tactile illusions occur in the absence of a delirium.

Coding note: The ICD-10-CM code depends on whether or not there is a comorbid other (or unknown) substance use disorder and whether or not there are perceptual disturbances.

For other (or unknown) substance withdrawal, without perceptual disturbances: If a mild other (or unknown) substance use disorder is comorbid, the ICD-10-CM code is **F19.130**, and if a moderate or severe other (or unknown) substance use disorder is comorbid, the ICD-10-CM code is **F19.230**. If there is no comorbid other (or unknown) substance use disorder (e.g., in a patient taking an other [or unknown] substance solely under appropriate medical supervision), then the ICD-10-CM code is **F19.930**.

For other (or unknown) substance withdrawal, with perceptual disturbances: If a mild other (or unknown) substance use disorder is comorbid, the ICD-10-CM code is **F19.132**, and if a moderate or severe other (or unknown) substance use disorder is comorbid, the ICD-10-CM code is **F19.232**. If there is no comorbid other (or unknown) substance use disorder (e.g., in a patient taking an other [or unknown] substance solely under appropriate medical supervision), then the ICD-10-CM code is **F19.932**.

Other (or Unknown) Substance–Induced Mental Disorders

Because the category of other or unknown substances is inherently ill-defined, the extent and range of these substance-induced mental disorders are uncertain. Nevertheless, other (or unknown) substance–induced mental disorders are possible and are described in other chapters of the book with disorders with which they share phenomenology (see the substance/medication-induced mental disorders in these chapters): other (or unknown) substance–induced psychotic disorder ("Schizophrenia Spectrum and Other Psychotic Disorders"); other (or unknown) substance–induced and related bipolar disorder ("Bipolar and Related Disorders"); other (or unknown) substance–induced depressive disorder ("Depressive Disorders"); other (or unknown) substance–induced anxiety disorders ("Anxiety Disorders"); other (or unknown) substance–induced obsessive-compulsive disorder ("Obsessive-Compulsive and Related Disorders"); other (or unknown) substance–induced sleep disorder ("Sleep-Wake Disorders"); other (or unknown) substance–induced sexual dysfunction ("Sexual Dysfunctions"); and other (or unknown) substance/medication–induced major or mild neurocognitive disorder ("Neurocognitive Disorders"). For other (or unknown) substance–induced intoxication delirium, other (or unknown) substance–induced withdrawal delirium, and delirium induced by other (or unknown) substance taken as prescribed, see the criteria and discussion of delirium in the chapter "Neurocognitive Disorders." These other (or unknown) substance–induced mental disorders are diagnosed instead of other (or unknown) substance intoxication or other (or unknown) substance withdrawal only when the symptoms are sufficiently severe to warrant independent clinical attention.

Unspecified Other (or Unknown) Substance–Related Disorder

F19.99

This category applies to presentations in which symptoms characteristic of an other (or unknown) substance–related disorder that cause clinically significant distress or impairment in social, occupational, or other important areas of functioning predominate but do not meet the full criteria for any specific other (or unknown) substance–related disorder or any of the disorders in the substance-related disorders diagnostic class.

Non-Substance-Related Disorders

Gambling Disorder

F63.0

A. Persistent and recurrent problematic gambling behavior leading to clinically significant impairment or distress, as indicated by the individual exhibiting four (or more) of the following in a 12-month period:

1. Needs to gamble with increasing amounts of money in order to achieve the desired excitement.
2. Is restless or irritable when attempting to cut down or stop gambling.
3. Has made repeated unsuccessful efforts to control, cut back, or stop gambling.
4. Is often preoccupied with gambling (e.g., having persistent thoughts of reliving past gambling experiences, handicapping or planning the next venture, thinking of ways to get money with which to gamble).
5. Often gambles when feeling distressed (e.g., helpless, guilty, anxious, depressed).
6. After losing money gambling, often returns another day to get even ("chasing" one's losses).
7. Lies to conceal the extent of involvement with gambling.
8. Has jeopardized or lost a significant relationship, job, or educational or career opportunity because of gambling.
9. Relies on others to provide money to relieve desperate financial situations caused by gambling.

B. The gambling behavior is not better explained by a manic episode.

Specify if:

   Episodic: Meeting diagnostic criteria at more than one time point, with symptoms subsiding between periods of gambling disorder for at least several months.

   Persistent: Experiencing continuous symptoms, to meet diagnostic criteria for multiple years.

Specify if:

   In early remission: After full criteria for gambling disorder were previously met, none of the criteria for gambling disorder have been met for at least 3 months but for less than 12 months.

   In sustained remission: After full criteria for gambling disorder were previously met, none of the criteria for gambling disorder have been met during a period of 12 months or longer.

Specify current severity:

   Mild: 4–5 criteria met.
   Moderate: 6–7 criteria met.
   Severe: 8–9 criteria met.

Neurocognitive Disorders

Neurocognitive Domains

The criteria for the various neurocognitive disorders are based on defined cognitive domains. Table 1 provides for each of the key domains a working definition, examples of symptoms or observations regarding impairments in everyday activities, and examples of assessments. The domains thus defined, along with guidelines for clinical thresholds, form the basis on which the neurocognitive disorders, their levels, and their subtypes may be diagnosed. Additional information is provided in DSM-5-TR.

TABLE 1 Neurocognitive domains

Cognitive domain	Examples of symptoms or observations	Examples of assessments
Complex attention (sustained attention, divided attention, selective attention, processing speed)	*Major:* Has increased difficulty in environments with multiple stimuli (TV, radio, conversation); is easily distracted by competing events in the environment. Is unable to attend unless input is restricted and simplified. Has difficulty holding new information in mind, such as recalling phone numbers or addresses just given, or reporting what was just said. Is unable to perform mental calculations. All thinking takes longer than usual, and components to be processed must be simplified to one or a few. *Mild:* Normal tasks take longer than previously. Begins to find errors in routine tasks; finds work needs more double-checking than previously. Thinking is easier when not competing with other things (radio, TV, other conversations, cell phone, driving).	*Sustained attention:* Maintenance of attention over time (e.g., pressing a button every time a tone is heard, and over a period of time). *Selective attention:* Maintenance of attention despite competing stimuli or distractors: hearing numbers and letters read and asked to count only letters. *Divided attention:* Attending to two tasks within the same time period: rapidly tapping while learning a story being read. Processing speed can be quantified on any task by timing it (e.g., time to put together a design of blocks; time to match symbols with numbers; speed in responding, such as counting speed or serial 3 speed).

TABLE 1 Neurocognitive domains (continued)

Cognitive domain	Examples of symptoms or observations	Examples of assessments
Executive function (planning, decision making, working memory, responding to feedback/error correction, overriding habits/inhibition, mental flexibility)	*Major:* Abandons complex projects. Needs to focus on one task at a time. Needs to rely on others to plan instrumental activities of daily living or make decisions. *Mild:* Increased effort required to complete multistage projects. Has increased difficulty multitasking or difficulty resuming a task interrupted by a visitor or phone call. May complain of increased fatigue from the extra effort required to organize, plan, and make decisions. May report that large social gatherings are more taxing or less enjoyable due to increased effort required to follow shifting conversations.	*Planning:* Ability to find the exit to a maze; interpret a sequential picture or object arrangement. *Decision making:* Performance of tasks that assess process of deciding in the face of competing alternatives (e.g., simulated gambling). *Working memory:* Ability to hold information for a brief period and to manipulate it (e.g., adding up a list of numbers or repeating a series of numbers or words backward). *Feedback/error utilization:* Ability to benefit from feedback to infer the rules for solving a problem. *Overriding habits/inhibition:* Ability to choose a more complex and effortful solution to be correct (e.g., looking away from the direction indicated by an arrow; naming the color of a word's font rather than naming the word). *Mental/cognitive flexibility:* Ability to shift between two concepts, tasks, or response rules (e.g., from number to letter, from verbal to key-press response, from adding numbers to ordering numbers, from ordering objects by size to ordering by color).

TABLE 1   Neurocognitive domains *(continued)*

Cognitive domain	Examples of symptoms or observations	Examples of assessments
Learning and memory (immediate memory, recent memory [including free recall, cued recall, and recognition memory], very-long-term memory [semantic; autobiographical], implicit learning)	*Major:* Repeats self in conversation, often within the same conversation. Cannot keep track of short list of items when shopping, or of plans for the day. Requires frequent reminders to orient to task at hand. *Mild:* Has difficulty recalling recent events, and relies increasingly on list making or calendar. Needs occasional reminders or re-reading to keep track of characters in a movie or novel. Occasionally may repeat self over a few weeks to the same person. Loses track of whether bills have already been paid. **Note:** Except in severe forms of major neurocognitive disorder, semantic, autobiographical, and implicit memory are relatively preserved, compared with recent memory.	*Immediate memory span:* Ability to repeat a list of words or digits. **Note:** Immediate memory sometimes subsumed under "working memory" (see "Executive Function"). *Recent memory:* Assesses the process of encoding new information (e.g., word lists, a short story, or diagrams). The aspects of recent memory that can be tested include 1) free recall (the person is asked to recall as many words, diagrams, or elements of a story as possible); 2) cued recall (examiner aids recall by providing semantic cues like "List all the food items on the list" or "Name all of the children from the story"); and 3) recognition memory (examiner asks about specific items—e.g., "Was 'apple' on the list?" or "Did you see this diagram or figure?"). Other aspects of memory that can be assessed include semantic memory (memory for facts), autobiographical memory (memory for personal events or people), and implicit (procedural) learning (unconscious learning of skills).

TABLE 1 Neurocognitive domains (continued)

Cognitive domain	Examples of symptoms or observations	Examples of assessments
Language (expressive language [including naming, word finding, fluency, and grammar and syntax] and receptive language)	*Major:* Has significant difficulties with expressive or receptive language. Often uses general use terms such as "that thing" and "you know what I mean," and prefers general pronouns rather than names. With severe impairment, may not even recall names of closer friends and family. Idiosyncratic word usage, grammatical errors, and spontaneity of output and economy of utterances occur. Stereotypy of speech occurs; echolalia and automatic speech typically precede mutism. *Mild:* Has noticeable word-finding difficulty. May substitute general for specific terms. May avoid use of specific names of acquaintances. Grammatical errors involve subtle omission or incorrect use of articles, prepositions, auxiliary verbs, etc.	*Expressive language:* Confrontational naming (identification of objects or pictures); fluency (e.g., name as many items as possible in a semantic [e.g., animals] or phonemic [e.g., words starting with "f"] category in 1 minute). *Grammar and syntax* (e.g., omission or incorrect use of articles, prepositions, auxiliary verbs): Errors observed during naming and fluency tests are compared with norms to assess frequency of errors and compare with normal slips of the tongue. *Receptive language:* Comprehension (word definition and object-pointing tasks involving animate and inanimate stimuli): performance of actions/activities according to verbal command.

TABLE 1 Neurocognitive domains (continued)

Cognitive domain	Examples of symptoms or observations	Examples of assessments
Perceptual-motor (includes abilities subsumed under the terms *visual perception, visuoconstructional, perceptual-motor, praxis,* and *gnosis*)	*Major:* Has significant difficulties with previously familiar activities (using tools, driving motor vehicle), navigating in familiar environments; is often more confused at dusk, when shadows and lowering levels of light change perceptions. *Mild:* May need to rely more on maps or others for directions. Uses notes and follows others to get to a new place. May find self lost or turned around when not concentrating on task. Is less precise in parking. Needs to expend greater effort for spatial tasks such as carpentry, assembly, sewing, or knitting.	*Visual perception:* Line bisection tasks can be used to detect basic visual defect or attentional neglect. Motor-free perceptual tasks (including facial recognition) require the identification and/or matching of figures—best when tasks cannot be verbally mediated (e.g., figures are not objects); some require the decision of whether a figure can be "real" or not based on dimensionality. *Visuoconstructional:* Assembly of items requiring hand-eye coordination, such as drawing, copying, and block assembly. *Perceptual-motor:* Integrating perception with purposeful movement (e.g., inserting blocks into a form board without visual cues; rapidly inserting pegs into a slotted board). *Praxis:* Integrity of learned movements, such as ability to imitate gestures (wave goodbye) or pantomime use of objects to command ("Show me how you would use a hammer"). *Gnosis:* Perceptual integrity of awareness and recognition, such as recognition of faces and colors.

TABLE 1   Neurocognitive domains (continued)

Cognitive domain	Examples of symptoms or observations	Examples of assessments
Social cognition (recognition of emotions, theory of mind)	*Major:* Behavior clearly out of acceptable social range; shows insensitivity to social standards of modesty in dress, or of political, religious, or sexual topics of conversation. Focuses excessively on a topic despite group's disinterest or direct feedback. Behavioral intention without regard to family or friends. Makes decisions without regard to safety (e.g., inappropriate clothing for weather or social setting). Typically, has little insight into these changes. *Mild:* Has subtle changes in behavior or attitude, often described as a change in personality, such as less ability to recognize social cues or read facial expressions, decreased empathy, increased extraversion or introversion, decreased inhibition, or subtle or episodic apathy or restlessness.	*Recognition of emotions:* Identification of emotion in images of faces representing a variety of both positive and negative emotions. *Theory of mind:* Ability to consider another person's mental state (thoughts, desires, intentions) or experience—story cards with questions to elicit information about the mental state of the individuals portrayed, such as "Where will the girl look for the lost bag?" or "Why is the boy sad?"

Delirium

A. A disturbance in attention (i.e., reduced ability to direct, focus, sustain, and shift attention) accompanied by reduced awareness of the environment.

B. The disturbance develops over a short period of time (usually hours to a few days), represents a change from baseline attention and awareness, and tends to fluctuate in severity during the course of a day.

C. An additional disturbance in cognition (e.g., memory deficit, disorientation, language, visuospatial ability, or perception).

D. The disturbances in Criteria A and C are not better explained by another preexisting, established, or evolving neurocognitive disorder and do not occur in the context of a severely reduced level of arousal, such as coma.

E. There is evidence from the history, physical examination, or laboratory findings that the disturbance is a direct physiological consequence of another medical condition, substance intoxication or withdrawal (i.e., due to a drug of abuse or to a medication), or exposure to a toxin, or is due to multiple etiologies.

Specify if:

Acute: Lasting a few hours or days.

Persistent: Lasting weeks or months.

Specify if:

Hyperactive: The individual has a hyperactive level of psychomotor activity that may be accompanied by mood lability, agitation, and/or refusal to cooperate with medical care.

Hypoactive: The individual has a hypoactive level of psychomotor activity that may be accompanied by sluggishness and lethargy that approaches stupor.

Mixed level of activity: The individual has a normal level of psychomotor activity even though attention and awareness are disturbed. Also includes individuals whose activity level rapidly fluctuates.

Specify whether:

Substance intoxication delirium: This diagnosis should be made instead of substance intoxication when the symptoms in Criteria A and C predominate in the clinical picture and when they are sufficiently severe to warrant clinical attention.

Coding note: The ICD-10-CM codes for the [specific substance] intoxication delirium are indicated in the table below. Note that the ICD-10-CM code depends on whether or not there is a comorbid substance use disorder present for the same class of substance. If a mild substance use disorder is comorbid with the substance intoxication delirium, the 4th position character is "1," and the clinician should record "mild [substance] use disorder" before the substance intoxication delirium (e.g., "mild cocaine use disorder with cocaine intoxication delirium"). If a moderate or severe substance use disorder is comorbid with the substance intoxication delirium, the 4th position character is "2," and the clinician should record "moderate [substance] use disorder" or "severe [substance] use disorder," depending on the severity of the comorbid substance use disorder. If there is no comorbid substance use disorder (e.g., after a one-time heavy use of the substance), then the 4th position character is "9," and the clinician should record only the substance intoxication delirium.

	ICD-10-CM		
Substance intoxication delirium	With mild use disorder	With moderate or severe use disorder	Without use disorder
Alcohol	F10.121	F10.221	F10.921
Cannabis	F12.121	F12.221	F12.921
Phencyclidine	F16.121	F16.221	F16.921
Other hallucinogen	F16.121	F16.221	F16.921
Inhalant	F18.121	F18.221	F18.921
Opioid	F11.121	F11.221	F11.921
Sedative, hypnotic, or anxiolytic	F13.121	F13.221	F13.921
Amphetamine-type substance (or other stimulant)	F15.121	F15.221	F15.921
Cocaine	F14.121	F14.221	F14.921
Other (or unknown) substance	F19.121	F19.221	F19.921

Substance withdrawal delirium: This diagnosis should be made instead of substance withdrawal when the symptoms in Criteria A and C predominate in the clinical picture and when they are sufficiently severe to warrant clinical attention.

Code: The ICD-10-CM codes for the [specific substance] withdrawal delirium are indicated in the table below. Note that the ICD-10-CM code depends on whether or not there is a comorbid substance use disorder present for the same class of substance. If a mild substance use disorder is comorbid with the substance withdrawal delirium, the 4th position character is "1," and the clinician should record "mild [substance] use disorder" before the substance withdrawal delirium (e.g., "mild alcohol use disorder with alcohol withdrawal delirium"). If a moderate or severe substance use disorder is comorbid with the substance withdrawal delirium, the 4th position character is "2," and the clinician should record "moderate [substance] use disorder" or "severe [substance] use disorder," depending on the severity of the comorbid substance use disorder. If there is no comorbid substance use disorder (e.g., after regular use of an anxiolytic substance taken as prescribed), then the 4th position character is "9," and the clinician should record only the substance withdrawal delirium.

	ICD-10-CM		
Substance withdrawal delirium	With mild use disorder	With moderate or severe use disorder	Without use disorder
Alcohol	F10.131	F10.231	F10.931
Opioid	F11.188	F11.288	F11.988
Sedative, hypnotic, or anxiolytic	F13.131	F13.231	F13.931
Other (or unknown) substance	F19.131	F19.231	F19.931

Medication-induced delirium: This diagnosis applies when the symptoms in Criteria A and C arise as a side effect of a medication taken as prescribed.

Code [specific medication]-induced delirium: **F11.921** opioid taken as prescribed (or **F11.988** if during withdrawal from opioid taken as prescribed); **F12.921** pharmaceutical cannabis receptor agonist taken as prescribed; **F13.921** sedative, hypnotic, or anxiolytic taken as prescribed (or **F13.931** if during withdrawal from sedative, hypnotic, or anxiolytic taken as prescribed); **F15.921** amphetamine-type substance or other stimulant taken as prescribed; **F16.921** ketamine or other hallucinogen taken as prescribed or for medical reasons; **F19.921** for medications that do not fit into any of the classes (e.g., dexamethasone) and in cases in which a substance is judged to be an etiological factor but the specific class of substance is unknown (or **F19.931** if during withdrawal from medications that do not fit into any of the classes, taken as prescribed).

F05 Delirium due to another medical condition: There is evidence from the history, physical examination, or laboratory findings that the disturbance is attributable to the physiological consequences of another medical condition.

Coding note: Include the name of the other medical condition in the name of the delirium (e.g., F05 delirium due to hepatic encephalopathy). The other medical condition should also be coded and listed separately immediately before the delirium due to another medical condition (e.g., K72.90 hepatic encephalopathy; F05 delirium due to hepatic encephalopathy).

F05 Delirium due to multiple etiologies: There is evidence from the history, physical examination, or laboratory findings that the delirium has more than one etiology (e.g., more than one etiological medical condition; another medical condition plus substance intoxication or medication side effect).

> **Coding note:** Use multiple separate codes reflecting specific delirium etiologies (e.g., K72.90 hepatic encephalopathy; F05 delirium due to hepatic failure; F10.231 alcohol withdrawal delirium). Note that the etiological medical condition both appears as a separate code that precedes the delirium code and is substituted into the delirium due to another medical condition rubric.

Recording Procedures

Substance Intoxication Delirium

The name of the substance intoxication delirium begins with the specific substance (e.g., cocaine) that is presumed to be causing the delirium. The diagnostic code is selected from the table included in the criteria set, which is based on the drug class and presence or absence of a comorbid substance use disorder. For substances that do not fit into any of the classes (e.g., dexamethasone), the code for "other substance" should be used; and in cases in which a substance is judged to be an etiological factor but the specific class of substance is unknown, the category "unknown substance" should be used.

When recording the name of the disorder, the comorbid substance use disorder (if any) is listed first, followed by the word "with," followed by the name of the substance intoxication delirium, followed by the course (i.e., acute, persistent), followed by the specifier indicating level of psychomotor activity (i.e., hyperactive, hypoactive, mixed level of activity). For example, in the case of acute hyperactive intoxication delirium occurring in a man with a severe cocaine use disorder, the diagnosis is F14.221 severe cocaine use disorder with cocaine intoxication delirium, acute, hyperactive. A separate diagnosis of the comorbid severe cocaine use disorder is not given. If the intoxication delirium occurs without a comorbid substance use disorder (e.g., after a one-time heavy use of the substance), no accompanying substance use disorder is noted (e.g., F16.921 phencyclidine intoxication delirium, acute, hypoactive).

Substance Withdrawal Delirium

The name of the substance withdrawal delirium begins with the specific substance (e.g., alcohol) that is presumed to be causing the withdrawal delirium. The diagnostic code is selected from substance-specific codes in the coding note included in the criteria set. When recording the name of the disorder, the comorbid substance use disorder (if any) is listed first, followed by the word "with," followed by the substance withdrawal delirium, followed by the course (i.e., acute, persistent), followed by the specifier indicating level of psychomotor activity (i.e., hyperactive, hypoactive, mixed level of activity). For example, in the case of acute hyperactive withdrawal delirium occurring in a man with a severe alcohol use disorder, the diagnosis is F10.231 severe alcohol use disorder with alcohol withdrawal delirium, acute, hyperactive. A separate diagnosis of the comorbid severe alcohol use disorder is not given.

Medication-Induced Delirium

The name of the medication-induced delirium begins with the specific substance (e.g., dexamethasone) that is presumed to be causing the delirium. The name of the disorder is followed by the course (i.e., acute, persistent), followed by the specifier indicating level of psychomotor activity (i.e., hyperactive, hypoactive, mixed level of activity). For example, in the case of acute hyperactive medication-induced delirium occurring in a man using dexamethasone as prescribed, the diagnosis is F19.921 dexamethasone-induced delirium, acute, hyperactive.

Other Specified Delirium

R41.0

This category applies to presentations in which symptoms characteristic of delirium that cause clinically significant distress or impairment in social, occupational, or other important areas of functioning predominate but do not meet the full criteria for delirium or any of the disorders in the neurocognitive disorders diagnostic class. The other specified delirium category is used in situations in which the clinician chooses to communicate the specific reason that the presentation does not meet the criteria for delirium or any specific neurocognitive disorder. This is done by recording "other specified delirium" followed by the specific reason (e.g., "subsyndromal delirium").

An example of a presentation that can be specified using the "other specified" designation is the following:

Subsyndromal delirium: A delirium-like presentation involving disturbances in attention, higher-level thought, and circadian rhythm, in which the severity of cognitive impairment falls short of that required for the diagnosis of delirium.

Unspecified Delirium

R41.0

This category applies to presentations in which symptoms characteristic of delirium that cause clinically significant distress or impairment in social, occupational, or other important areas of functioning predominate but do not meet the full criteria for delirium or any of the disorders in the neurocognitive disorders diagnostic class. The unspecified delirium category is used in situations in which the clinician chooses *not* to specify the reason that the criteria are not met for delirium, and includes presentations for which there is insufficient information to make a more specific diagnosis (e.g., in emergency room settings).

Major and Mild Neurocognitive Disorders

Major Neurocognitive Disorder

A. Evidence of significant cognitive decline from a previous level of performance in one or more cognitive domains (complex attention, executive function, learning and memory, language, perceptual-motor, or social cognition) based on:

1. Concern of the individual, a knowledgeable informant, or the clinician that there has been a significant decline in cognitive function; and

2. . A substantial impairment in cognitive performance, preferably documented by standardized neuropsychological testing or, in its absence, another quantified clinical assessment.

B. The cognitive deficits interfere with independence in everyday activities (i.e., at a minimum, requiring assistance with complex instrumental activities of daily living such as paying bills or managing medications).

C. The cognitive deficits do not occur exclusively in the context of a delirium.

D. The cognitive deficits are not better explained by another mental disorder (e.g., major depressive disorder, schizophrenia).

Specify whether due to:
  Note: Each subtype listed has specific diagnostic criteria and corresponding text, which follow the general discussion of major and mild neurocognitive disorders.
  Alzheimer's disease
  Frontotemporal degeneration
  Lewy body disease
  Vascular disease
  Traumatic brain injury
  Substance/medication use
  HIV infection
  Prion disease
  Parkinson's disease
  Huntington's disease
  Another medical condition
  Multiple etiologies
  Unspecified etiology

Coding note: Code based on medical or substance etiology. In most cases of major neurocognitive disorder, there is need for an additional code for the etiological medical condition, which must immediately precede the diagnostic code for major neurocognitive disorder, as noted in coding table on pp. 251–253.

Specify (see coding table for details):

Without behavioral disturbance: If the cognitive disturbance is not accompanied by any clinically significant behavioral disturbance.

With behavioral disturbance *(specify disturbance):* If the cognitive disturbance is accompanied by a clinically significant behavioral disturbance (e.g., psychotic symptoms, mood disturbance, agitation, apathy, or other behavioral symptoms).

Coding note: Use additional code(s) to indicate clinically significant psychiatric symptoms due to the same medical condition causing the major neurocognitive disorder (e.g., **F06.2** psychotic disorder due to Alzheimer's disease, with delusions; **F06.32** depressive disorder due to Parkinson's disease, with major depressive–like episode). **Note:** Mental disorders due to another medical condition are included with disorders with which they share phenomenology (e.g., for depressive disorders due to another medical condition, see the chapter "Depressive Disorders").

Specify current severity:

Mild: Difficulties with instrumental activities of daily living (e.g., housework, managing money).

Moderate: Difficulties with basic activities of daily living (e.g., feeding, dressing).

Severe: Fully dependent.

Coding and Recording Procedures

The following are examples of coding and recording major neurocognitive disorders due to an etiological subtype (*for more information, see coding table on pp. 251–253 and coding notes in the specific diagnostic criteria for each major and mild neurocognitive disorder subtype*):

Major neurocognitive disorder due to probable Alzheimer's disease, without behavioral disturbance, mild: G30.9 Alzheimer's disease, F02.80 major neurocognitive disorder due to probable Alzheimer's disease, without behavioral disturbance, mild.

Major neurocognitive disorder due to traumatic brain injury, with behavioral disturbance, moderate: S06.2X9S diffuse traumatic brain injury with loss of consciousness of unspecified duration, sequela; F02.81 major neurocognitive disorder due to traumatic brain injury, with behavioral disturbance, moderate; F06.34 bipolar and related disorder due to traumatic brain injury, with mixed features.

Mild Neurocognitive Disorder

A. Evidence of modest cognitive decline from a previous level of performance in one or more cognitive domains (complex attention, executive function, learning and memory, language, perceptual-motor, or social cognition) based on:

1. Concern of the individual, a knowledgeable informant, or the clinician that there has been a mild decline in cognitive function; and

2. A modest impairment in cognitive performance, preferably documented by standardized neuropsychological testing or, in its absence, another quantified clinical assessment.

B. The cognitive deficits do not interfere with capacity for independence in everyday activities (i.e., complex instrumental activities of daily living such as paying bills or managing medications are preserved, but greater effort, compensatory strategies, or accommodation may be required).

C. The cognitive deficits do not occur exclusively in the context of a delirium.

D. The cognitive deficits are not better explained by another mental disorder (e.g., major depressive disorder, schizophrenia).

Specify whether due to:
Note: Each subtype listed has specific diagnostic criteria and corresponding text, which follow the general discussion of major and mild neurocognitive disorders.

Alzheimer's disease
Frontotemporal degeneration
Lewy body disease
Vascular disease
Traumatic brain injury
Substance/medication use
HIV infection
Prion disease
Parkinson's disease
Huntington's disease
Another medical condition
Multiple etiologies
Unspecified etiology

Coding note: For mild neurocognitive disorder due to any of the medical etiologies listed above, code **G31.84.** Do *not* use additional codes for the presumed etiological medical conditions. For substance/medication-induced mild neurocognitive disorder, code based on type of substance; see "Substance/Medication-Induced Major or Mild Neurocognitive Disorder." For unspecified mild neurocognitive disorder, code **R41.9.**

Specify (behavioral disturbance cannot be coded but should still be recorded):

Without behavioral disturbance: If the cognitive disturbance is not accompanied by any clinically significant behavioral disturbance.

With behavioral disturbance *(specify disturbance):* If the cognitive disturbance is accompanied by a clinically significant behavioral disturbance (e.g., psychotic symptoms, mood disturbance, agitation, apathy, or other behavioral symptoms).

Coding note: Use additional code(s) to indicate clinically significant psychiatric symptoms due to the same medical condition causing the mild neurocognitive disorder (e.g., **F06.2** psychotic disorder due to traumatic brain injury, with delusions; or **F06.32** depressive disorder due to HIV disease, with major depressive–like episode). **Note:** Mental disorders due to another medical condition are included with disorders with which they share phenomenology (e.g., for depressive disorders due to another medical condition, see the chapter "Depressive Disorders").

Coding and Recording Procedures

The following are examples of coding and recording mild neurocognitive disorders due to an etiological subtype (*for more information, see coding table on pp. 251–253 and coding notes in the specific diagnostic criteria for each major and mild neurocognitive disorder subtype*):

G31.84 Mild neurocognitive disorder due to Alzheimer's disease, without behavioral disturbance.

G31.84 Mild neurocognitive disorder due to traumatic brain injury, with behavioral disturbance; F06.34 bipolar and related disorder due to traumatic brain injury, with mixed features.

Etiological subtype	Associated etiological medical code for major neurocognitive disorder[a]	Major neurocognitive disorder code	Mild neurocognitive disorder code
Alzheimer's disease	G30.9	F02.8x[b]	G31.84[c] Do not use additional code for Alzheimer's disease.
Frontotemporal degeneration	G31.09	F02.8x[b]	G31.84[c] Do not use additional code for frontotemporal degeneration.
Lewy body disease	G31.83	F02.8x[b]	G31.84[c] Do not use additional code for Lewy body disease.
Vascular disease	No additional medical code.	F01.5x[b] Do not use additional code for the vascular disease.	G31.84[c] Do not use additional code for the vascular disease.
Traumatic brain injury	S06.2X9S	F02.8x[b]	G31.84[c] Do not use additional code for the traumatic brain injury.
Substance/medication-induced	No additional medical code.	Code based on the type of substance causing the major neurocognitive disorder.[d]	Code based on the type of substance causing the mild neurocognitive disorder.[d]

Etiological subtype	Associated etiological medical code for major neurocognitive disorder[a]	Major neurocognitive disorder code	Mild neurocognitive disorder code
HIV infection	B20	F02.8x[b]	G31.84[c] Do not use additional code for HIV infection.
Prion disease	A81.9	F02.8x[b]	G31.84[c] Do not use additional code for prion disease.
Parkinson's disease	G20	F02.8x[b]	G31.84[c] Do not use additional code for Parkinson's disease.
Huntington's disease	G10	F02.8x[b]	G31.84[c] Do not use additional code for Huntington's disease.
Due to another medical condition	Code the other medical condition first (e.g., G35 multiple sclerosis).	F02.8x[b]	G31.84[c] Do not use additional codes for the presumed etiological medical conditions.

Etiological subtype	Associated etiological medical code for major neurocognitive disorder[a]	Major neurocognitive disorder code	Mild neurocognitive disorder code
Due to multiple etiologies	Code all of the etiological medical conditions first (with the exception of vascular disease).	F02.8x[b] (code once for major neurocognitive disorder due to all etiologies that apply) Code also major vascular NCD (F01.5x), if present. Code also the relevant substance/medication-induced major neurocognitive disorders if substances or medications play a role in the etiology.	G31.84[c] Do not use additional codes for the presumed etiological medical conditions. Code also the relevant substance/medication-induced mild neurocognitive disorders if substances or medications play a role in the etiology.
Unspecified neurocognitive disorder	No additional medical code.	R41.9[c]	R41.9[c]

[a]Code first, before code for major neurocognitive disorder.

[b]Code fifth character based on symptom specifier: .x0 without behavioral disturbance; .x1 with behavioral disturbance (e.g., psychotic symptoms, mood disturbance, agitation, apathy, or other behavioral symptoms). **Note:** The severity specifiers "mild," "moderate," and "severe" cannot be coded for major neurocognitive disorder but should still be recorded.

[c]**Note:** "With behavioral disturbance" and "without behavioral disturbance" cannot be coded but should still be recorded.

[d]See coding table in "Substance/Medication-Induced Major or Mild Neurocognitive Disorder" for ICD-10-CM code. **Note:** The severity specifiers "mild," "moderate," and "severe" (for substance/medication-induced major neurocognitive disorder) and the accompanying symptom specifiers "with behavioral disturbance" and "without behavioral disturbance" (for substance/medication-induced major or mild neurocognitive disorder) cannot be coded but should still be recorded.

Major or Mild Neurocognitive Disorder
Due to Alzheimer's Disease

A. The criteria are met for major or mild neurocognitive disorder.
B. There is insidious onset and gradual progression of impairment in one or more cognitive domains (for major neurocognitive disorder, at least two domains must be impaired).
C. Criteria are met for either probable or possible Alzheimer's disease as follows:

For major neurocognitive disorder:

Probable Alzheimer's disease is diagnosed if either of the following is present; otherwise, **possible Alzheimer's disease** should be diagnosed.

1. Evidence of a causative Alzheimer's disease genetic mutation from family history or genetic testing.
2. All three of the following are present:
   a. Clear evidence of decline in memory and learning and at least one other cognitive domain (based on detailed history or serial neuropsychological testing).
   b. Steadily progressive, gradual decline in cognition, without extended plateaus.
   c. No evidence of mixed etiology (i.e., absence of other neurodegenerative or cerebrovascular disease, or another neurological, mental, or systemic disease or condition likely contributing to cognitive decline).

For mild neurocognitive disorder:

Probable Alzheimer's disease is diagnosed if there is evidence of a causative Alzheimer's disease genetic mutation from either genetic testing or family history.

Possible Alzheimer's disease is diagnosed if there is no evidence of a causative Alzheimer's disease genetic mutation from either genetic testing or family history, and all three of the following are present:

1. Clear evidence of decline in memory and learning.
2. Steadily progressive, gradual decline in cognition, without extended plateaus.
3. No evidence of mixed etiology (i.e., absence of other neurodegenerative or cerebrovascular disease, or another neurological or systemic disease or condition likely contributing to cognitive decline).

D. The disturbance is not better explained by cerebrovascular disease, another neurodegenerative disease, the effects of a substance, or another mental, neurological, or systemic disorder.

Coding note (see coding table on pp. 251–253):

For major neurocognitive disorder due to probable or possible Alzheimer's disease, with behavioral disturbance, code first **G30.9** Alzheimer's disease, followed by **F02.81**.

For major neurocognitive disorder due to probable or possible Alzheimer's disease, without behavioral disturbance, code first **G30.9** Alzheimer's disease, followed by **F02.80**.

Note: The severity specifiers "mild," "moderate," and "severe" cannot be coded for major neurocognitive disorder but should still be recorded.

For mild neurocognitive disorder due to Alzheimer's disease, code **G31.84**. (**Note:** Do *not* use the additional code for Alzheimer's disease. "With behavioral disturbance" and "without behavioral disturbance" cannot be coded but should still be recorded.)

For major or mild neurocognitive disorder due to Alzheimer's disease: Use additional code(s) to indicate clinically significant psychiatric symptoms due to Alzheimer's disease (e.g., **F06.2** psychotic disorder due to Alzheimer's disease, with delusions; **F06.32** depressive disorder due to Alzheimer's disease, with major depressive–like episode).

Major or Mild Frontotemporal Neurocognitive Disorder

A. The criteria are met for major or mild neurocognitive disorder.

B. The disturbance has insidious onset and gradual progression.

C. Either (1) or (2):

   1. Behavioral variant:

       a. Three or more of the following behavioral symptoms:

           i.   Behavioral disinhibition.
           ii. Apathy or inertia.
           iii. Loss of sympathy or empathy.
           iv. Perseverative, stereotyped or compulsive/ritualistic behavior.
           v.   Hyperorality and dietary changes.

       b. Prominent decline in social cognition and/or executive abilities.

   2. Language variant:

       a. Prominent decline in language ability, in the form of speech production, word finding, object naming, grammar, or word comprehension.

D. Relative sparing of learning and memory and perceptual-motor function.

E. The disturbance is not better explained by cerebrovascular disease, another neurodegenerative disease, the effects of a substance, or another mental, neurological, or systemic disorder.

Probable frontotemporal neurocognitive disorder is diagnosed if either of the following is present; otherwise, **possible frontotemporal neurocognitive disorder** should be diagnosed:

1. Evidence of a causative frontotemporal neurocognitive disorder genetic mutation, from either family history or genetic testing.
2. Evidence of disproportionate frontal and/or temporal lobe involvement from neuroimaging.

Possible frontotemporal neurocognitive disorder is diagnosed if there is no evidence of a genetic mutation, and neuroimaging has not been performed.

Coding note (see coding table on pp. 251–253):

For major neurocognitive disorder due to probable or possible frontotemporal degeneration, with behavioral disturbance, code first **G31.09** frontotemporal degeneration, followed by **F02.81**.

For major neurocognitive disorder due to probable or possible frontotemporal degeneration, without behavioral disturbance, code first **G31.09** frontotemporal degeneration, followed by **F02.80**.

Note: The severity specifiers "mild," "moderate," and "severe" cannot be coded for major neurocognitive disorder but should still be recorded.

For mild neurocognitive disorder due to frontotemporal degeneration, code **G31.84**. (**Note:** Do *not* use the additional code for frontotemporal degeneration. "With behavioral disturbance" and "without behavioral disturbance" cannot be coded but should still be recorded.)

For major or mild frontotemporal neurocognitive disorder: Use additional code(s) to indicate clinically significant psychiatric symptoms due to frontotemporal degeneration (e.g., **F06.33** bipolar and related disorder due to frontotemporal degeneration, with manic features; **F07.0** personality change due to frontotemporal degeneration, disinhibited type).

Major or Mild Neurocognitive Disorder With Lewy Bodies

A. The criteria are met for major or mild neurocognitive disorder.
B. The disorder has an insidious onset and gradual progression.
C. The disorder meets a combination of core diagnostic features and suggestive diagnostic features for either probable or possible neurocognitive disorder with Lewy bodies.

   For probable major or mild neurocognitive disorder with Lewy bodies, the individual has two core features, or one suggestive feature with one or more core features. For **possible major or mild neurocognitive disorder with Lewy bodies,** the individual has only one core feature, or one or more suggestive features.

1. Core diagnostic features:

    a. Fluctuating cognition with pronounced variations in attention and alertness.

    b. Recurrent visual hallucinations that are well formed and detailed.

    c. Spontaneous features of parkinsonism, with onset subsequent to the development of cognitive decline.

2. Suggestive diagnostic features:

    a. Meets criteria for rapid eye movement sleep behavior disorder.

    b. Severe neuroleptic sensitivity.

D. The disturbance is not better explained by cerebrovascular disease, another neurodegenerative disease, the effects of a substance, or another mental, neurological, or systemic disorder.

Coding note (see coding table on pp. 251–253):

For major neurocognitive disorder with probable or possible Lewy bodies, with behavioral disturbance, code first **G31.83** Lewy body disease, followed by **F02.81**.

For major neurocognitive disorder with probable or possible Lewy bodies, without behavioral disturbance, code first **G31.83** Lewy body disease, followed by **F02.80**.

Note: The severity specifiers "mild," "moderate," and "severe" cannot be coded for major neurocognitive disorder but should still be recorded.

For mild neurocognitive disorder with Lewy bodies, code **G31.84**. (**Note:** Do *not* use the additional code for Lewy body disease. "With behavioral disturbance" and "without behavioral disturbance" cannot be coded but should still be recorded.)

For major or mild neurocognitive disorder with Lewy bodies: Use additional code(s) to indicate clinically significant psychiatric symptoms due to Lewy body disease (e.g., **F06.0** psychotic disorder due to Lewy body disease, with hallucinations; **F06.31** depressive disorder due to Lewy body disease, with depressive features).

Major or Mild Vascular Neurocognitive Disorder

A. The criteria are met for major or mild neurocognitive disorder.

B. The clinical features are consistent with a vascular etiology, as suggested by either of the following:

1. Onset of the cognitive deficits is temporally related to one or more cerebrovascular events.

2. Evidence for decline is prominent in complex attention (including processing speed) and frontal-executive function.

C. There is evidence of the presence of cerebrovascular disease from history, physical examination, and/or neuroimaging considered sufficient to account for the neurocognitive deficits.

D. The symptoms are not better explained by another brain disease or systemic disorder.

Probable vascular neurocognitive disorder is diagnosed if one of the following is present; otherwise **possible vascular neurocognitive disorder** should be diagnosed:

1. Clinical criteria are supported by neuroimaging evidence of significant parenchymal injury attributed to cerebrovascular disease (neuroimaging-supported).
2. The neurocognitive syndrome is temporally related to one or more documented cerebrovascular events.
3. Both clinical and genetic (e.g., cerebral autosomal dominant arteriopathy with subcortical infarcts and leukoencephalopathy) evidence of cerebrovascular disease is present.

Possible vascular neurocognitive disorder is diagnosed if the clinical criteria are met but neuroimaging is not available and the temporal relationship of the neurocognitive syndrome with one or more cerebrovascular events is not established.

Coding note (see coding table on pp. 251–253):
For major neurocognitive disorder probably or possibly due to vascular disease, with behavioral disturbance, code **F01.51**.
For major neurocognitive disorder probably or possibly due to vascular disease, without behavioral disturbance, code **F01.50**.
An additional medical code for the vascular disease is not used.
Note: The severity specifiers "mild," "moderate," and "severe" cannot be coded for major neurocognitive disorder but should still be recorded.

For mild vascular neurocognitive disorder, code **G31.84**. (*Note:* Do *not* use an additional code for the vascular disease. "With behavioral disturbance" and "without behavioral disturbance" cannot be coded but should still be recorded.)
For major or mild vascular neurocognitive disorder: Use additional code(s) to indicate clinically significant psychiatric symptoms due to cerebrovascular disease (e.g., **F06.31** depressive disorder due to the cerebrovascular disease, with depressive features).

Major or Mild Neurocognitive Disorder Due to Traumatic Brain Injury

A. The criteria are met for major or mild neurocognitive disorder.
B. There is evidence of a traumatic brain injury—that is, an impact to the head or other mechanisms of rapid movement or displacement of the brain within the skull, with one or more of the following:

1. Loss of consciousness.
2. Posttraumatic amnesia.
3. Disorientation and confusion.
4. Neurological signs (e.g., neuroimaging demonstrating injury; visual field cuts; anosmia; hemiparesis; hemisensory loss;

cortical blindness; aphasia; apraxia; weakness; loss of balance; other sensory loss that cannot be accounted for by peripheral or other causes).

C. The neurocognitive disorder presents immediately after the occurrence of the traumatic brain injury or immediately after recovery of consciousness and persists past the acute post-injury period.

Coding note (see coding table on pp. 251–253):

For major neurocognitive disorder due to traumatic brain injury, with behavioral disturbance: code first **S06.2X9S** diffuse traumatic brain injury with loss of consciousness of unspecified duration, sequela; followed by **F02.81** major neurocognitive disorder due to traumatic brain injury, with behavioral disturbance.

For major neurocognitive disorder due to traumatic brain injury, without behavioral disturbance: code first **S06.2X9S** diffuse traumatic brain injury with loss of consciousness of unspecified duration, sequela; followed by **F02.80** major neurocognitive disorder due to traumatic brain injury, without behavioral disturbance.

Note: The severity specifiers "mild," "moderate," and "severe" cannot be coded for major neurocognitive disorder but should still be recorded.

For mild neurocognitive disorder due to traumatic brain injury, code **G31.84**. (*Note:* Do *not* use the additional code for traumatic brain injury. "With behavioral disturbance" and "without behavioral disturbance" cannot be coded but should still be recorded.)

For major or mild neurocognitive disorder due to traumatic brain injury: Use additional code(s) to indicate clinically significant psychiatric symptoms due to the traumatic brain injury (e.g., **F06.34** bipolar and related disorder due to traumatic brain injury, with mixed features; **F07.0** personality change due to traumatic brain injury, apathetic type).

Substance/Medication-Induced Major or Mild Neurocognitive Disorder

A. The criteria are met for major or mild neurocognitive disorder.
B. The neurocognitive impairments do not occur exclusively during the course of a delirium and persist beyond the usual duration of intoxication and acute withdrawal.
C. The involved substance or medication and duration and extent of use are capable of producing the neurocognitive impairment.
D. The temporal course of the neurocognitive deficits is consistent with the timing of substance or medication use and abstinence (e.g., the deficits remain stable or improve after a period of abstinence).
E. The neurocognitive disorder is not attributable to another medical condition or is not better explained by another mental disorder.

Coding note (see also coding table on pp. 251–253): The ICD-10-CM codes for the [specific substance/medication]-induced neurocognitive disorders are indicated in the table below. Note that the ICD-10-CM code depends on whether or not there is a comorbid substance use disorder present for the same class of substance. In any case, an additional separate diagnosis of a substance use disorder is not given.

Substance-induced major neurocognitive disorder: If a mild substance use disorder is comorbid with the substance-induced major neurocognitive disorder, the 4th position character is "1," and the clinician should record "mild [substance] use disorder" before the substance-induced major neurocognitive disorder (e.g., "mild inhalant use disorder with inhalant-induced major neurocognitive disorder"). For alcohol and sedative, hypnotic, or anxiolytic substances, a mild substance use disorder is insufficient to cause a substance-induced major neurocognitive disorder; thus, there are no available ICD-10-CM codes for this combination. If a moderate or severe substance use disorder is comorbid with the substance-induced major neurocognitive disorder, the 4th position character is "2," and the clinician should record "moderate [substance] use disorder" or "severe [substance] use disorder," depending on the severity of the comorbid substance use disorder. If there is no comorbid substance use disorder, then the 4th position character is "9," and the clinician should record only the substance-induced major neurocognitive disorder.

Substance-induced mild neurocognitive disorder: If a mild substance use disorder is comorbid with the substance-induced mild neurocognitive disorder, the 4th position character is "1," and the clinician should record "mild [substance] use disorder" before the substance-induced mild neurocognitive disorder (e.g., "mild cocaine use disorder with cocaine-induced mild neurocognitive disorder"). If a moderate or severe substance use disorder is comorbid with the substance-induced mild neurocognitive disorder, the 4th position character is "2," and the clinician should record "moderate [substance] use disorder" or "severe [substance] use disorder," depending on the severity of the comorbid substance use disorder. If there is no comorbid substance use disorder, then the 4th position character is "9," and the clinician should record only the substance-induced mild neurocognitive disorder.

The severity specifiers "mild," "moderate," and "severe" (for major neurocognitive disorder) and the accompanying symptom specifiers "with behavioral disturbance" and "without behavioral disturbance" (for major or mild neurocognitive disorder) cannot be coded but should still be recorded.

	ICD-10-CM		
	With mild use disorder	With moderate or severe use disorder	Without use disorder
Substance-induced major neurocognitive disorder (NCD)			
Alcohol (major NCD), nonamnestic-confabulatory type	NA	F10.27	F10.97

	ICD-10-CM		
	With mild use disorder	With moderate or severe use disorder	Without use disorder
Alcohol (major NCD), amnestic-confabulatory type	NA	F10.26	F10.96
Inhalant (major NCD)	F18.17	F18.27	F18.97
Sedative, hypnotic, or anxiolytic (major NCD)	NA	F13.27	F13.97
Other (or unknown) substance (major NCD)	F19.17	F19.27	F19.97
Substance-induced mild neurocognitive disorder (NCD)			
Alcohol (mild NCD)	F10.188	F10.288	F10.988
Inhalant (mild NCD)	F18.188	F18.288	F18.988
Sedative, hypnotic, or anxiolytic (mild NCD)	F13.188	F13.288	F13.988
Amphetamine-type substance or other stimulant (mild NCD)	F15.188	F15.288	F15.988
Cocaine (mild NCD)	F14.188	F14.288	F14.988
Other (or unknown) substance (mild NCD)	F19.188	F19.288	F19.988

Specify if:

Persistent: Neurocognitive impairment continues to be significant after an extended period of abstinence.

Recording Procedures

The name of the substance/medication-induced neurocognitive disorder begins with the specific substance (e.g., alcohol) that is presumed to be causing the neurocognitive symptoms. The ICD-10-CM code that corresponds to the applicable drug class is selected from the table included in the criteria set. For substances that do not fit into any of the classes (e.g., intrathecal methotrexate), the ICD-10-CM code for the other (or unknown) substance class should be used and the name of the specific substance recorded (e.g., F19.988 intrathecal methotrexate-induced mild neurocognitive disorder). In cases in which a substance is judged to be an etiological factor but the specific substance is unknown, the ICD-10-CM code for the other (or unknown) substance class is used, and the fact that the substance is unknown is recorded (e.g., F19.97 unknown substance-induced major neurocognitive disorder).

When recording the name of the disorder, the comorbid substance use disorder (if any) is listed first, followed by the word "with," followed by the name of the disorder (i.e., [specific substance]–induced major neurocognitive disorder or [specific substance]–induced mild neurocognitive disorder), followed by the type in the case of alcohol (i.e., nonamnestic-confabulatory type, amnestic-confabulatory type), followed by specification of duration (i.e., persistent). For example, in the case of persistent amnestic-confabulatory symptoms in a man with a severe alcohol use disorder, the diagnosis is F10.26 severe alcohol use disorder with alcohol-induced major neurocognitive disorder, amnestic-confabulatory type, persistent. A separate diagnosis of the comorbid severe alcohol use disorder is not given. If the substance-induced neurocognitive disorder occurs without a comorbid substance use disorder (e.g., after a sporadic heavy use of inhalants), no accompanying substance use disorder is noted (e.g., F18.988 [specific inhalant]–induced mild neurocognitive disorder).

Major or Mild Neurocognitive Disorder Due to HIV Infection

A. The criteria are met for major or mild neurocognitive disorder.
B. There is documented infection with human immunodeficiency virus (HIV).
C. The neurocognitive disorder is not better explained by non-HIV conditions, including secondary brain diseases such as progressive multifocal leukoencephalopathy or cryptococcal meningitis.
D. The neurocognitive disorder is not attributable to another medical condition and is not better explained by a mental disorder.

Coding note (see coding table on pp. 251–253):

For major neurocognitive disorder due to HIV infection, with behavioral disturbance, code first **B20** HIV infection, followed by **F02.81** major neurocognitive disorder due to HIV infection, with behavioral disturbance.

For major neurocognitive disorder due to HIV infection, without behavioral disturbance, code first **B20** HIV infection, followed by **F02.80** major neurocognitive disorder due to HIV infection, without behavioral disturbance.

Note: The severity specifiers "mild," "moderate," and "severe" cannot be coded for major neurocognitive disorder but should still be recorded.

For mild neurocognitive disorder due to HIV infection, code **G31.84**. (**Note:** Do *not* use the additional code for HIV infection. "With behavioral disturbance" and "without behavioral disturbance" cannot be coded but should still be recorded.)

For major or mild neurocognitive disorder due to HIV infection: Use additional code(s) to indicate clinically significant psychiatric symptoms due to HIV infection (e.g., **F06.34** bipolar and related disorder due to HIV infection, with mixed features; **F07.0** personality change due to traumatic brain injury, apathetic type).

Major or Mild Neurocognitive Disorder Due to Prion Disease

A. The criteria are met for major or mild neurocognitive disorder.
B. There is insidious onset, and rapid progression of impairment is common.
C. There are motor features of prion disease, such as myoclonus or ataxia, or biomarker evidence.
D. The neurocognitive disorder is not attributable to another medical condition and is not better explained by another mental disorder.

Coding note (see coding table on pp. 251–253):

For major neurocognitive disorder due to prion disease, with behavioral disturbance, code first **A81.9** prion disease, followed by **F02.81** major neurocognitive disorder due to prion disease, with behavioral disturbance.

For major neurocognitive disorder due to prion disease, without behavioral disturbance, code first **A81.9** prion disease, followed by **F02.80** major neurocognitive disorder due to prion disease, without behavioral disturbance.

Note: The severity specifiers "mild," "moderate," and "severe" cannot be coded for major neurocognitive disorder but should still be recorded.

For mild neurocognitive disorder due to prion disease, code **G31.84**. (**Note:** Do *not* use the additional code for prion disease. "With behavioral disturbance" and "without behavioral disturbance" cannot be coded but should still be recorded.)

For major or mild neurocognitive disorder due to prion disease: Use additional code(s) to indicate clinically significant psychiatric symptoms due to prion disease (e.g., **F06.2** psychotic disorder due to prion disease, with delusions; **F06.32** depressive disorder due to prion disease with major depressive–like episode).

Major or Mild Neurocognitive Disorder Due to Parkinson's Disease

A. The criteria are met for major or mild neurocognitive disorder.
B. The disturbance occurs in the setting of established Parkinson's disease.
C. There is insidious onset and gradual progression of impairment.
D. The neurocognitive disorder is not attributable to another medical condition and is not better explained by another mental disorder.

Major or mild neurocognitive disorder probably due to Parkinson's disease should be diagnosed if 1 and 2 are both met. **Major or mild neurocognitive disorder possibly due to Parkinson's disease** should be diagnosed if 1 or 2 is met:

1. There is no evidence of mixed etiology (i.e., absence of other neurodegenerative or cerebrovascular disease or another neurological, mental, or systemic disease or condition likely contributing to cognitive decline).
2. The Parkinson's disease clearly precedes the onset of the neurocognitive disorder.

Coding note (see coding table on pp. 251–253):

For major neurocognitive disorder probably or possibly due to Parkinson's disease, with behavioral disturbance, code first **G20** Parkinson's disease, followed by **F02.81**.

For major neurocognitive disorder probably or possibly due to Parkinson's disease, without behavioral disturbance, code first **G20** Parkinson's disease, followed by **F02.80**.

Note: The severity specifiers "mild," "moderate," and "severe" cannot be coded for major neurocognitive disorder but should still be recorded.

For mild neurocognitive disorder due to Parkinson's disease, code **G31.84.** (**Note:** Do *not* use the additional code for Parkinson's disease. "With behavioral disturbance" and "without behavioral disturbance" cannot be coded but should still be recorded.)

For major or mild neurocognitive disorder due to Parkinson's disease: Use additional code(s) to indicate clinically significant psychiatric symptoms due to Parkinson's disease (e.g., **F06.0** psychotic disorder due to Parkinson's disease, with hallucinations; **F06.31** depressive disorder due to Parkinson's disease, with depressive features; **F07.0** personality change due to traumatic brain injury, apathetic type).

Major or Mild Neurocognitive Disorder Due to Huntington's Disease

A. The criteria are met for major or mild neurocognitive disorder.
B. There is insidious onset and gradual progression.
C. There is clinically established Huntington's disease, or risk for Huntington's disease based on family history or genetic testing.
D. The neurocognitive disorder is not attributable to another medical condition and is not better explained by another mental disorder.

Coding note (see coding table on pp. 251–253):

For major neurocognitive disorder due to Huntington's disease, with behavioral disturbance, code first **G10** Huntington's disease, followed by **F02.81** major neurocognitive disorder due to Huntington's disease, with behavioral disturbance.

For major neurocognitive disorder due to Huntington's disease, without behavioral disturbance, code first **G10** Huntington's disease, followed by **F02.80** major neurocognitive disorder due to Huntington's disease, without behavioral disturbance.

Note: The severity specifiers "mild," "moderate," and "severe" cannot be coded for major neurocognitive disorder but should still be recorded.

For mild neurocognitive disorder due to Huntington's disease, code **G31.84**. (**Note:** Do *not* use the additional code for Huntington's disease. "With behavioral disturbance" and "without behavioral disturbance" cannot be coded but should still be recorded.)

For major or mild neurocognitive disorder due to Huntington's disease: Use additional code(s) to indicate clinically significant psychiatric symptoms due to Huntington's disease (e.g., **F06.31** depressive disorder due to Huntington's disease, with depressive features; **F06.4** anxiety disorder due to Huntington's disease).

Major or Mild Neurocognitive Disorder Due to Another Medical Condition

A. The criteria are met for major or mild neurocognitive disorder.
B. There is evidence from the history, physical examination, or laboratory findings that the neurocognitive disorder is the pathophysiological consequence of another medical condition (e.g., multiple sclerosis).
C. The cognitive deficits are not better explained by another mental disorder (e.g., major depressive disorder) or another specific neurocognitive disorder (e.g., major neurocognitive disorder due to Alzheimer's disease).

Coding note (see coding table on pp. 251–253):

For major neurocognitive disorder due to another medical condition, with behavioral disturbance, code first the other medical condition, followed by the major neurocognitive disorder due to another medical condition, with behavioral disturbance (e.g., **G35** multiple sclerosis, **F02.81** major neurocognitive disorder due to multiple sclerosis, with behavioral disturbance).

For major neurocognitive disorder due to another medical condition, without behavioral disturbance, code first the other medical condition, followed by the major neurocognitive disorder due to another medical condition, without behavioral disturbance (e.g., **G35** multiple sclerosis, **F02.80** major neurocognitive disorder due to multiple sclerosis, without behavioral disturbance).

Note: The severity specifiers "mild," "moderate," and "severe" cannot be coded for major neurocognitive disorder but should still be recorded.

For mild neurocognitive disorder due to another medical condition, code **G31.84**. (**Note:** Do *not* use the additional code for the other medical condition. "With behavioral disturbance" and "without behavioral disturbance" cannot be coded but should still be recorded.)

For major or mild neurocognitive disorder due to another medical condition: Use additional code(s) to indicate clinically significant psychiatric symptoms due to another medical condition (e.g., **F06.32** depressive disorder due to multiple sclerosis with major depressive–like episode).

Major or Mild Neurocognitive Disorder Due to Multiple Etiologies

A. The criteria are met for major or mild neurocognitive disorder.
B. There is evidence from the history, physical examination, or laboratory findings that the neurocognitive disorder is the pathophysiological consequence of more than one etiological process, excluding substances (e.g., neurocognitive disorder due to Alzheimer's disease with subsequent development of vascular neurocognitive disorder).

   Note: Refer to the diagnostic criteria for the various neurocognitive disorders due to specific medical conditions for guidance on establishing the particular etiologies.

C. The cognitive deficits are not better explained by another mental disorder and do not occur exclusively during the course of a delirium.

Coding note (see coding table on pp. 251–253):

For major neurocognitive disorder due to multiple etiologies, code first all of the etiological medical conditions (with the exception of vascular disease, which is not coded), followed by either **F02.81** for major neurocognitive disorder due to multiple etiologies, with behavioral disturbance; or **F02.80** for major neurocognitive disorder due to multiple etiologies, without behavioral disturbance.

If vascular disease is among the multiple etiological medical conditions, code next either **F01.51** for major vascular neurocognitive disorder, with behavioral disturbance; or **F01.50** for major vascular neurocognitive disorder, without behavioral disturbance.

Note: The severity specifiers "mild," "moderate," and "severe" cannot be coded for major neurocognitive disorder but should still be recorded.

For example, for a presentation of major neurocognitive disorder, moderate, with a behavioral disturbance, that is judged to be due to Alzheimer's disease, vascular disease, and HIV infection, and in which heavy chronic alcohol use is judged to be a contributing factor, code the following: **G30.9** Alzheimer's disease, **B20** HIV infection; **F02.81** major neurocognitive disorder due to Alzheimer's disease and HIV infection, moderate, with behavioral disturbance; **F01.51** major vascular neurocognitive disorder, moderate, with behavioral disturbance; and **F10.27** severe alcohol use disorder with alcohol-induced major neurocognitive disorder, moderate, nonamnestic-confabulatory type.

For mild neurocognitive disorder due to multiple etiologies, code **G31.84**. (**Note:** Do *not* use the additional codes for the etiologies. "With behavioral disturbance" and "without behavioral disturbance" cannot be coded but should still be recorded.)

For major or mild neurocognitive disorder due to multiple etiologies: Use additional code(s) to indicate clinically significant psychiatric symptoms due to the various etiologies (e.g., **F06.2** psychotic disorder due to Alzheimer's disease, with delusions; **F06.31** depressive disorder due to cerebrovascular disease, with depressive features).

Unspecified Neurocognitive Disorder

R41.9

This category applies to presentations in which symptoms characteristic of a neurocognitive disorder that cause clinically significant distress or impairment in social, occupational, or other important areas of functioning predominate but do not meet the full criteria for any of the disorders in the neurocognitive disorders diagnostic class. The unspecified neurocognitive disorder category is used in situations in which the precise etiology cannot be determined with sufficient certainty to make an etiological attribution.

Coding note: For unspecified major or mild neurocognitive disorder, code **R41.9**. (**Note:** Do *not* use additional codes for any presumed etiological medical conditions. "With behavioral disturbance" and "without behavioral disturbance" cannot be coded but should still be recorded.)

General Personality Disorder

A. An enduring pattern of inner experience and behavior that devi-
    ates markedly from the expectations of the individual's culture.
    This pattern is manifested in two (or more) of the following areas:

    1. Cognition (i.e., ways of perceiving and interpreting self, other
        people, and events).
    2. Affectivity (i.e., the range, intensity, lability, and appropriateness
        of emotional response).
    3. Interpersonal functioning.
    4. Impulse control.

B. The enduring pattern is inflexible and pervasive across a broad
    range of personal and social situations.
C. The enduring pattern leads to clinically significant distress or
    impairment in social, occupational, or other important areas of
    functioning.
D. The pattern is stable and of long duration, and its onset can be
    traced back at least to adolescence or early adulthood.
E. The enduring pattern is not better explained as a manifestation or
    consequence of another mental disorder.
F. The enduring pattern is not attributable to the physiological effects
    of a substance (e.g., a drug of abuse, a medication) or another med-
    ical condition (e.g., head trauma).

Cluster A Personality Disorders

Paranoid Personality Disorder

F60.0

A. A pervasive distrust and suspiciousness of others such that their
    motives are interpreted as malevolent, beginning by early adult-
    hood and present in a variety of contexts, as indicated by four (or
    more) of the following:

    1. Suspects, without sufficient basis, that others are exploiting,
        harming, or deceiving him or her.

    2. Is preoccupied with unjustified doubts about the loyalty or trustworthiness of friends or associates.

    3. Is reluctant to confide in others because of unwarranted fear that the information will be used maliciously against him or her.

    4. Reads hidden demeaning or threatening meanings into benign remarks or events.

    5. Persistently bears grudges (i.e., is unforgiving of insults, injuries, or slights).

    6. Perceives attacks on his or her character or reputation that are not apparent to others and is quick to react angrily or to counterattack.

    7. Has recurrent suspicions, without justification, regarding fidelity of spouse or sexual partner.

B. Does not occur exclusively during the course of schizophrenia, a bipolar disorder or depressive disorder with psychotic features, or another psychotic disorder and is not attributable to the physiological effects of another medical condition.

Note: If criteria are met prior to the onset of schizophrenia, add "premorbid," i.e., "paranoid personality disorder (premorbid)."

Schizoid Personality Disorder

F60.1

A. A pervasive pattern of detachment from social relationships and a restricted range of expression of emotions in interpersonal settings, beginning by early adulthood and present in a variety of contexts, as indicated by four (or more) of the following:

    1. Neither desires nor enjoys close relationships, including being part of a family.

    2. Almost always chooses solitary activities.

    3. Has little, if any, interest in having sexual experiences with another person.

    4. Takes pleasure in few, if any, activities.

    5. Lacks close friends or confidants other than first-degree relatives.

    6. Appears indifferent to the praise or criticism of others.

    7. Shows emotional coldness, detachment, or flattened affectivity.

B. Does not occur exclusively during the course of schizophrenia, a bipolar disorder or depressive disorder with psychotic features, another psychotic disorder, or autism spectrum disorder and is not attributable to the physiological effects of another medical condition.

Note: If criteria are met prior to the onset of schizophrenia, add "premorbid," i.e., "schizoid personality disorder (premorbid)."

Schizotypal Personality Disorder

F21

A. A pervasive pattern of social and interpersonal deficits marked by acute discomfort with, and reduced capacity for, close relationships as well as by cognitive or perceptual distortions and eccentricities of behavior, beginning by early adulthood and present in a variety of contexts, as indicated by five (or more) of the following:

1. Ideas of reference (excluding delusions of reference).
2. Odd beliefs or magical thinking that influences behavior and is inconsistent with subcultural norms (e.g., superstitiousness, belief in clairvoyance, telepathy, or "sixth sense"; in children and adolescents, bizarre fantasies or preoccupations).
3. Unusual perceptual experiences, including bodily illusions.
4. Odd thinking and speech (e.g., vague, circumstantial, metaphorical, overelaborate, or stereotyped).
5. Suspiciousness or paranoid ideation.
6. Inappropriate or constricted affect.
7. Behavior or appearance that is odd, eccentric, or peculiar.
8. Lack of close friends or confidants other than first-degree relatives.
9. Excessive social anxiety that does not diminish with familiarity and tends to be associated with paranoid fears rather than negative judgments about self.

B. Does not occur exclusively during the course of schizophrenia, a bipolar disorder or depressive disorder with psychotic features, another psychotic disorder, or autism spectrum disorder.

Note: If criteria are met prior to the onset of schizophrenia, add "premorbid," e.g., "schizotypal personality disorder (premorbid)."

Cluster B Personality Disorders

Antisocial Personality Disorder

F60.2

A. A pervasive pattern of disregard for and violation of the rights of others, occurring since age 15 years, as indicated by three (or more) of the following:

1. Failure to conform to social norms with respect to lawful behaviors, as indicated by repeatedly performing acts that are grounds for arrest.

2. Deceitfulness, as indicated by repeated lying, use of aliases, or conning others for personal profit or pleasure.
3. Impulsivity or failure to plan ahead.
4. Irritability and aggressiveness, as indicated by repeated physical fights or assaults.
5. Reckless disregard for safety of self or others.
6. Consistent irresponsibility, as indicated by repeated failure to sustain consistent work behavior or honor financial obligations.
7. Lack of remorse, as indicated by being indifferent to or rationalizing having hurt, mistreated, or stolen from another.

B. The individual is at least age 18 years.
C. There is evidence of conduct disorder with onset before age 15 years.
D. The occurrence of antisocial behavior is not exclusively during the course of schizophrenia or bipolar disorder.

Borderline Personality Disorder

F60.3

A pervasive pattern of instability of interpersonal relationships, self-image, and affects, and marked impulsivity, beginning by early adulthood and present in a variety of contexts, as indicated by five (or more) of the following:

1. Frantic efforts to avoid real or imagined abandonment. (**Note:** Do not include suicidal or self-mutilating behavior covered in Criterion 5.)
2. A pattern of unstable and intense interpersonal relationships characterized by alternating between extremes of idealization and devaluation.
3. Identity disturbance: markedly and persistently unstable self-image or sense of self.
4. Impulsivity in at least two areas that are potentially self-damaging (e.g., spending, sex, substance abuse, reckless driving, binge eating). (**Note:** Do not include suicidal or self-mutilating behavior covered in Criterion 5.)
5. Recurrent suicidal behavior, gestures, or threats, or self-mutilating behavior.
6. Affective instability due to a marked reactivity of mood (e.g., intense episodic dysphoria, irritability, or anxiety usually lasting a few hours and only rarely more than a few days).
7. Chronic feelings of emptiness.
8. Inappropriate, intense anger or difficulty controlling anger (e.g., frequent displays of temper, constant anger, recurrent physical fights).
9. Transient, stress-related paranoid ideation or severe dissociative symptoms.

Histrionic Personality Disorder

F60.4

A pervasive pattern of excessive emotionality and attention seeking, beginning by early adulthood and present in a variety of contexts, as indicated by five (or more) of the following:

1. Is uncomfortable in situations in which he or she is not the center of attention.
2. Interaction with others is often characterized by inappropriate sexually seductive or provocative behavior.
3. Displays rapidly shifting and shallow expression of emotions.
4. Consistently uses physical appearance to draw attention to self.
5. Has a style of speech that is excessively impressionistic and lacking in detail.
6. Shows self-dramatization, theatricality, and exaggerated expression of emotion.
7. Is suggestible (i.e., easily influenced by others or circumstances).
8. Considers relationships to be more intimate than they actually are.

Narcissistic Personality Disorder

F60.81

A pervasive pattern of grandiosity (in fantasy or behavior), need for admiration, and lack of empathy, beginning by early adulthood and present in a variety of contexts, as indicated by five (or more) of the following:

1. Has a grandiose sense of self-importance (e.g., exaggerates achievements and talents, expects to be recognized as superior without commensurate achievements).
2. Is preoccupied with fantasies of unlimited success, power, brilliance, beauty, or ideal love.
3. Believes that he or she is "special" and unique and can only be understood by, or should associate with, other special or high-status people (or institutions).
4. Requires excessive admiration.
5. Has a sense of entitlement (i.e., unreasonable expectations of especially favorable treatment or automatic compliance with his or her expectations).
6. Is interpersonally exploitative (i.e., takes advantage of others to achieve his or her own ends).
7. Lacks empathy: is unwilling to recognize or identify with the feelings and needs of others.
8. Is often envious of others or believes that others are envious of him or her.
9. Shows arrogant, haughty behaviors or attitudes.

Cluster C Personality Disorders

Avoidant Personality Disorder

F60.6

A pervasive pattern of social inhibition, feelings of inadequacy, and hypersensitivity to negative evaluation, beginning by early adulthood and present in a variety of contexts, as indicated by four (or more) of the following:

1. Avoids occupational activities that involve significant interpersonal contact because of fears of criticism, disapproval, or rejection.
2. Is unwilling to get involved with people unless certain of being liked.
3. Shows restraint within intimate relationships because of the fear of being shamed or ridiculed.
4. Is preoccupied with being criticized or rejected in social situations.
5. Is inhibited in new interpersonal situations because of feelings of inadequacy.
6. Views self as socially inept, personally unappealing, or inferior to others.
7. Is unusually reluctant to take personal risks or to engage in any new activities because they may prove embarrassing.

Dependent Personality Disorder

F60.7

A pervasive and excessive need to be taken care of that leads to submissive and clinging behavior and fears of separation, beginning by early adulthood and present in a variety of contexts, as indicated by five (or more) of the following:

1. Has difficulty making everyday decisions without an excessive amount of advice and reassurance from others.
2. Needs others to assume responsibility for most major areas of his or her life.
3. Has difficulty expressing disagreement with others because of fear of loss of support or approval. (**Note:** Do not include realistic fears of retribution.)
4. Has difficulty initiating projects or doing things on his or her own (because of a lack of self-confidence in judgment or abilities rather than a lack of motivation or energy).
5. Goes to excessive lengths to obtain nurturance and support from others, to the point of volunteering to do things that are unpleasant.
6. Feels uncomfortable or helpless when alone because of exaggerated fears of being unable to care for himself or herself.

7. Urgently seeks another relationship as a source of care and support when a close relationship ends.
8. Is unrealistically preoccupied with fears of being left to take care of himself or herself.

Obsessive-Compulsive Personality Disorder

F60.5

A pervasive pattern of preoccupation with orderliness, perfectionism, and mental and interpersonal control, at the expense of flexibility, openness, and efficiency, beginning by early adulthood and present in a variety of contexts, as indicated by four (or more) of the following:

1. Is preoccupied with details, rules, lists, order, organization, or schedules to the extent that the major point of the activity is lost.
2. Shows perfectionism that interferes with task completion (e.g., is unable to complete a project because his or her own overly strict standards are not met).
3. Is excessively devoted to work and productivity to the exclusion of leisure activities and friendships (not accounted for by obvious economic necessity).
4. Is overconscientious, scrupulous, and inflexible about matters of morality, ethics, or values (not accounted for by cultural or religious identification).
5. Is unable to discard worn-out or worthless objects even when they have no sentimental value.
6. Is reluctant to delegate tasks or to work with others unless they submit to exactly his or her way of doing things.
7. Adopts a miserly spending style toward both self and others; money is viewed as something to be hoarded for future catastrophes.
8. Shows rigidity and stubbornness.

Other Personality Disorders

Personality Change Due to Another Medical Condition

F07.0

A. A persistent personality disturbance that represents a change from the individual's previous characteristic personality pattern.

Note: In children, the disturbance involves a marked deviation from normal development or a significant change in the child's usual behavior patterns, lasting at least 1 year.

B. There is evidence from the history, physical examination, or laboratory findings that the disturbance is the direct pathophysiological consequence of another medical condition.
C. The disturbance is not better explained by another mental disorder (including another mental disorder due to another medical
condition).
D. The disturbance does not occur exclusively during the course of
a delirium.
E. The disturbance causes clinically significant distress or impairment
in social, occupational, or other important areas of functioning.

Specify whether:

Labile type: If the predominant feature is affective lability.

Disinhibited type: If the predominant feature is poor impulse control as evidenced by sexual indiscretions, etc.

Aggressive type: If the predominant feature is aggressive behavior.

Apathetic type: If the predominant feature is marked apathy and
indifference.

Paranoid type: If the predominant feature is suspiciousness or
paranoid ideation.

Other type: If the presentation is not characterized by any of the
above subtypes.

Combined type: If more than one feature predominates in the clinical picture.

Unspecified type

Coding note: Include the name of the other medical condition (e.g.,
F07.0 personality change due to temporal lobe epilepsy). The other
medical condition should be coded and listed separately immediately
before the personality change due to another medical condition (e.g.,
G40.209 temporal lobe epilepsy; F07.0 personality change due to temporal lobe epilepsy).

Other Specified Personality Disorder

F60.89

This category applies to presentations in which symptoms characteristic
of a personality disorder that cause clinically significant distress or impairment in social, occupational, or other important areas of functioning
predominate but do not meet the full criteria for any of the disorders in
the personality disorders diagnostic class. The other specified personality disorder category is used in situations in which the clinician chooses
to communicate the specific reason that the presentation does not
meet the criteria for any specific personality disorder. This is done by
recording "other specified personality disorder" followed by the specific
reason (e.g., "mixed personality features").

Unspecified Personality Disorder

F60.9

This category applies to presentations in which symptoms characteristic of a personality disorder that cause clinically significant distress or impairment in social, occupational, or other important areas of functioning predominate but do not meet the full criteria for any of the disorders in the personality disorders diagnostic class. The unspecified personality disorder category is used in situations in which the clinician chooses *not* to specify the reason that the criteria are not met for a specific personality disorder and includes presentations in which there is insufficient information to make a more specific diagnosis.

Paraphilic Disorders

Voyeuristic Disorder

F65.3

A. Over a period of at least 6 months, recurrent and intense sexual arousal from observing an unsuspecting person who is naked, in the process of disrobing, or engaging in sexual activity, as manifested by fantasies, urges, or behaviors.

B. The individual has acted on these sexual urges with a nonconsenting person, or the sexual urges or fantasies cause clinically significant distress or impairment in social, occupational, or other important areas of functioning.

C. The individual experiencing the arousal and/or acting on the urges is at least 18 years of age.

Specify if:

In a controlled environment: This specifier is primarily applicable to individuals living in institutional or other settings where opportunities to engage in voyeuristic behavior are restricted.

In full remission: The individual has not acted on the urges with a nonconsenting person, and there has been no distress or impairment in social, occupational, or other areas of functioning, for at least 5 years while in an uncontrolled environment.

Exhibitionistic Disorder

F65.2

A. Over a period of at least 6 months, recurrent and intense sexual arousal from the exposure of one's genitals to an unsuspecting person, as manifested by fantasies, urges, or behaviors.

B. The individual has acted on these sexual urges with a nonconsenting person, or the sexual urges or fantasies cause clinically significant distress or impairment in social, occupational, or other important areas of functioning.

Specify whether:

Sexually aroused by exposing genitals to prepubertal children
Sexually aroused by exposing genitals to physically mature individuals
Sexually aroused by exposing genitals to prepubertal children and to physically mature individuals

Specify if:

In a controlled environment: This specifier is primarily applicable to individuals living in institutional or other settings where opportunities to expose one's genitals are restricted.

In full remission: The individual has not acted on the urges with a nonconsenting person, and there has been no distress or impairment in social, occupational, or other areas of functioning, for at least 5 years while in an uncontrolled environment.

Frotteuristic Disorder

F65.81

A. Over a period of at least 6 months, recurrent and intense sexual arousal from touching or rubbing against a nonconsenting person, as manifested by fantasies, urges, or behaviors.
B. The individual has acted on these sexual urges with a nonconsenting person, or the sexual urges or fantasies cause clinically significant distress or impairment in social, occupational, or other important areas of functioning.

Specify if:

In a controlled environment: This specifier is primarily applicable to individuals living in institutional or other settings where opportunities to touch or rub against a nonconsenting person are restricted.

In full remission: The individual has not acted on the urges with a nonconsenting person, and there has been no distress or impairment in social, occupational, or other areas of functioning, for at least 5 years while in an uncontrolled environment.

Sexual Masochism Disorder

F65.51

A. Over a period of at least 6 months, recurrent and intense sexual arousal from the act of being humiliated, beaten, bound, or otherwise made to suffer, as manifested by fantasies, urges, or behaviors.
B. The fantasies, sexual urges, or behaviors cause clinically significant distress or impairment in social, occupational, or other important areas of functioning.

Specify if:

With asphyxiophilia: If the individual engages in the practice of achieving sexual arousal related to restriction of breathing.

Specify if:

In a controlled environment: This specifier is primarily applicable to individuals living in institutional or other settings where opportunities to engage in masochistic sexual behaviors are restricted.

In full remission: There has been no distress or impairment in social, occupational, or other areas of functioning for at least 5 years while in an uncontrolled environment.

Sexual Sadism Disorder
F65.52

A. Over a period of at least 6 months, recurrent and intense sexual arousal from the physical or psychological suffering of another person, as manifested by fantasies, urges, or behaviors.
B. The individual has acted on these sexual urges with a nonconsenting person, or the sexual urges or fantasies cause clinically significant distress or impairment in social, occupational, or other important areas of functioning.

Specify if:
In a controlled environment: This specifier is primarily applicable to individuals living in institutional or other settings where opportunities to engage in sadistic sexual behaviors are restricted.
In full remission: The individual has not acted on the urges with a nonconsenting person, and there has been no distress or impairment in social, occupational, or other areas of functioning, for at least 5 years while in an uncontrolled environment.

Pedophilic Disorder
F65.4

A. Over a period of at least 6 months, recurrent, intense sexually arousing fantasies, sexual urges, or behaviors involving sexual activity with a prepubescent child or children (generally age 13 years or younger).
B. The individual has acted on these sexual urges, or the sexual urges or fantasies cause marked distress or interpersonal difficulty.
C. The individual is at least age 16 years and at least 5 years older than the child or children in Criterion A.
   Note: Do not include an individual in late adolescence involved in an ongoing sexual relationship with a 12- or 13-year-old.

Specify whether:
Exclusive type (attracted only to children)
Nonexclusive type

Specify if:
Sexually attracted to males
Sexually attracted to females
Sexually attracted to both

Specify if:
Limited to incest

Fetishistic Disorder

F65.0

A. Over a period of at least 6 months, recurrent and intense sexual arousal from either the use of nonliving objects or a highly specific focus on nongenital body part(s), as manifested by fantasies, urges, or behaviors.

B. The fantasies, sexual urges, or behaviors cause clinically significant distress or impairment in social, occupational, or other important areas of functioning.

C. The fetish objects are not limited to articles of clothing used in cross-dressing (as in transvestic disorder) or devices specifically designed for the purpose of tactile genital stimulation (e.g., vibrator).

Specify:

Body part(s)
Nonliving object(s)
Other

Specify if:

In a controlled environment: This specifier is primarily applicable to individuals living in institutional or other settings where opportunities to engage in fetishistic behaviors are restricted.
In full remission: There has been no distress or impairment in social, occupational, or other areas of functioning for at least 5 years while in an uncontrolled environment.

Transvestic Disorder

F65.1

A. Over a period of at least 6 months, recurrent and intense sexual arousal from cross-dressing, as manifested by fantasies, urges, or behaviors.

B. The fantasies, sexual urges, or behaviors cause clinically significant distress or impairment in social, occupational, or other important areas of functioning.

Specify if:

With fetishism: If sexually aroused by fabrics, materials, or garments.
With autogynephilia: If sexually aroused by thoughts or images of self as a woman.

Specify if:

In a controlled environment: This specifier is primarily applicable to individuals living in institutional or other settings where opportunities to cross-dress are restricted.

In full remission: There has been no distress or impairment in social, occupational, or other areas of functioning for at least 5 years while in an uncontrolled environment.

Other Specified Paraphilic Disorder

F65.89

This category applies to presentations in which symptoms characteristic of a paraphilic disorder that cause clinically significant distress or impairment in social, occupational, or other important areas of functioning predominate but do not meet the full criteria for any of the disorders in the paraphilic disorders diagnostic class. The other specified paraphilic disorder category is used in situations in which the clinician chooses to communicate the specific reason that the presentation does not meet the criteria for any specific paraphilic disorder. This is done by recording "other specified paraphilic disorder" followed by the specific reason (e.g., "zoophilia").

Examples of presentations that can be specified using the "other specified" designation include, but are not limited to, recurrent and intense sexual arousal involving *telephone scatologia* (obscene phone calls), *necrophilia* (corpses), *zoophilia* (animals), *coprophilia* (feces), *klismaphilia* (enemas), or *urophilia* (urine) that has been present for at least 6 months and causes marked distress or impairment in social, occupational, or other important areas of functioning. Other specified paraphilic disorder can be specified as in remission and/or as occurring in a controlled environment.

Unspecified Paraphilic Disorder

F65.9

This category applies to presentations in which symptoms characteristic of a paraphilic disorder that cause clinically significant distress or impairment in social, occupational, or other important areas of functioning predominate but do not meet the full criteria for any of the disorders in the paraphilic disorders diagnostic class. The unspecified paraphilic disorder category is used in situations in which the clinician chooses *not* to specify the reason that the criteria are not met for a specific paraphilic disorder, and includes presentations in which there is insufficient information to make a more specific diagnosis.

Other Specified Mental Disorder Due to Another Medical Condition

F06.8

This category applies to presentations in which symptoms characteristic of a mental disorder due to another medical condition that cause clinically significant distress or impairment in social, occupational, or other important areas of functioning predominate but do not meet the full criteria for any specific mental disorder attributable to another medical condition. The other specified mental disorder due to another medical condition category is used in situations in which the clinician chooses to communicate the specific reason that the presentation does not meet the criteria for any specific mental disorder attributable to another medical condition. This is done by recording the name of the disorder, with the specific etiological medical condition inserted in place of "another medical condition," followed by the specific symptomatic manifestation that does not meet the criteria for any specific mental disorder due to another medical condition. Furthermore, the diagnostic code for the specific medical condition must be listed immediately before the code for the other specified mental disorder due to another medical condition. For example, dissociative symptoms due to complex partial seizures would be coded and recorded as G40.209 complex partial seizures, F06.8 other specified mental disorder due to complex partial seizures, dissociative symptoms.

An example of a presentation that can be specified using the "other specified" designation is the following:

Dissociative symptoms: This includes symptoms occurring, for example, in the context of complex partial seizures.

Unspecified Mental Disorder Due to Another Medical Condition

F09

This category applies to presentations in which symptoms characteristic of a mental disorder due to another medical condition that cause clinically significant distress or impairment in social, occupational, or other important areas of functioning predominate but do not meet the full criteria for any specific mental disorder due to another medical condition. The unspecified mental disorder due to another medical condition category is used in situations in which the clinician chooses *not* to specify the reason that the criteria are not met for a specific mental disorder due to another medical condition, and includes presentations for which there is insufficient information to make a more specific diagnosis (e.g., in emergency room settings). This is done by recording the name of the disorder, with the specific etiological medical condition inserted in place of "another medical condition." Furthermore, the diagnostic code for the specific medical condition must be listed immediately before the code for the unspecified mental disorder due to another medical condition. For example, dissociative symptoms due to complex partial seizures would be coded and recorded as G40.209 complex partial seizures, F09 unspecified mental disorder due to complex partial seizures.

Other Specified Mental Disorder

F99

This category applies to presentations in which symptoms characteristic of a mental disorder that cause clinically significant distress or impairment in social, occupational, or other important areas of functioning predominate but do not meet the full criteria for any specific mental disorder. The other specified mental disorder category is used in situations in which the clinician chooses to communicate the specific reason that the presentation does not meet the criteria for any specific mental disorder. This is done by recording "other specified mental disorder" followed by the specific reason.

Unspecified Mental Disorder

F99

This category applies to presentations in which symptoms characteristic of a mental disorder that cause clinically significant distress or impairment in social, occupational, or other important areas of functioning predominate but do not meet the full criteria for any mental disorder. The unspecified mental disorder category is used in situations in which the clinician chooses *not* to specify the reason that the criteria are not met for a specific mental disorder, and includes presentations for which there is insufficient information to make a more specific diagnosis (e.g., in emergency room settings).

Additional Codes

Z03.89   No Diagnosis or Condition

This code applies to situations in which the individual has been evaluated and it is determined that no mental disorder or condition is present.

Medication-induced movement disorders are included in Section II of DSM-5-TR because of their frequent importance in 1) the management by medication of mental disorders or other medical conditions and 2) the differential diagnosis of mental disorders (e.g., anxiety disorder vs. medication-induced akathisia; malignant catatonia [a particularly severe and potentially life-threatening form of catatonia] vs. neuroleptic malignant syndrome; tardive dyskinesia vs. chorea). Although these movement disorders are labeled "medication induced," it is often difficult to establish the causal relationship between medication exposure and the development of the movement disorder, especially because some of these movement disorders also occur in the absence of medication exposure. The conditions and problems listed in this chapter are not mental disorders.

The term *neuroleptic* is becoming outdated because it highlights the propensity of antipsychotic medications to cause abnormal movements, and it is being replaced with the term *antipsychotic medications and other dopamine receptor blocking agents* in many contexts. Although newer antipsychotic medications may be less likely to cause some medication-induced movement disorders, those disorders still occur. Antipsychotic medications and other dopamine receptor blocking agents include so-called conventional, "typical," or first-generation antipsychotic agents (e.g., chlorpromazine, haloperidol, fluphenazine); "atypical" or second-generation antipsychotic agents (e.g., clozapine, risperidone, olanzapine, quetiapine); certain dopamine receptor blocking drugs used in the treatment of symptoms such as nausea and gastroparesis (e.g., prochlorperazine, promethazine, trimethobenzamide, thiethylperazine, metoclopramide); and amoxapine, which is indicated for the treatment of depression.

Medication-Induced Parkinsonism

G21.11 Antipsychotic Medication– and Other Dopamine Receptor Blocking Agent– Induced Parkinsonism

G21.19 Other Medication-Induced Parkinsonism

Medication-induced parkinsonism (MIP), the second most common cause of parkinsonism after Parkinson's disease, is associated with significant morbidity, disability, and treatment nonadherence, particularly in individuals with psychiatric disorders. Because early recognition is important, any new case of parkinsonism should prompt a thorough medication history, which is essential for diagnosis of MIP. A temporal relationship between medication initiation and onset of parkinsonism should be evident. A host of agents that may be prescribed in individuals with psychiatric disorders may also induce parkinsonism, but MIP is most often seen upon exposure to antipsychotic medications that block dopamine D_2 receptors. MIP occurs at higher rates with antipsychotics that have higher potency for the dopamine D_2 receptor, such as haloperidol, fluphenazine, and risperidone, but there are no differences in the clinical features of parkinsonism between first- and second-generation antipsychotics.

Other medications that can cause MIP include calcium channel antagonists (e.g., flunarizine, cinnarizine), dopamine depleters (e.g., reserpine, tetrabenazine), antiepileptics (e.g., phenytoin, valproate, levetiracetam), antidepressants (e.g., selective serotonin reuptake inhibitors, monoamine oxidase inhibitors), lithium, chemotherapeutic drugs (e.g., cystosine arabinoside, cyclophosphamide, vincristine, doxorubicin, paclitaxel, etoposide), and immunosuppressants (e.g., cyclosporine, tacrolimus). Toxins (e.g., 1-methyl-4-phenyl-1,2,3,6-tetra-hydropyridine [MPTP], organophosphate pesticides, manganese, methanol, cyanide, carbon monoxide, and carbon disulfide) may also cause MIP.

The time course for development of MIP varies. Usually, MIP develops a few weeks after starting or raising the dose of a medication known to cause parkinsonism or after reducing an antiparkinsonian medication (e.g., an anticholinergic agent) that is being used to treat or prevent medication-induced dystonia or parkinsonian symptoms. However, MIP may also develop rapidly after starting or raising the dose of a medication or have an insidious onset after many months of exposure. With antipsychotic medications or other dopamine receptor blocking agents, MIP typically develops 2–4 weeks after starting the medication and usually by 3 months. Mainly with calcium channel blockers, a second peak of symptom onset is reported after about 1 year.

Reported rates of MIP are affected by absence of standard diagnostic criteria, incorrect diagnosis or misattribution of MIP signs to Lewy body disease (e.g., Parkinson's disease), or a psychiatric condition, and overall lack of recognition, especially in milder cases. It is estimated that at least 50% of outpatients receiving long-term antipsychotic treatment with typical agents develop parkinsonian signs or symptoms at some point in their course of treatment.

There are no clinical characteristics that distinguish MIP reliably from Parkinson's disease. Because motor signs and symptoms in Parkinson's disease begin unilaterally and progress asymmetrically, the subacute onset of bilateral parkinsonism within weeks of starting an antipsychotic or other MIP-causing agent is highly suggestive for MIP. Parkinsonian signs are often symmetric in MIP, but asymmetric patterns are not uncommon and should not exclude a diagnosis of MIP. In addition, the course and presentation of parkinsonism should not be better accounted for by psychiatric phenomena, such as catatonia, negative symptoms of schizophrenia, or psychomotor retardation in a major depressive episode; other nonparkinsonian medication-induced movement disorders; another neurological or general medical condition (e.g., Parkinson's disease, Wilson's disease); or antipsychotic-exacerbated Parkinson's disease.

In MIP, rigidity and bradykinesia are more often present, whereas tremor is somewhat less common and may be absent. Parkinsonian tremor, also referred to as a "pill-rolling tremor," is a steady, rhythmic oscillatory movement (3–6 cycles per second) that is apparent at rest and is typically slower than other tremors. It may be intermittent, unilateral or bilateral, or dependent on limb position (i.e., positional tremor). The tremor may involve the limbs, head, jaw, mouth, lip ("rabbit syndrome"), or tongue. As it is present at rest, the tremor can be suppressed, especially when the individual attempts to perform a task with the tremulous limb. Individuals may describe the tremor as "shaking" and report that it may worsen with anxiety, stress, or fatigue.

Parkinsonian rigidity is experienced as an involuntary stiffness and inflexibility of the muscles of the limbs, shoulders, neck, or trunk. Rigidity is evaluated by assessing muscle tone, or the amount of resistance present when the examiner moves a limb (and stretches the muscles) passively around a joint. In lead-pipe rigidity, increased tone is constant throughout range of motion (in contrast to the clasp-knife rigidity spasticity). Cogwheel rigidity is thought to represent a tremor superimposed on rigidity. Most common in the wrists and elbows, it is experienced as a rhythmic, ratchet-like resistance (cogwheeling) when the muscles are passively moved around a joint. Individuals with parkinsonian rigidity may complain of generalized muscle tenderness or stiffness, tightness in their limbs, muscle or joint pain, body aching, or lack of coordination.

Bradykinesia and akinesia are observable states of decreased or absent spontaneous motor activity, respectively. There is global slowing as well as slowness in initiating and executing movements. Everyday behaviors (e.g., grooming) can be difficult to perform normally and may be reduced. Individuals may complain of listlessness, lack of spontaneity and drive, or fatigue. Parkinsonian rigidity and bradykinesia manifest as gait abnormalities, including decreased stride length, arm swing, or overall spontaneity of walking. Other signs include a hunched posture with bent-over neck and stooped shoulders, a staring facial expression, and small shuffling steps. Drooling can arise as a result of reduced pharyngeal motor activity and swallowing, but because of anticholinergic properties of these medications, it may be less common in antipsychotic-induced parkinsonism as compared with other medications that cause MIP.

MIP is associated with increased gait dysfunction, falls, and nursing home placement. As such, MIP is a serious iatrogenic movement disorder in older individuals that warrants recognition and early diagnosis. Associated behavioral symptoms may include depression and worsening of negative signs of schizophrenia. Other parkinsonian signs and symptoms include small handwriting (micrographia), reduced motor dexterity, hypophonia, decreased gag reflex, dysphagia, postural instability, reduced facial expression and blinking, and seborrhea. When parkinsonism is associated with severe decreased motor activity, medical complications of parkinsonism include contractures, bedsores, pulmonary emboli, urinary incontinence, aspiration pneumonia, weight loss, and hip fractures.

Consistent risk factors are female gender, older age, cognitive impairment, other concurrent neurological conditions, HIV infection, family history of Parkinson's disease, and severe psychiatric disease. MIP secondary to antipsychotic use is also reported in children. The risk of MIP is reduced if individuals are taking anticholinergic medications.

Differential Diagnosis

Parkinson's disease and Parkinson's-plus conditions such as multiple system atrophy, progressive supranuclear palsy, and Wilson's disease are distinguished from MIP by their other signs and symptoms that accompany parkinsonism. For example, Parkinson's disease is suggested by evidence of three or more cardinal features of Parkinson's disease (e.g., resting tremor, rigidity, bradykinesia, postural instability), hyposmia, sleep disturbances such as rapid eye movement (REM) sleep behavior disorder, and urinary and other autonomic symptoms common to Parkinson's disease. These features are less likely to be present in MIP. Individuals with primary neurological causes of parkinsonism are also susceptible to worsening symptoms if treated with medications causing MIP.

Nonparkinsonian tremors tend to be finer (e.g., smaller amplitude) and faster (10 cycles per second) and worsen on intention (e.g., when reaching out to grab an object). With substance withdrawal, there is usually associated hyperreflexia and increased autonomic signs. In cerebellar disease, tremor worsens on intention and may be associated with nystagmus, ataxia, or scanning speech. Choreiform movements associated with tardive dyskinesia lack the steady rhythmicity of a parkinsonian tremor. Strokes and other central nervous system lesions can cause focal neurological signs or immobility from flaccid or spastic paralysis, which is characterized by decreased muscle strength and increased tone on passive movement that gives away with further pressure (i.e., clasp-knife rigidity). This contrasts with the lead-pipe rigidity and normal muscle strength in MIP.

Diagnostic alternatives to MIP are also suggested by a family history of an inherited neurological condition, rapidly progressive parkinsonism not accounted for by recent psychopharmacological changes, or presence of focal neurological signs (e.g., frontal release signs, cranial nerve abnormalities, a positive Babinski sign), Neuroleptic malignant syndrome involves severe akinesia and rigidity, but also characteristic physical and laboratory findings (e.g., fever, increased creatine phosphokinase).

Psychomotor slowing, inactivity, and apathy seen in major depressive disorder can be indistinguishable from the motor slowness or akinesia of MIP, but major depressive disorder is more likely to include vegetative signs (e.g., early-morning awakening), hopelessness, and despair. Negative symptoms of schizophrenia, catatonia associated with schizophrenia, or mood disorders with catatonic features may also be difficult to distinguish from medication-induced akinesia. Rigidity may also manifest in psychotic disorders, delirium, major neurocognitive disorder, anxiety disorders, and functional neurological symptom disorder (conversion disorder). In parkinsonian rigidity, resistance to passive motion is constant through the full range of motion, whereas it is inconsistent in psychiatric disorders or other neurological conditions presenting with rigidity. In general, the constellation of associated physical signs on examination and symptoms associated with the tremor, rigidity, and bradykinesia of parkinsonism helps distinguish MIP-related rigidity and bradykinesia from other primary psychiatric causes of rigidity and decreased movement.

Neuroleptic Malignant Syndrome

G21.0   Neuroleptic Malignant Syndrome

Individuals with neuroleptic malignant syndrome have generally been exposed to a dopamine antagonist within 72 hours prior to symptom development. Hyperthermia (>100.4°F or >38.0°C on at least two occasions, measured orally), associated with profuse diaphoresis, is a distinguishing feature of neuroleptic malignant syndrome, setting it apart from other neurological side effects of antipsychotic medications and other dopamine receptor blocking agents. Extreme elevations in temperature, reflecting a breakdown in central thermoregulation, are more likely to support the diagnosis of neuroleptic malignant syndrome. Generalized rigidity, described as "lead pipe" in its most severe form and usually unresponsive to antiparkinsonian agents, is a cardinal feature of the disorder and may be associated with other neurological symptoms (e.g., tremor, sialorrhea, akinesia, dystonia, trismus, myoclonus, dysarthria, dysphagia, rhabdomyolysis). Creatine kinase elevation of at least four times the upper limit of normal is commonly seen. Changes in mental status, characterized by delirium or altered consciousness ranging from stupor to coma, are often an early sign of neuroleptic malignant syndrome. Affected individuals may appear alert but dazed and unresponsive, consistent with catatonic stupor. Autonomic activation and instability—manifested by tachycardia (rate>25% above baseline), diaphoresis, blood pressure elevation (systolic or diastolic ≥25% above baseline) or fluctuation (≥20 mmHg diastolic change or ≥25 mmHg systolic change within 24 hours), urinary incontinence, and pallor—may be seen at any time but provide an early clue to the diagnosis. Tachypnea (rate >50% above baseline) is common, and respiratory distress—resulting from metabolic acidosis, hypermetabolism, chest wall restriction, aspiration pneumonia, or pulmonary emboli—can occur and lead to sudden respiratory arrest.

Although several laboratory abnormalities are associated with neuroleptic malignant syndrome, no single abnormality is specific to the diagnosis. Individuals with neuroleptic malignant syndrome may have leukocytosis, metabolic acidosis, hypoxia, decreased serum iron concentrations, and elevations in serum muscle enzymes and catecholamines. Findings from cerebrospinal fluid analysis and neuroimaging studies are generally normal, whereas electroencephalography shows generalized slowing. Autopsy findings in fatal cases have been nonspecific and variable, depending on complications.

Evidence from database studies suggests incidence rates for neuroleptic malignant syndrome of 0.01%–0.02% among individuals treated with antipsychotics. A population-based study conducted in Hong Kong found an incidence risk of 0.11% in individuals treated with antipsychotic medication.

The temporal progression of signs and symptoms provides important clues to the diagnosis and prognosis of neuroleptic malignant syndrome. Alteration in mental status and other neurological signs typically precede systemic signs. The onset of symptoms varies from hours to days after drug initiation. Some cases develop within 24 hours after drug initiation, most within the first week, and virtually all cases within 30 days. Once the syndrome is diagnosed and oral antipsychotic drugs and other dopamine receptor blocking agents are discontinued, neuroleptic malignant syndrome is self-limited in most cases. The mean recovery time after drug discontinuation is 7–10 days, with most individuals recovering within 1 week and nearly all within 30 days. The duration may be prolonged when long-acting antipsychotic medications are implicated. There have been reports of individuals in whom residual neurological signs persisted for weeks after the acute hypermetabolic symptoms resolved. Total resolution of symptoms can be obtained in most cases of neuroleptic malignant syndrome; however, fatality rates of 10%–20% have been reported when the disorder is not recognized. Although many individuals do not experience a recurrence of neuroleptic malignant syndrome when rechallenged with antipsychotic medication, some do, especially when antipsychotic medications are reinstituted soon after an episode.

Neuroleptic malignant syndrome is a potential risk in any individual after administration of an antipsychotic medication or other dopamine receptor blocking agent. It is not specific to any neuropsychiatric diagnosis and may occur in persons without a diagnosable mental disorder who receive dopamine antagonists. Clinical, systemic, and metabolic factors associated with a heightened risk of neuroleptic malignant syndrome include agitation, exhaustion, dehydration, and iron deficiency. A prior episode associated with antipsychotic medication and other dopamine receptor blocking agents has been described in 15%–20% of index cases, suggesting underlying vulnerability in some individuals; however, genetic findings based on neurotransmitter receptor polymorphisms have not been replicated consistently.

Nearly all antipsychotic medication and other dopamine receptor blocking agents have been associated with neuroleptic malignant syndrome, although high-potency antipsychotics pose a greater risk compared with low-potency agents and atypical antipsychotics. Partial or milder forms may be associated with newer antipsychotics, but neuroleptic malignant syndrome varies in severity even with older drugs. Dopamine receptor blocking agents used in medical settings (e.g., metoclopramide, prochlorperazine) have also been implicated. Parenteral administration routes, rapid titration rates, and higher total drug dosages have been associated with increased risk; however, neuroleptic malignant syndrome usually occurs within the therapeutic dosage range of antipsychotic medications and other dopamine receptor blocking agents.

Differential Diagnosis

Neuroleptic malignant syndrome should be distinguished from other serious neurological or medical conditions, including central nervous system infections, inflammatory or autoimmune conditions, status epilepticus, subcortical structural lesions, and systemic conditions (e.g., pheochromocytoma, thyrotoxicosis, tetanus, heat stroke).

Neuroleptic malignant syndrome also should be distinguished from similar syndromes resulting from the use of other substances or medications, such as serotonin syndrome; parkinsonian hyperthermia syndrome following abrupt discontinuation of dopamine agonists; alcohol or sedative withdrawal; malignant hyperthermia occurring during anesthesia; hyperthermia associated with misuse of stimulants and hallucinogens; and atropine poisoning from anticholinergics.

In rare instances, individuals with schizophrenia or a mood disorder may present with malignant catatonia, which may be indistinguishable from neuroleptic malignant syndrome. Some investigators consider neuroleptic malignant syndrome to be a drug-induced form of malignant catatonia.

Medication-Induced Acute Dystonia

G24.02   Medication-Induced Acute Dystonia

The essential features of medication-induced acute dystonia are sustained abnormal muscle contractions (increased muscle tone) and postures that develop in association with use of a medication known to cause acute dystonia. Any medication that blocks dopamine D_2-like receptors can induce an acute dystonic reaction (ADR). Most commonly, ADRs occur after exposure to antipsychotics and antiemetic and promotility agents. A variety of other medication classes are also reported to have induced ADRs, including selective serotonin reuptake inhibitors, cholinesterase inhibitors, opioids, and methylphenidate.

Dystonic reactions vary greatly in severity and location and can be focal, segmented, or generalized. They most often affect head and neck muscles, but can extend to upper and lower limbs or trunk. A common presentation is acute oro-mandibular (jaw) dystonia involving the tongue and mouth with tongue protrusion, or gaping or grimacing postures that can impair speech (dysarthria) and swallowing (dysphagia) and may evolve into frank trismus (lockjaw). Involvement of ocular muscles (oculogyric crisis) manifests as involuntary forced and sustained conjugate deviations of eyes upward, downward, or sideways that can last minutes to hours. Blepharospasm can also occur. Cervical (neck) dystonia presents as abnormal forward, backward, lateral, or twisting positions of the head and neck in relation to the body (e.g., antecollis, retrocollis, laterocollis, and torticollis). Focal limb dystonia, generally more distal than proximal, Pisa syndrome (lateral bending of the trunk with a tendency to lean to one side), and back arching that may evolve into opisthotonos (backward arching of head, neck, and spine) can also occur. Acute laryngeal dystonia is life-threatening, causing airway obstruction, and manifests as a "clutching of the throat," stridor, dysphonia, dysphagia, dyspnea, and respiratory distress from the medication effects on vocal cords and laryngeal muscles.

At least 50% of patients develop ADR signs or symptoms within 24–48 hours of starting or rapidly raising the dose of antipsychotic medication or other dopamine receptor blocking agent or of reducing a medication being used to treat or prevent acute extrapyramidal symptoms (e.g., anticholinergic agents). Approximately 90% of affected individuals have onset of ADRs within 5 days. The symptoms must not be better accounted for by a mental disorder (e.g., catatonia) and must not be due to a primary neurological or other medical condition, or a tardive medication-induced movement disorder.

Fear and anxiety often accompany ADRs given their intense nature, inability of the individual to control or stop the movements, and, when present, difficulty breathing, speaking, or swallowing. Some individuals experience pain or cramps in affected muscles. Individuals who are unaware of the possibility of developing a medication-induced dystonia can be especially distressed, increasing the likelihood of subsequent medication nonadherence. Thought disorder, delusions, or mannerisms in an individual with psychosis may cause the affected individual or others to mistakenly regard his or her dystonic symptoms as a feature of the psychiatric condition, which could lead to increased doses of the causative medication. The risk of developing ADRs is greatest in children and in adults younger than age 40 with psychosis, with a greater incidence in males than females in both children and adults. Other risk factors for developing ADRs include prior dystonic reactions to antipsychotic medications or other dopamine receptor blocking agents and use of high-potency typical antipsychotic medications.

Differential Diagnosis

It is important to distinguish between medication-induced ADRs and other causes of dystonia, especially in individuals being treated with antipsychotic or other dopamine receptor blocking medications. A primary neurological or other medical condition is evident based on the time course and evolution of the dystonic phenomena (e.g., dystonia precedes exposure to the antipsychotic medication or progresses in the absence of change in medication) and, possibly, other evidence of focal neurological signs. Idiopathic focal or segmental dystonias usually persist for several days or weeks independent of medication. A family history of dystonia may also be present. Tardive dystonia secondary to medication exposure, including antipsychotic medication or other dopamine receptor blocking agents, does not have acute onset and may become evident when the dose of an antipsychotic medication is lowered. Other neurological conditions (e.g., epileptic seizures, viral and bacterial infections, trauma, space-occupying lesions in the peripheral or central nervous system) and endocrinopathies (e.g., hypoparathyroidism) can also produce symptoms (e.g., tetany) that resemble a medication-induced acute dystonia. Other diagnoses that mimic an acute medication-induced dystonia include anaphylaxis, tardive laryngeal dystonia, and respiratory dyskinesia. Neuroleptic malignant syndrome can produce dystonia but differs in that it is also accompanied by fever and generalized rigidity.

Catatonia associated with a mood disorder or schizophrenia can be distinguished by the temporal relationship between the symptoms and the exposure to antipsychotic treatment (e.g., dystonia preceding exposure to antipsychotic medication) and response to pharmacological intervention (e.g., no improvement after lowering of dose of the antipsychotic medication or in response to anticholinergic administration). Furthermore, individuals with medication-induced acute dystonia are generally distressed about the dystonic reaction and usually seek intervention. In contrast, individuals with the retarded type of catatonia are typically mute and withdrawn and do not express subjective distress about their condition.

Medication-Induced Acute Akathisia

G25.71   Medication-Induced Acute Akathisia

The essential features of medication-induced acute akathisia are subjective complaints of restlessness and at least one of the following observed movements: fidgety movements or swinging of the legs while seated, rocking from foot to foot or "walking on the spot" while standing, pacing to relieve the restlessness, or an inability to sit or stand still for at least several minutes. Individuals experiencing the most severe form of medication-induced acute akathisia may be unable to maintain any position for more than a few seconds. The subjective complaints include a sense of inner restlessness, most often in the legs; a compulsion to move one's legs; distress if one is asked not to move one's legs; and dysphoria and anxiety. The symptoms typically occur within 4 weeks of initiating or increasing the dose of a medication that can cause akathisia, which includes antipsychotic medications and other dopamine receptor blocking agents, tricyclic antidepressants, selective serotonin reuptake inhibitors, dopamine agonists, and calcium channel blockers, and can occasionally follow the reduction of medication used to treat or prevent acute extrapyramidal symptoms (e.g., anticholinergic agents). The symptoms are not better explained by a mental disorder (e.g., schizophrenia, substance withdrawal, agitation from a major depressive or manic episode, hyperactivity in attention-deficit/hyperactivity disorder) and are not due to a neurological or other medical condition (e.g., Parkinson's disease, iron-deficiency anemia).

The subjective distress resulting from akathisia is significant and can lead to noncompliance with antipsychotic or antidepressant treatment. Akathisia may be associated with dysphoria, irritability, aggression, or suicide attempts. Worsening of psychotic symptoms or behavioral dyscontrol may lead to an increase in medication dose, which may exacerbate the problem. Akathisia can develop very rapidly after initiating or increasing the causative medication. The development of akathisia appears to be dose dependent and to be more frequently associated with particular high-potency antipsychotic medications or drugs with higher affinity for central dopamine receptors. Acute akathisia tends to persist for as long as the causative medication is continued, although the intensity may fluctuate over time. The reported prevalence of akathisia among individuals receiving antipsychotic medication or other dopamine receptor blocking agents has varied widely (20%–75%). Variations in reported prevalence may be attributable to a lack of consistency in the definition, antipsychotic prescribing practices, study design, and the demographics of the population being studied.

Differential Diagnosis

Medication-induced acute akathisia may be clinically indistinguishable from syndromes of restlessness due to certain neurological or other medical conditions, and to agitation presenting as part of a mental disorder (e.g., a manic episode). The akathisia of Parkinson's disease and iron-deficiency anemia is phenomenologically similar to medication-induced acute akathisia. The frequently abrupt appearance of restlessness soon after initiation or increase in medication usually distinguishes medication-induced acute akathisia.

Serotonin-specific reuptake inhibitor antidepressant medications may produce akathisia that appears to be identical in phenomenology and treatment response to akathisia induced by antipsychotic medication or other dopamine receptor blocking agents. Tardive dyskinesia also often has a component of generalized restlessness that may coexist with akathisia in an individual receiving antipsychotic medications or other dopamine blocking agents. Antipsychotic medication and other dopamine blocking agent–induced acute akathisia is differentiated from antipsychotic medication and other dopamine blocking agent–induced tardive dyskinesia by the nature of the movements and their relationship to the initiation of medication. The time course of symptomatic presentation relative to medication dose changes may aid in this distinction. An increase in antipsychotic medication will often exacerbate akathisia, whereas it often temporarily relieves the symptoms of tardive dyskinesia.

Medication-induced acute akathisia should be distinguished from symptoms that are better accounted for by a mental disorder. Individuals with depressive episodes, manic episodes, generalized anxiety disorder, schizophrenia spectrum and other psychotic disorders, attention-deficit/hyperactivity disorder, major neurocognitive disorder, delirium, substance intoxication (e.g., with cocaine), or substance withdrawal (e.g., from an opioid) may also display agitation that is difficult to distinguish from akathisia. Some of these individuals are able to differentiate akathisia from the anxiety, restlessness, and agitation characteristic of a mental disorder by their experience of akathisia as being different from previously experienced feelings. Other evidence that restlessness or agitation may be better accounted for by a mental disorder includes the onset of agitation prior to exposure to the causative medication, absence of increasing restlessness with increasing doses of the causative medication, and absence of relief with pharmacological interventions (e.g., no improvement after decreasing the dose of the causative medication or treatment with another medication intended to treat the akathisia).

Tardive Dyskinesia

G24.01   Tardive Dyskinesia

The essential features of tardive dyskinesia are abnormal, involuntary movements of the tongue, jaw, trunk, or extremities that develop in association with the use of medications that block postsynaptic dopamine receptors, such as first- and second-generation antipsychotic medications and other medications such as metoclopramide for gastrointestinal disorders. The movements are present over a period of at least 4 weeks and may be choreiform (rapid, jerky, nonrepetitive), athetoid (slow, sinuous, continual), or semirhythmic (e.g., stereotypies) in nature; however, the movements are distinctly different from the rhythmic (3-6 Hz) tremors commonly seen in medication-induced parkinsonism. Signs or symptoms of tardive dyskinesia develop during exposure to the antipsychotic medication or other dopamine blocking agent, or within 4 weeks of withdrawal from an oral agent (or within 8 weeks of withdrawal from a long-acting injectable agent). There must be a history of the use of the offending agent for at least 3 months (or 1 month in individuals age 60 years or older). Although a large number of epidemiological studies have established the etiological relationship between dopamine blocking drug use and tardive dyskinesia, any dyskinesia in an individual who is receiving antipsychotic medication is not necessarily tardive dyskinesia.

Abnormal orofacial movements are the most obvious manifestations of tardive dyskinesia and have been observed in most individuals afflicted with tardive dyskinesia; however, approximately one-half can have limb involvement, and up to one-quarter can have axial dyskinesia of the neck, shoulders, or trunk. Involvement of other muscle groups (e.g., pharyngeal, diaphragm, abdominal) may occur but is uncommon, especially in the absence of dyskinesia of the orofacial region, limbs, or trunk. Limb or truncal dyskinesia without orofacial involvement may be more common in younger individuals, whereas orofacial dyskinesias are typical in older individuals.

The symptoms of tardive dyskinesia tend to be worsened by stimulants, antipsychotic medication withdrawal, and anticholinergic medications (such as benztropine, commonly used to manage medication-induced parkinsonism) and may be transiently worsened by emotional arousal, stress, and distraction during voluntary movements in unaffected parts of the body. The abnormal movements of dyskinesia are transiently reduced by relaxation and by voluntary movements in affected parts of the body. They are generally absent during sleep. Dyskinesia may be suppressed, at least temporarily, by increased doses of antipsychotic medication.

The overall prevalence of tardive dyskinesia in individuals who have received long-term antipsychotic medication treatment ranges from 20% to 30%. The overall incidence among younger individuals ranges from 3% to 5% per year. Middle-age and elderly individuals appear to develop tardive dyskinesia more often, with prevalence figures reported up to 50% and an incidence of 25%–30% after an average of 1 year's cumulative exposure to antipsychotic medication. Prevalence also varies depending on setting, with tardive dyskinesia tending to be more common among chronically institutionalized individuals. Variations in reported prevalence may be attributable to a lack of consistency in the definition of tardive dyskinesia, antipsychotic prescribing practices, study design, and the demographics of the population being studied.

There is no obvious gender difference in the susceptibility to tardive dyskinesia, although the risk may be somewhat greater in postmenopausal women. Greater cumulative amounts of antipsychotic medications and early development of acute extrapyramidal side effects (such as medication-induced parkinsonism) are two of the most consistent risk factors for tardive dyskinesia. Mood disorders (especially major depressive disorder), neurological conditions, and alcohol use disorder have also been found to be risk factors in some groups of individuals. Second-generation antipsychotics are associated with a somewhat lower incidence of tardive dyskinesia compared with first-generation antipsychotics, but the difference is not as large as once thought, especially when the dose of the first-generation antipsychotic is taken into account; the most important risk factors are age and cumulative exposure.

Onset of tardive dyskinesia may occur at any age and is almost always insidious. The signs are typically minimal to mild at onset and escape notice except by a keen observer. In many cases, tardive dyskinesia is objectively mild but, although it has been thought of as a cosmetic problem, can be associated with significant distress and social avoidance. In severe cases, it may be associated with medical complications (e.g., ulcers in cheeks and tongue; loss of teeth; macroglossia; difficulty in walking, swallowing, or breathing; muffled speech; weight loss; depression; suicidal ideation). In older individuals there is a greater likelihood that tardive dyskinesia may become more severe or more generalized with continued antipsychotic medication use. When antipsychotic medications are discontinued, some patients experience symptom improvement over time; however, for others tardive dyskinesia can be enduring.

Differential Diagnosis

It is imperative to distinguish medication-induced parkinsonism from tardive dyskinesia because the treatments commonly used to manage medication-induced parkinsonism (i.e., anticholinergic medications) may worsen the abnormal motor movements associated with tardive dyskinesia. Moreover, treatments used to manage tardive dyskinesia (i.e., VMAT2 inhibitors) may worsen the symptoms of medication-induced parkinsonism.

Dyskinesia that emerges during withdrawal from an antipsychotic medication or other dopamine receptor blocking agent may remit with continued withdrawal from the medication. If the dyskinesia persists for at least 4 weeks, a diagnosis of tardive dyskinesia may be warranted. Tardive dyskinesia must be distinguished from other causes of orofacial and body dyskinesia. These conditions include Huntington's disease, Wilson's disease, Sydenham's (rheumatic) chorea, systemic lupus erythematosus, thyrotoxicosis, heavy metal poisoning, ill-fitting dentures, dyskinesia due to other medications such as L-dopa or bromocriptine, and spontaneous dyskinesias. Factors that may be helpful in making the distinction are evidence that the symptoms preceded the exposure to the antipsychotic medication or other dopamine receptor blocking agent or that other focal neurological signs are present. It should be noted that other movement disorders may coexist with tardive dyskinesia. Because spontaneous dyskinesia can occur in more than 5% of individuals and is also more common in elderly persons, it may be difficult to prove that antipsychotic medications produced tardive dyskinesia in a given individual. Tardive dyskinesia must be distinguished from symptoms that are due to a medication-induced acute movement disorder (e.g., medication-induced parkinsonism, acute dystonia, acute akathisia). Acute dystonia and acute akathisia can develop quickly within hours to days, and medication-induced parkinsonism develops within weeks of initiating or increasing the dose of an antipsychotic medication or other dopamine receptor blocking agent (or reducing the dose of a medication used to treat the acute extrapyramidal symptoms). Tardive dyskinesia, on the other hand, generally develops after more prolonged exposure to antipsychotic medication (months to years) and can appear after the withdrawal of antipsychotic medication; the minimum exposure history required for the diagnosis of tardive dyskinesia is antipsychotic medication use for at least 3 months (or 1 month in middle-age and elderly individuals).

Tardive Dystonia
Tardive Akathisia

G24.09   Tardive Dystonia
G25.71   Tardive Akathisia

This category is for tardive syndromes involving other types of movement problems, such as dystonia or akathisia, which are distinguished by their late emergence in the course of treatment and their potential persistence for months to years, even in the face of discontinuation of an antipsychotic medication or other dopamine receptor blocking agent or dosage reduction.

Medication-Induced Postural Tremor

G25.1   Medication-Induced Postural Tremor

The essential feature of this condition is a fine tremor occurring during attempts to maintain a posture, which develops in association with the use of medication. Medications with which such a tremor may be associated include lithium, β-adrenergic medications (e.g., isoproterenol), stimulants (e.g., amphetamine), dopaminergic medications, anticonvulsant medications (e.g., valproic acid), antidepressant medications, and methylxanthines (e.g., caffeine, theophylline). The tremor is a regular, rhythmic oscillation of the limbs (most commonly hands and fingers), head, mouth, or tongue, most commonly with a frequency of between 8 and 12 cycles per second. It is most easily observed when the affected body part is held in a sustained posture (e.g., hands outstretched, mouth held open). The tremor may worsen in severity when the affected body part is moved intentionally (kinetic or action tremor). When an individual describes a tremor that is consistent with postural tremor but the clinician does not directly observe the tremor, it may be helpful to try to re-create the situation in which the tremor occurred (e.g., drinking from a cup and saucer).

Most available information concerns lithium-induced tremor. Lithium tremor is a common, usually benign, and well-tolerated side effect of therapeutic doses. However, it may cause social embarrassment, occupational difficulties, and noncompliance in some individuals. As serum lithium levels approach toxic levels, the tremor may become coarser and be accompanied by muscle twitching, fasciculations, or ataxia. Nontoxic lithium tremor may improve spontaneously over time. A variety of factors may increase the risk of lithium tremor (e.g., increasing age, high serum lithium levels, concurrent antidepressant or antipsychotic medication or another dopamine receptor blocking agent, excessive caffeine intake, personal or family history of tremor, presence of alcohol use disorder, and associated anxiety). The frequency of complaints about tremor appears to decrease with duration of lithium treatment. Factors that may exacerbate the tremor include anxiety, stress, fatigue, hypoglycemia, thyrotoxicosis, pheochromocytoma, hypothermia, and alcohol withdrawal. Tremor can also be an early feature of serotonin syndrome.

Differential Diagnosis

Medication-induced postural tremor should be distinguished from a preexisting tremor that is not caused by the effects of a medication. Factors that help to establish that the tremor was preexisting include its temporal relationship to the initiation of medication, lack of correlation with serum levels of the medication, and persistence after the medication is discontinued. If a preexisting, nonpharmacologically induced tremor is present (e.g., essential tremor) that worsens with medication, such a tremor would not be considered to be medication-induced postural tremor. The factors described above that may contribute to the severity of a medication-induced postural tremor (e.g., anxiety, stress, fatigue, hypoglycemia, thyrotoxicosis, pheochromocytoma, hypothermia, alcohol withdrawal) may also be a cause of tremor independent of the medication.

Medication-induced postural tremor is not diagnosed if the tremor is better accounted for by medication-induced parkinsonism. A medication-induced postural tremor is usually absent at rest and intensifies when the affected part is brought into action or held in a sustained position. In contrast, the tremor related to medication-induced parkinsonism is usually lower in frequency (3–6 Hz), worse at rest, and suppressed during intentional movement and usually occurs in association with other symptoms of medication-induced parkinsonism (e.g., akinesia, rigidity).

Other Medication-Induced Movement Disorder

G25.79   Other Medication-Induced Movement Disorder

This category is for medication-induced movement disorders not captured by any of the specific disorders listed earlier. Examples include 1) presentations resembling neuroleptic malignant syndrome that are associated with medications other than antipsychotic medications and other dopamine receptor blocking agents and 2) other medication-induced tardive conditions.

Antidepressant Discontinuation Syndrome

T43.205A   Initial encounter
T43.205D   Subsequent encounter
T43.205S   Sequelae

Discontinuation symptoms may occur following treatment with all types of antidepressants. The incidence of this syndrome depends on the dosage and half-life of the medication being taken, as well as the rate at which the medication is tapered. Short half-life medications that are abruptly discontinued (or when the dose is significantly reduced) rather than tapered gradually may pose the greatest risk. The short-acting antidepressants paroxetine and venlafaxine are the agents most commonly associated with discontinuation symptoms. Antidepressant discontinuation syndrome may occur in the context of intermittent nonadherence to treatment and therefore may be irregularly present in some individuals who have not actually stopped taking the medication. This is especially true for very short half-life medications (e.g., venlafaxine). By contrast, long half-life medications like fluoxetine seldom produce significant discontinuation effects.

Unlike withdrawal syndromes associated with opioids, alcohol, and other substances, antidepressant discontinuation syndrome has no pathognomonic symptoms. Instead, the symptoms tend to be vague and variable. Symptoms typically begin 2–4 days after the last dose of the antidepressant. For selective serotonin reuptake inhibitors, symptoms such as dizziness, tinnitus, "electric shock"–like sensations, insomnia, and acute anxiety are described. The antidepressant use before discontinuation must not have incurred hypomania or mixed state (i.e., there should be confidence that the discontinuation syndrome is not the result of fluctuations in mood stability associated with the previous treatment). For the tricyclic antidepressants, sudden discontinuation has been associated with gastrointestinal symptoms (cramping—reflecting cholinergic overactivity after stopping an anticholinergic tricyclic antidepressant) as well as rebound hypomania.

The antidepressant discontinuation syndrome is based solely on pharmacological factors and is not related to the reinforcing effects of an antidepressant. Unlike the discontinuation of substances with reinforcing effects like opioids, drug craving does not occur. Also, when a stimulant is used to augment an antidepressant, abrupt cessation may result in stimulant withdrawal symptoms (see "Stimulant Withdrawal" in the chapter "Substance-Related and Addictive Disorders") rather than the antidepressant discontinuation syndrome described here.

The prevalence of antidepressant discontinuation syndrome is unknown but is thought to vary according to any of the following factors: the dosage before discontinuation, the half-life (i.e., occurring more commonly with short half-life medications) and receptor-binding affinity of the medication (e.g., more likely to occur with serotonin reuptake inhibitors), and possibly the individual's genetically influenced rate of metabolism for this medication. Therefore, discontinuation reactions occur more frequently with short half-life medications, but may also be influenced by rapid or ultrarapid metabolizer status of cytochrome enzymes that metabolize the antidepressant.

Because longitudinal studies are lacking, little is known about the clinical course of antidepressant discontinuation syndrome. Symptoms appear to abate over time with very gradual dosage reductions. Symptoms are usually short-lived, lasting no more than 2 weeks, and are seldom present more than 3 weeks after discontinuation.

Differential Diagnosis

The differential diagnosis of antidepressant discontinuation syndrome includes a relapse of the disorder for which the medication was prescribed (e.g., depression or panic disorder), somatic symptom disorder, bipolar I or bipolar II disorder with mixed features, substance use disorders, migraine, or cerebrovascular accident. Discontinuation symptoms often resemble symptoms of a persistent anxiety disorder or a return of somatic symptoms of depression for which the medication was initially given. It is important not to confuse discontinuation syndrome with a relapse of the original depressive or anxiety disorder for which the medication was being prescribed. Antidepressant discontinuation syndrome differs from substance withdrawal in that antidepressants themselves have no reinforcing or euphoric effects. Individuals typically do not escalate the dose of medications on their own, and they generally do not engage in drug-seeking behavior to obtain additional medication. Criteria for a substance use disorder are not met.

Other Adverse Effect of Medication

T50.905A   Initial encounter
T50.905D   Subsequent encounter
T50.905S   Sequelae

This category is available for optional use by clinicians to code side effects of medication (other than movement symptoms) when these adverse effects become a main focus of clinical attention. Examples include severe hypotension, cardiac arrhythmias, and priapism.

Other Conditions That May Be a Focus of Clinical Attention

This chapter includes conditions and psychosocial or environmental problems that may be a focus of clinical attention or otherwise affect the diagnosis, course, prognosis, or treatment of an individual's mental disorder. These conditions are presented with their corresponding codes from ICD-10-CM (usually Z codes). A condition or problem in this chapter may be coded 1) if it is a reason for the current visit; 2) if it helps to explain the need for a test, procedure, or treatment; 3) if it plays a role in the initiation or exacerbation of a mental disorder; or 4) if it constitutes a problem that should be considered in the overall management plan.

The conditions and problems listed in this chapter are not mental disorders. Their inclusion in DSM-5-TR is meant to draw attention to the scope of additional issues that may be encountered in routine clinical practice and to provide a systematic listing that may be useful to clinicians in documenting these issues.

For quick reference to all codes in this section, see the DSM-5-TR Classification. Conditions and problems that may be a focus of clinical attention are listed in the subsequent text as follows:

1. **Suicidal behavior** (potentially self-injurious behavior with at least some intent to die) **and nonsuicidal self-injury** (intentional self-inflicted damage to the body in the absence of suicidal intent).
2. **Abuse and neglect** (e.g., child and adult maltreatment and neglect problems, including physical abuse, sexual abuse, neglect, and psychological abuse).
3. **Relational problems** (e.g., parent-child relational problem, sibling relational problem, relationship distress with spouse or intimate partner, disruption by separation or divorce).
4. **Educational problems** (e.g., illiteracy or low-level literacy, schooling unavailable or unattainable, failed school examinations, underachievement in school).
5. **Occupational problems** (e.g., unemployment, change of job, threat of job loss, stressful work schedule, discord with boss and workmates).
6. **Housing problems** (e.g., homelessness; inadequate housing; discord with neighbor, lodger, or landlord).
7. **Economic problems** (e.g., lack of adequate food or safe drinking water, extreme poverty, low income).
8. **Problems related to the social environment** (e.g., problem related to living alone, acculturation difficulty, social exclusion or rejection).

9. **Problems related to interaction with the legal system** (e.g., conviction in criminal proceedings, imprisonment or other incarceration, problems related to release from prison, problems related to other legal circumstances).

10. **Problems related to other psychosocial, personal, and environmental circumstances** (e.g., problems related to unwanted pregnancy, victim of crime, victim of terrorism).

11. **Problems related to access to medical and other health care** (e.g., unavailability or inaccessibility of health care facilities).

12. **Circumstances of personal history** (e.g., personal history of psychological trauma, military deployment).

13. **Other health service encounters for counseling and medical advice** (e.g., sex counseling, other counseling or consultation).

14. **Additional conditions or problems that may be a focus of clinical attention** (e.g., wandering associated with a mental disorder, uncomplicated bereavement, phase of life problem).

Suicidal Behavior and Nonsuicidal Self-Injury

Coding Note for ICD-10-CM Suicidal Behavior
For T codes only, the 6th character should be coded as follows:

A (initial encounter)—Use while the individual is receiving active treatment for the condition (e.g., emergency department encounter, evaluation and treatment by a new clinician); or
D (subsequent encounter)—Use for encounters after the individual has received active treatment for the condition and when he or she is receiving routine care for the condition during the healing or recovery phase (e.g., medication adjustment, other aftercare and follow-up visits).

Suicidal Behavior

This category may be used for individuals who have engaged in potentially self-injurious behavior with at least some intent to die as a result of the act. Evidence of intent to end one's life can be explicit or inferred from the behavior or circumstances. A suicide attempt may or may not result in actual self-injury. If the individual is dissuaded by another person or changes his or her mind before initiating the behavior, this category does not apply.

Current Suicidal Behavior

T14.91A   Initial encounter: If suicidal behavior is part of the initial encounter with the clinical presentation

T14.91D   Subsequent encounter: If suicidal behavior is part of subsequent encounters with the clinical presentation

Z91.51   **History of Suicidal Behavior**
If suicidal behavior has occurred during the individual's lifetime

Nonsuicidal Self-Injury

This category may be used for individuals who have engaged in intentional self-inflicted damage to their body of a sort likely to induce bleeding, bruising, or pain (e.g., cutting, burning, stabbing, hitting, excessive rubbing) in the absence of suicidal intent.

R45.88   **Current Nonsuicidal Self-Injury**
If nonsuicidal self-injurious behavior is part of the clinical presentation

Z91.52   **History of Nonsuicidal Self-Injury**
If nonsuicidal self-injurious behavior has occurred during the individual's lifetime

Abuse and Neglect

Maltreatment by a family member (e.g., caregiver, intimate adult partner) or by a nonrelative can be the area of current clinical focus, or such maltreatment can be an important factor in the assessment and treatment of individuals with mental disorders or other medical conditions. Because of the legal implications of abuse and neglect, care should be used in assessing these conditions and assigning these codes. Having a past history of abuse or neglect can influence diagnosis and treatment response in a number of mental disorders, and may also be noted along with the diagnosis.

For the following categories, in addition to listings of the confirmed or suspected event of abuse or neglect, other codes are provided for use if the current clinical encounter is to provide mental health services to either the victim or the perpetrator of the abuse or neglect. A separate code is also provided for designating a past history of abuse or neglect.

Coding Note for ICD-10-CM Abuse and Neglect Conditions
For T codes only, the 7th character should be coded as follows:

A (initial encounter)—Use while the individual is receiving active treatment for the condition (e.g., surgical treatment, emergency department encounter, evaluation and treatment by a new clinician); or

D (subsequent encounter)—Use for encounters after the individual has received active treatment for the condition and when he or she is receiving routine care for the condition during the healing or recovery phase (e.g., cast change or removal, removal of external or internal fixation device, medication adjustment, other aftercare and follow-up visits).

Child Maltreatment and Neglect Problems

Child Physical Abuse

This category may be used when physical abuse of a child is a focus of clinical attention. Child physical abuse is nonaccidental physical injury to a child—ranging from minor bruises to severe fractures or death—occurring as a result of punching, beating, kicking, biting, shaking, throwing, stabbing, choking, hitting (with a hand, stick, strap, or other object), burning, or any other method that is inflicted by a parent, caregiver, or other individual who has responsibility for the child. Such injury is considered abuse regardless of whether the caregiver intended to hurt the child. Physical discipline, such as spanking or paddling, is not considered abuse as long as it is reasonable and causes no bodily injury to the child.

Child Physical Abuse, Confirmed
T74.12XA Initial encounter
T74.12XD Subsequent encounter

Child Physical Abuse, Suspected
T76.12XA Initial encounter
T76.12XD Subsequent encounter

Other Circumstances Related to Child Physical Abuse
Z69.010   Encounter for mental health services for victim of child physical abuse by parent
Z69.020   Encounter for mental health services for victim of nonparental child physical abuse
Z62.810   Personal history (past history) of physical abuse in childhood
Z69.011   Encounter for mental health services for perpetrator of parental child physical abuse
Z69.021   Encounter for mental health services for perpetrator of nonparental child physical abuse

Child Sexual Abuse

This category may be used when sexual abuse of a child is a focus of clinical attention. Child sexual abuse encompasses any sexual act involving a child that is intended to provide sexual gratification to a parent, caregiver, or other individual who has responsibility for the child. Sexual abuse includes activities such as fondling a child's genitals, penetration, incest, rape, sodomy, and indecent exposure. Sexual abuse also includes noncontact exploitation of a child by a parent or caregiver—for example, forcing, tricking, enticing, threatening, or pressuring a child to participate in acts for the sexual gratification of others, without direct physical contact between child and abuser.

Child Sexual Abuse, Confirmed
T74.22XA Initial encounter
T74.22XD Subsequent encounter

Child Sexual Abuse, Suspected

T76.22XA Initial encounter
T76.22XD Subsequent encounter

Other Circumstances Related to Child Sexual Abuse

Z69.010 Encounter for mental health services for victim of child sexual abuse by parent
Z69.020 Encounter for mental health services for victim of nonparental child sexual abuse
Z62.810 Personal history (past history) of sexual abuse in childhood
Z69.011 Encounter for mental health services for perpetrator of parental child sexual abuse
Z69.021 Encounter for mental health services for perpetrator of nonparental child sexual abuse

Child Neglect

This category may be used when child neglect is a focus of clinical attention. Child neglect is defined as any confirmed or suspected egregious act or omission by a child's parent or other caregiver that deprives the child of basic age-appropriate needs and thereby results, or has reasonable potential to result, in physical or psychological harm to the child. Child neglect encompasses abandonment; lack of appropriate supervision; failure to attend to necessary emotional or psychological needs; and failure to provide necessary education, medical care, nourishment, shelter, and/or clothing.

Child Neglect, Confirmed

T74.02XA Initial encounter
T74.02XD Subsequent encounter

Child Neglect, Suspected

T76.02XA Initial encounter
T76.02XD Subsequent encounter

Other Circumstances Related to Child Neglect

Z69.010 Encounter for mental health services for victim of child neglect by parent
Z69.020 Encounter for mental health services for victim of nonparental child neglect
Z62.812 Personal history (past history) of neglect in childhood
Z69.011 Encounter for mental health services for perpetrator of parental child neglect
Z69.021 Encounter for mental health services for perpetrator of nonparental child neglect

Child Psychological Abuse

This category may be used when psychological abuse of a child is a focus of clinical attention. Child psychological abuse is nonaccidental verbal or symbolic acts by a child's parent or caregiver that result, or have reasonable potential to result, in significant psychological harm to the child. (Physical and sexual abusive acts are not included in this category.) Examples of psychological abuse of a child include berating, disparaging, or humiliating the child; threatening the child; harming/abandoning—or indicating that the alleged offender will harm/abandon—people or things that the child cares about; confining the child (as by tying a child's arms or legs together or binding a child to furniture or another object, or confining a child to a small enclosed area [e.g., a closet]); egregious scapegoating of the child; coercing the child to inflict pain on himself or herself; and disciplining the child excessively (i.e., at an extremely high frequency or duration, even if not at a level of physical abuse) through physical or nonphysical means.

Child Psychological Abuse, Confirmed

T74.32XA   Initial encounter
T74.32XD   Subsequent encounter

Child Psychological Abuse, Suspected

T76.32XA   Initial encounter
T76.32XD   Subsequent encounter

Other Circumstances Related to Child Psychological Abuse

Z69.010   Encounter for mental health services for victim of child psychological abuse by parent
Z69.020   Encounter for mental health services for victim of nonparental child psychological abuse
Z62.811   Personal history (past history) of psychological abuse in childhood
Z69.011   Encounter for mental health services for perpetrator of parental child psychological abuse
Z69.021   Encounter for mental health services for perpetrator of nonparental child psychological abuse

Adult Maltreatment and Neglect Problems

Spouse or Partner Violence, Physical

This category may be used when spouse or partner physical violence is a focus of clinical attention. Spouse or partner physical violence is nonaccidental acts of physical force that result, or have reasonable potential to result, in physical harm to an intimate partner or that evoke significant fear in the partner. Nonaccidental acts of physical force include shoving, slapping, hair pulling, pinching, restraining, shaking, throwing, biting, kicking, hitting with the fist or an object, burning, poisoning, applying force to the throat, cutting off the air supply, holding the head under water, and using a weapon. Acts for the purpose of physically protecting oneself or one's partner are excluded.

Spouse or Partner Violence, Physical, Confirmed

T74.11XA Initial encounter

T74.11XD Subsequent encounter

Spouse or Partner Violence, Physical, Suspected

T76.11XA Initial encounter

T76.11XD Subsequent encounter

Other Circumstances Related to Spouse or Partner Violence, Physical

Z69.11 Encounter for mental health services for victim of spouse or partner violence, physical

Z91.410 Personal history (past history) of spouse or partner violence, physical

Z69.12 Encounter for mental health services for perpetrator of spouse or partner violence, physical

Spouse or Partner Violence, Sexual

This category may be used when spouse or partner sexual violence is a focus of clinical attention. Spouse or partner sexual violence involves the use of physical force or psychological coercion to compel the partner to engage in a sexual act against his or her will, whether or not the act is completed. Also included in this category are sexual acts with an intimate partner who is unable to consent.

Spouse or Partner Violence, Sexual, Confirmed

T74.21XA Initial encounter

T74.21XD Subsequent encounter

Spouse or Partner Violence, Sexual, Suspected

T76.21XA Initial encounter

T76.21XD Subsequent encounter

Other Circumstances Related to Spouse or Partner Violence, Sexual

Z69.81 Encounter for mental health services for victim of spouse or partner violence, sexual

Z91.410 Personal history (past history) of spouse or partner violence, sexual

Z69.12 Encounter for mental health services for perpetrator of spouse or partner violence, sexual

Spouse or Partner Neglect

This category may be used when spouse or partner neglect is a focus of clinical attention. Spouse or partner neglect is any egregious act or omission by one partner that deprives a dependent partner of basic needs and thereby results, or has reasonable potential to result, in physical or psychological harm to the dependent partner. This category may be used in the context of relationships in which one partner is extremely dependent on the other partner for care or for assistance in navigating ordinary daily activities—for example, a partner who is incapable of self-care because of substantial physical, psychological/intellectual, or cultural limitations (e.g., inability to communicate with others and manage everyday activities as a result of living in a foreign culture).

Spouse or Partner Neglect, Confirmed

T74.01XA   Initial encounter
T74.01XD   Subsequent encounter

Spouse or Partner Neglect, Suspected

T76.01XA   Initial encounter
T76.01XD   Subsequent encounter

Other Circumstances Related to Spouse or Partner Neglect

Z69.11   Encounter for mental health services for victim of spouse or partner neglect
Z91.412   Personal history (past history) of spouse or partner neglect
Z69.12   Encounter for mental health services for perpetrator of spouse or partner neglect

Spouse or Partner Abuse, Psychological

This category may be used when spouse or partner psychological abuse is a focus of clinical attention. Spouse or partner psychological abuse encompasses nonaccidental verbal or symbolic acts by one partner that result, or have reasonable potential to result, in significant harm to the other partner. Acts of psychological abuse include berating or humiliating the victim; interrogating the victim; restricting the victim's ability to come and go freely; obstructing the victim's access to assistance (e.g., law enforcement; legal, protective, or medical resources); threatening the victim with physical harm or sexual assault; harming, or threatening to harm, people or things that the victim cares about; unwarranted restriction of the victim's access to or use of economic resources; isolating the victim from family, friends, or social support resources; stalking the victim; and trying to make the victim question his or her sanity ("gaslighting").

Spouse or Partner Abuse, Psychological, Confirmed

T74.31XA   Initial encounter
T74.31XD   Subsequent encounter

Spouse or Partner Abuse, Psychological, Suspected

T76.31XA   Initial encounter
T76.31XD   Subsequent encounter

Other Circumstances Related to Spouse or Partner Abuse, Psychological

Z69.11 Encounter for mental health services for victim of spouse or partner psychological abuse

Z91.411 Personal history (past history) of spouse or partner psychological abuse

Z69.12 Encounter for mental health services for perpetrator of spouse or partner psychological abuse

Adult Abuse by Nonspouse or Nonpartner

This category may be used when the abuse of an adult by another adult who is not an intimate partner is a focus of clinical attention. Such maltreatment may involve acts of physical, sexual, or emotional abuse. Examples of adult abuse include nonaccidental acts of physical force (e.g., pushing/shoving, scratching, slapping, throwing something that could hurt, punching, biting) that have resulted—or have reasonable potential to result—in physical harm or have caused significant fear; forced or coerced sexual acts; and verbal or symbolic acts with the potential to cause psychological harm (e.g., berating or humiliating the person; interrogating the person; restricting the person's ability to come and go freely; obstructing the person's access to assistance; threatening the person; harming or threatening to harm people or things that the person cares about; restricting the person's access to or use of economic resources; isolating the person from family, friends, or social support resources; stalking the person; trying to make the person think that he or she is crazy). Acts for the purpose of physically protecting oneself or the other person are excluded.

Adult Physical Abuse by Nonspouse or Nonpartner, Confirmed
T74.11XA Initial encounter
T74.11XD Subsequent encounter

Adult Physical Abuse by Nonspouse or Nonpartner, Suspected
T76.11XA Initial encounter
T76.11XD Subsequent encounter

Adult Sexual Abuse by Nonspouse or Nonpartner, Confirmed
T74.21XA Initial encounter
T74.21XD Subsequent encounter

Adult Sexual Abuse by Nonspouse or Nonpartner, Suspected
T76.21XA Initial encounter
T76.21XD Subsequent encounter

Adult Psychological Abuse by Nonspouse or Nonpartner, Confirmed
T74.31XA Initial encounter
T74.31XD Subsequent encounter

Adult Psychological Abuse by Nonspouse or Nonpartner, Suspected
T76.31XA Initial encounter
T76.31XD Subsequent encounter

Other Circumstances Related to Adult Abuse by Nonspouse or Nonpartner
Z69.81   Encounter for mental health services for victim of non-spousal or nonpartner adult abuse
Z69.82   Encounter for mental health services for perpetrator of nonspousal or nonpartner adult abuse

Relational Problems

Key relationships, especially intimate adult partner relationships and parent/caregiver-child relationships, have a significant impact on the health of the individuals in these relationships. These relationships can be health promoting and protective, neutral, or detrimental to health outcomes. In the extreme, these close relationships can be associated with maltreatment or neglect, which has significant medical and psychological consequences for the affected individual. A relational problem may come to clinical attention either as the reason that the individual seeks health care or as a problem that affects the course, prognosis, or treatment of the individual's mental disorder or other medical condition.

Parent-Child Relational Problem
Z62.820   Parent–Biological Child
Z62.821   Parent–Adopted Child
Z62.822   Parent–Foster Child
Z62.898   Other Caregiver–Child

For this category, the term *parent* is used to refer to one of the child's primary caregivers, who may be a biological, adoptive, or foster parent or may be another relative (such as a grandparent) who fulfills a parental role for the child. This category may be used when the main focus of clinical attention is to address the quality of the parent-child relationship or when the quality of the parent-child relationship is affecting the course, prognosis, or treatment of a mental disorder or other medical condition. Typically, the parent-child relational problem is associated with impaired functioning in behavioral, cognitive, or affective domains. Examples of behavioral problems include inadequate parental control, supervision, and involvement with the child; parental overprotection; excessive parental pressure; arguments that escalate to threats of physical violence; and avoidance without resolution of problems. Cognitive problems may include negative attributions of the other's intentions, hostility toward or scapegoating of the other, and unwarranted feelings of estrangement. Affective problems may include feelings of sadness, apathy, or anger about the other individual in the relationship. Clinicians should take into account the developmental needs of the child and the cultural context.

Z62.891   Sibling Relational Problem

This category may be used when the focus of clinical attention is a pattern of interaction among siblings that is associated with significant impairment in individual or family functioning or with development of symptoms in one or more of the siblings, or when a sibling relational problem is affecting the course, prognosis, or treatment of a sibling's mental disorder or other medical condition. This category may be used for either children or adults if the focus is on the sibling relationship. Siblings in this context include full, half-, step-, foster, and adopted siblings.

Z63.0   Relationship Distress With Spouse or Intimate Partner

This category may be used when the major focus of the clinical contact is to address the quality of the intimate (spouse or partner) relationship or when the quality of that relationship is affecting the course, prognosis, or treatment of a mental disorder or other medical condition. Partners can be of the same or different genders. Typically, the relationship distress is associated with impaired functioning in behavioral, cognitive, or affective domains. Examples of behavioral problems include conflict resolution difficulty, withdrawal, and overinvolvement. Cognitive problems can manifest as chronic negative attributions of the other's intentions or dismissals of the partner's positive behaviors. Affective problems would include chronic sadness, apathy, and/or anger about the other partner.

Problems Related to the Family Environment

Z62.29   Upbringing Away From Parents

This category may be used when the main focus of clinical attention pertains to issues regarding a child being raised away from the parents or when this separate upbringing affects the course, prognosis, or treatment of a mental disorder or other medical condition. The child could be one who is under state custody and placed in kin care or foster care. The child could also be one who is living in a nonparental relative's home, or with friends, but whose out-of-home placement is not mandated or sanctioned by the courts. Problems related to a child living in a group home or orphanage are also included. This category excludes issues related to Z59.3 Problem Related to Living in a Residential Institution.

Z62.898   Child Affected by Parental Relationship Distress

This category may be used when the focus of clinical attention is the negative effects of parental relationship discord (e.g., high levels of conflict, distress, or disparagement) on a child in the family, including effects on the child's mental disorder or other medical condition.

Z63.5   Disruption of Family by Separation or Divorce

This category may be used when partners in an intimate adult couple are living apart because of relationship problems or are in the process of divorce.

Z63.8   High Expressed Emotion Level Within Family

Expressed emotion is a construct used as a qualitative measure of the "amount" of emotion—in particular, hostility, emotional overinvolvement, and criticism directed toward a family member who is an identified patient—displayed in the family environment. This category may be used when a family's high level of expressed emotion is the focus of clinical attention or is affecting the course, prognosis, or treatment of a family member's mental disorder or other medical condition.

Educational Problems

These categories may be used when an academic or educational problem is the focus of clinical attention or has an impact on the individual's diagnosis, treatment, or prognosis. Problems to be considered include illiteracy or low-level literacy; lack of access to schooling owing to unavailability or unattainability; problems with academic performance (e.g., failing school examinations, receiving failing marks or grades) or underachievement (below what would be expected given the individual's intellectual capacity); discord with teachers, school staff, or other students; problems related to inadequate teaching; and any other problems related to education and/or literacy.

Z55.0   **Illiteracy and Low-Level Literacy**
Z55.1   **Schooling Unavailable and Unattainable**
Z55.2   **Failed School Examinations**
Z55.3   **Underachievement in School**
Z55.4   **Educational Maladjustment and Discord With Teachers and Classmates**
Z55.8   **Problems Related to Inadequate Teaching**
Z55.9   **Other Problems Related to Education and Literacy**

Occupational Problems

These categories may be used when an occupational problem is the focus of clinical attention or has an impact on the individual's treatment or prognosis. Areas to be considered include problems with employment or in the work environment, including problems related to current military deployment status; unemployment; recent change of job; threat of job loss; stressful work schedule; uncertainty about career choices; sexual harassment on the job; other discord with boss, supervisor, co-workers, or others in the work environment; uncongenial or hostile work environments; other physical or mental strain related to work; sexual harassment on the job; and any other problems related to employment and/or occupation.

Z56.82   **Problem Related to Current Military Deployment Status**
This category may be used when an occupational problem directly related to an individual's military deployment status is the focus of clinical attention or has an impact on the individual's diagnosis, treatment, or prognosis. Psychological reactions to deployment are not included in this category; such reactions would be better captured as an adjustment disorder or another mental disorder.

Z56.0   Unemployment
Z56.1   Change of Job
Z56.2   Threat of Job Loss
Z56.3   Stressful Work Schedule
Z56.4   Discord With Boss and Workmates
Z56.5   Uncongenial Work Environment
Z56.6   Other Physical and Mental Strain Related to Work
Z56.81   Sexual Harassment on the Job
Z56.9   Other Problem Related to Employment

Housing Problems

Z59.01   Sheltered Homelessness

This category may be used when sheltered homelessness has an impact on an individual's treatment or prognosis. An individual is considered to be experiencing sheltered homelessness if the primary nighttime residence is a homeless shelter, a warming shelter, a domestic violence shelter, a motel, or in a temporary or transitional living situation.

Z59.02   Unsheltered Homelessness

This category may be used when unsheltered homelessness has an impact on an individual's treatment or prognosis. An individual is considered to be experiencing unsheltered homelessness if residing in a place not meant for human habitation, such as a public space (e.g., tunnel, transportation station, mall), a building not intended for residential use (e.g., abandoned structure, unused factory), a car, a cave, a cardboard box, or some other ad hoc housing situation.

Z59.1   Inadequate Housing

This category may be used when lack of adequate housing has an impact on an individual's treatment or prognosis. Examples of inadequate housing conditions include lack of heat (in cold temperatures) or electricity, infestation by insects or rodents, inadequate plumbing and toilet facilities, overcrowding, lack of adequate sleeping space, and excessive noise. It is important to consider cultural norms before assigning this category.

Z59.2   Discord With Neighbor, Lodger, or Landlord

This category may be used when discord with neighbors, lodgers, or a landlord is a focus of clinical attention or has an impact on the individual's treatment or prognosis.

Z59.3   Problem Related to Living in a Residential Institution

This category may be used when a problem (or problems) related to living in a residential institution is a focus of clinical attention or has an impact on the individual's treatment or prognosis. Psychological reactions to a change in living situation are not included in this category; such reactions would be better captured as an adjustment disorder.

Z59.9   Other Housing Problem

This category may be used when there is a problem related to housing circumstances other than as specified above.

Economic Problems

These categories may be used when an economic problem is the focus of clinical attention or has an impact on the individual's treatment or prognosis. Areas to be considered include lack of adequate food (food insecurity) or safe drinking water, extreme poverty, low income, insufficient social or health insurance or welfare support, or any other economic problems.

Z59.41   Food Insecurity

Z58.6   Lack of Safe Drinking Water

Z59.5   Extreme Poverty

Z59.6   Low Income

Z59.7   Insufficient Social or Health Insurance or Welfare Support

This category may be used for individuals who meet eligibility criteria for social or welfare support but are not receiving such support, who receive support that is insufficient to address their needs, or who otherwise lack access to needed insurance or support programs. Examples include inability to qualify for welfare support because of lack of proper documentation or evidence of address, inability to obtain adequate health insurance because of age or a preexisting condition, and denial of support owing to excessively stringent income or other requirements.

Z59.9   Other Economic Problem

This category may be used when there is a problem related to economic circumstances other than as specified above.

Problems Related to the Social Environment

Z60.2   Problem Related to Living Alone

This category may be used when a problem associated with living alone is the focus of clinical attention or has an impact on the individual's treatment or prognosis. Examples of such problems include chronic feelings of loneliness, isolation, and lack of structure in carrying out activities of daily living (e.g., irregular meal and sleep schedules, inconsistent performance of home maintenance chores).

Z60.3   Acculturation Difficulty

This category may be used when difficulty in adjusting to a new culture (e.g., following migration) is the focus of clinical attention or has an impact on the individual's treatment or prognosis.

Z60.4   Social Exclusion or Rejection

This category may be used when there is an imbalance of social power such that there is recurrent social exclusion or rejection by others. Examples of social rejection include bullying, teasing, and intimidation by others; being targeted by others for verbal abuse and humiliation; and being purposefully excluded from the activities of peers, workmates, or others in one's social environment.

Z60.5   Target of (Perceived) Adverse Discrimination or Persecution

This category may be used when there is perceived or experienced discrimination against or persecution of the individual based on his or her membership (or perceived membership) in a specific category. Typically, such categories include gender or gender identity, race, ethnicity, religion, sexual orientation, country of origin, political beliefs, disability status, caste, social status, weight, and physical appearance.

Z60.9   Other Problem Related to Social Environment
This category may be used when there is a problem related to the individual's social environment other than as specified above.

Problems Related to Interaction With the Legal System

These categories may be used when a problem related to interaction with the legal system is the focus of clinical attention or has an impact on the individual's treatment or prognosis. Areas to be considered include conviction in criminal proceedings, imprisonment or other incarceration, problems related to release from prison, and problems related to other legal circumstances (e.g., civil litigation, child custody or support proceedings).

Z65.0   Conviction in Criminal Proceedings Without Imprisonment

Z65.1   Imprisonment or Other Incarceration

Z65.2   Problems Related to Release From Prison

Z65.3   Problems Related to Other Legal Circumstances (e.g., civil litigation, child custody or support proceedings)

Problems Related to Other Psychosocial, Personal, and Environmental Circumstances

Z72.9   Problem Related to Lifestyle
This category may be used when a lifestyle problem is a specific focus of treatment or directly affects the course, prognosis, or treatment of a mental disorder or other medical condition. Examples of lifestyle problems include lack of physical exercise, inappropriate diet, high-risk sexual behavior, and poor sleep hygiene. A problem that is attributable to a symptom of a mental disorder should not be coded unless that problem is a specific focus of treatment or directly affects the course, prognosis, or treatment of the individual. In such cases, both the mental disorder and the lifestyle problem should be coded.

Z64.0   Problems Related to Unwanted Pregnancy

Z64.1   Problems Related to Multiparity

Z64.4   Discord With Social Service Provider, Including Probation Officer, Case Manager, or Social Services Worker

Z65.4   Victim of Crime

Z65.4   Victim of Terrorism or Torture

Z65.5   Exposure to Disaster, War, or Other Hostilities

Problems Related to Access to Medical and Other Health Care

These categories may be used when a problem related to access to medical or other health care is the focus of clinical attention or has an impact on the individual's treatment or prognosis.

Z75.3   Unavailability or Inaccessibility of Health Care Facilities

Z75.4   Unavailability or Inaccessibility of Other Helping Agencies

Circumstances of Personal History

Z91.49   Personal History of Psychological Trauma

Z91.82   Personal History of Military Deployment

Other Health Service Encounters for Counseling and Medical Advice

Z31.5   **Genetic Counseling**

This category may be used for individuals seeking genetic counseling to understand the risks of developing a mental disorder with a significant genetic component (e.g., bipolar disorder) for themselves and other family members, including their existing children, as well as the risks for their future children.

Z70.9   **Sex Counseling**

This category may be used when the individual seeks counseling related to sex education, sexual behavior, sexual orientation, sexual attitudes (embarrassment, timidity), others' sexual behavior or orientation (e.g., spouse, partner, child), sexual enjoyment, or any other sex-related issue.

Z71.3   **Dietary Counseling**

This category may be used when the individual seeks counseling related to dietary issues like weight management.

Z71.9   **Other Counseling or Consultation**

This category may be used when counseling is provided or advice/consultation is sought for a problem that is not specified above or elsewhere in this chapter (e.g., counseling regarding drug abuse prevention in an adolescent).

Additional Conditions or Problems That May Be a Focus of Clinical Attention

Z91.83   **Wandering Associated With a Mental Disorder**

This category may be used for individuals with a mental disorder whose desire to walk about leads to significant clinical management or safety concerns. For example, individuals with major neurocognitive or neurodevelopmental disorders may experience a restless urge to wander that places them at risk for falls and causes them to leave supervised settings without needed accompaniment. This category excludes individuals whose intent is to escape an unwanted housing situation (e.g., children who are running away from home, individuals who no longer wish to remain in the hospital) or those who walk or pace as a result of medication-induced akathisia.

Coding note: First code associated mental disorder (e.g., major neurocognitive disorder, autism spectrum disorder), then code Z91.83 wandering associated with [specific mental disorder].

Z63.4   Uncomplicated Bereavement

This category may be used when the focus of clinical attention is a normal reaction to the death of a loved one. As part of their reaction to such a loss, some grieving individuals present with symptoms characteristic of a major depressive episode—for example, feelings of sadness and associated symptoms such as insomnia, poor appetite, and weight loss. The bereaved individual typically regards the depressed mood as "normal," although the individual may seek professional help for relief of associated symptoms such as insomnia or anorexia. The duration and expression of "normal" bereavement vary considerably among different cultural groups. Further guidance in distinguishing grief from a major depressive episode and from prolonged grief disorder is provided in their respective texts.

Z60.0   Phase of Life Problem

This category may be used when a problem adjusting to a life-cycle transition (a particular developmental phase) is the focus of clinical attention or has an impact on the individual's treatment or prognosis. Examples of such transitions include entering or completing school, leaving parental control, getting married, starting a new career, becoming a parent, adjusting to an "empty nest" after children leave home, and retiring.

Z65.8   Religious or Spiritual Problem

This category may be used when the focus of clinical attention is a religious or spiritual problem. Examples include distressing experiences that involve loss or questioning of faith, problems associated with conversion to a new faith, or questioning of spiritual values that may not necessarily be related to an organized church or religious institution.

Z72.811   Adult Antisocial Behavior

This category may be used when the focus of clinical attention is adult antisocial behavior that is not attributable to a mental disorder (e.g., conduct disorder, antisocial personality disorder). Examples include the behavior of some professional thieves, racketeers, or dealers in illegal substances.

Z72.810   Child or Adolescent Antisocial Behavior

This category may be used when the focus of clinical attention is antisocial behavior in a child or adolescent that is not attributable to a mental disorder (e.g., intermittent explosive disorder, conduct disorder). Examples include isolated antisocial acts by children or adolescents (not a pattern of antisocial behavior).

Z91.19   Nonadherence to Medical Treatment

This category may be used when the focus of clinical attention is non-adherence to an important aspect of treatment for a mental disorder or another medical condition. Reasons for such nonadherence may include discomfort resulting from treatment (e.g., medication side effects), expense of treatment, personal value judgments or religious or cultural beliefs about the proposed treatment, age-related debility, and the presence of a mental disorder (e.g., schizophrenia, personality disorder). This category may be used only when the problem is sufficiently severe to warrant independent clinical attention and does not meet diagnostic criteria for psychological factors affecting other medical conditions.

E66.9   Overweight or Obesity

This category may be used when overweight or obesity is a focus of clinical attention.

Z76.5   Malingering

The essential feature of malingering is the intentional production of false or grossly exaggerated physical or psychological symptoms, motivated by external incentives such as avoiding military duty, avoiding work, obtaining financial compensation, evading criminal prosecution, or obtaining drugs. Under some circumstances, malingering may represent adaptive behavior—for example, feigning illness while a captive of the enemy during wartime. Malingering should be strongly considered if any combination of the following is noted:

1. Medicolegal context of presentation (e.g., the individual is referred by an attorney to the clinician for examination, or the individual self-refers while litigation or criminal charges are pending).
2. Marked discrepancy between the individual's claimed stress or disability and the objective findings and observations.
3. Lack of cooperation during the diagnostic evaluation and in complying with the prescribed treatment regimen.
4. The presence of antisocial personality disorder.

Malingering differs from factitious disorder in that the motivation for the symptom production in malingering is an external incentive, whereas in factitious disorder external incentives are absent. Malingering is differentiated from functional neurological symptom disorder (conversion disorder) and other somatic symptom–related mental disorders by the intentional production of symptoms and by the obvious external incentives associated with it. Definite evidence of feigning (such as clear evidence that loss of function is present during the examination but not at home) would suggest a diagnosis of factitious disorder if the individual's apparent aim is to assume the sick role, or malingering if it is to obtain an incentive, such as money.

R41.81   Age-Related Cognitive Decline

This category may be used when the focus of clinical attention is an objectively identified decline in cognitive functioning consequent to the aging process that is within normal limits given the individual's age. Individuals with this condition may report problems remembering names or appointments or may experience difficulty in solving complex problems. This category should be considered only after it has been determined that the cognitive impairment is not better explained by a specific mental disorder or attributable to a neurological condition.

R41.83   Borderline Intellectual Functioning

This category may be used when an individual's borderline intellectual functioning is the focus of clinical attention or has an impact on the individual's treatment or prognosis. Differentiating borderline intellectual functioning and mild intellectual developmental disorder (intellectual disability) requires careful assessment of intellectual and adaptive functions and their discrepancies, particularly in the presence of co-occurring mental disorders that may affect patient compliance with standardized testing procedures (e.g., schizophrenia or attention-deficit/hyperactivity disorder, with severe impulsivity).

Index

Page numbers printed in **boldface** type refer to tables or figures.